ASWB Clinical Exam Prep 2026-2027

Complete LCSW Study Guide with 850+ Practice Questions, DSM-5-TR Diagnosis, Therapeutic Interventions, NASW Ethics & Case-Based Learning for Social Work Licensure

Elisabeta Chelsea Wade

ASWB Clinical Exam Prep 2026-2027

Complete LCSW Study Guide with 850+ Practice Questions, DSM-5-TR Diagnosis, Therapeutic Interventions, NASW Ethics & Case-Based Learning for Social Work Licensure

ISBN: 978-1-923604-86-5

First Edition, 2025

DISCLAIMER

This book is designed to provide information and practice materials to assist candidates preparing for the Association of Social Work Boards (ASWB) Clinical licensure examination. It is sold with the understanding that the publisher and author are not engaged in rendering legal, accounting, medical, psychological, or other professional services.

Exam Preparation Notice: While this study guide is designed to align with the ASWB Clinical exam content outline, it does not guarantee passage of the examination. Exam content, format, and requirements may change. Candidates should verify current exam specifications with ASWB and their state licensing board.

Clinical Practice Notice: The clinical scenarios, case examples, and practice questions presented in this book are fictional composites created for educational purposes. Any resemblance to actual persons, living or deceased, or actual clinical cases is purely coincidental. All client names, identifying details, and circumstances have been created solely for illustration of clinical concepts and exam preparation.

Professional Disclaimer: This book provides educational content for exam preparation purposes only and does not constitute clinical supervision, professional consultation, or therapeutic intervention. Readers should not use this material as a substitute for appropriate clinical supervision, consultation with licensed professionals, or adherence to applicable laws, regulations, and professional standards in their jurisdiction.

Trademark Notice: ASWB®, Association of Social Work Boards®, and LCSW® are registered trademarks of the Association of Social Work Boards. DSM-5-TR® is a registered trademark of the American Psychiatric Association. This book is an independent publication and has not been authorized, sponsored, or otherwise approved by ASWB, APA, or NASW.

Medical and Mental Health Disclaimer: The information provided in this book regarding mental health conditions, diagnostic criteria, and therapeutic interventions is for educational and exam preparation purposes only. This content is not intended to diagnose, treat, cure, or prevent any disease or mental health condition. Readers should consult qualified healthcare professionals for medical or mental health concerns.

Ethical and Legal Notice: While this book discusses NASW Code of Ethics, confidentiality regulations, and legal requirements, it does not constitute legal advice. Laws, regulations, and ethical standards vary by jurisdiction and change over time. Practitioners should consult current regulations, state licensing boards, legal counsel, and professional ethics resources for guidance on specific situations.

Names and Scenarios Disclaimer: All individual names used in case examples, practice scenarios, and clinical illustrations are entirely fictional. These include but are not limited to: client names, therapist names, family member names, facility names, and organizational names. Any similarity to real persons or entities is unintentional and coincidental.

The following fictional names appear in educational scenarios throughout this text: Maria, John, Sarah, Marcus, Jennifer, Emma, James, Tom, Amanda, Dr. Chen, Dr. Martinez, Dr. Johnson, Dr. Thompson, Dr. Lee, Michael, Rosa, Fatima, Lisa, and others. These are composite characters created solely for instructional purposes.

Updates and Revisions: Clinical standards, diagnostic criteria, ethical guidelines, and exam content evolve. Readers are responsible for staying current with professional developments, continuing education requirements, and changes to licensure examination content.

For questions, corrections, or updates, please contact: [Your Contact Information]

Acknowledgment: This book references the DSM-5-TR (Diagnostic and Statistical Manual of Mental Disorders, Fifth Edition, Text Revision), NASW Code of Ethics, and ASWB exam content outlines for educational purposes. Readers should consult original source materials for complete and current information.

Table of Contents

Introduction

This book was written for one reason: to get you ready for the ASWB Clinical examination. The exam tests more than your ability to memorize facts. It tests your clinical judgment, your ethical reasoning, and your capacity to apply social work principles in real situations. You'll face scenario-based questions that mirror what you'll encounter in actual practice. That's exactly what this book prepares you for.

The 850-plus questions here aren't random. They're organized by the four content domains the ASWB uses to structure the exam. Each domain gets the attention it deserves based on how heavily it's weighted on the actual test. You'll find questions that range from straightforward recall to complex clinical scenarios requiring you to analyze, synthesize, and apply multiple concepts at once.

What makes this book different? Three things. First, the explanations don't just tell you the right answer—they explain why the other options are wrong. That's how you learn to think like the test-makers. Second, the questions reflect current practice standards, including recent DSM-5-TR criteria and updated NASW Code of Ethics guidelines. Third, you get three full-length practice exams that simulate the actual testing experience. No shortcuts, no gimmicks.

You'll also find quick-reference guides, charts, and summaries that condense complex information into formats you can review quickly. Use them. They're designed to reinforce what you've learned and help you spot patterns in how questions are constructed

How to Use This Study Guide

Start by taking one of the practice exams. Don't prepare first—just take it. This diagnostic approach shows you where you stand right now. Mark the questions you miss, but more importantly, mark the ones you guessed on, even if you guessed correctly. Those represent gaps in your knowledge.

Review your results by domain. If you missed 60% of the questions in Assessment and Diagnosis, that domain needs your immediate attention. Don't spread yourself thin trying to study everything at once. Focus on your weakest areas first.

Work through the domain-specific chapters in order of your weakest to strongest areas. Read each chapter completely before attempting the practice questions. When you do answer questions, don't just check if you got them right. Read every explanation, even for questions you answered correctly. You might discover you got the right answer for the wrong reason.

Here's a method that works: Answer a set of 25 questions, then immediately review the explanations. Don't wait until you've finished 100 questions to check your work. The feedback needs to be fresh. When you miss a question, write out in your own words why you missed it and what the correct reasoning should have been. This active processing helps cement the information in your memory.

Create a running list of concepts you struggle with. Maybe you consistently miss questions about duty to warn, or you can't distinguish between different personality disorders. Whatever patterns emerge, those become your focus areas. Go back to the relevant chapter sections and work through them again.

Use the practice exams strategically. Space them out—don't take all three in one week. After your initial diagnostic exam, study for several weeks, then take the second practice exam. Use the results to adjust your study plan. Save the third exam for the week before your test date. This gives you a final check on your readiness.

Case Example 1: Maria, an MSW graduate, started her exam prep by reading through all the chapters first, then taking practice questions. She failed her first attempt. On her second try, she changed her approach. She took a diagnostic practice exam first, discovered she was weakest in Human Development and Ethics, and spent 70% of her study time on those domains. She passed with a comfortable margin. The lesson? Let your actual performance, not your assumptions, guide your study plan.

Case Example 2: James felt confident because he'd been practicing clinical social work for five years. He skipped the study guide chapters and went straight to practice questions. He passed, but barely. Later, he admitted he'd guessed on at least 30 questions and got lucky. His overconfidence nearly cost him. Experience matters, but exam preparation requires specific knowledge of how the ASWB frames questions and what they're testing.

Case Example 3: Chen used a scattered approach, jumping between topics based on what felt interesting each day. She'd study crisis intervention one day, psychopharmacology the next, then ethics. After six weeks, she took a practice exam and scored poorly across all domains. She couldn't understand why until she realized she'd never mastered any single area—she'd just skimmed the surface of everything. She restructured her plan, mastered one domain at a time, and her scores improved dramatically.

The ASWB Clinical Exam Format

The ASWB Clinical examination contains 170 questions. You'll have four hours to complete it. That breaks down to roughly 1.4 minutes per question, though you'll move faster through some and slower through others. Of those 170 questions, 150 are scored and 20 are pretest questions that don't count toward your final score. You won't know which questions are pretest items, so treat every question as if it counts.

The exam is computer-based. You'll take it at a testing center, not at home. You'll use a computer mouse to select answers—no pencil, no paper, no ability to flag questions and return to them later in some testing software versions. Some centers allow you to mark questions for review, but don't count on it. Answer each question as you encounter it.

Questions appear one at a time on the screen. Most are multiple-choice with four options. You'll see standalone questions that present a scenario or ask about a concept, followed by four possible answers. Your job is to select the best answer. Note that word: best. Sometimes more than one answer might seem partially correct, but only one represents the best response according to social work standards and the ASWB's interpretation of those standards.

The scenarios you'll face are brief—usually a paragraph or two. They describe a client situation, a practice dilemma, or an ethical question. Then you're asked what you should do next, what the symptoms suggest, which intervention is most appropriate, or how you should handle the situation. These aren't academic exercises. They're designed to reflect real practice decisions.

You won't need to know obscure details or memorize long lists verbatim. The exam tests application, not just recall. You might see a question about a client presenting with specific symptoms, and you'll need to determine the most likely diagnosis. Or you'll read about a boundary situation and decide what action aligns with the NASW Code of Ethics. The focus stays on clinical judgment and ethical practice.

The testing center provides a basic calculator for questions that might require simple calculations, though these are rare on the clinical exam. You'll also get scratch paper or an erasable board for notes. Use it. Jot down key details from complex scenarios, work through elimination processes, or sketch out decision trees if that helps you think.

No breaks are scheduled during the exam, but you can request one if needed. The clock keeps running, though, so plan accordingly. Most test-takers find they don't need breaks if they've practiced pacing themselves.

Exam Content Distribution and Weighting

The ASWB organizes exam content into four domains. Each domain carries a specific weight, meaning a set percentage of the 150 scored questions come from that area. Understanding this distribution helps you allocate study time appropriately.

Human Development, Diversity, and Behavior in the Environment accounts for roughly 27% of scored questions. That's approximately 41 questions. This domain covers developmental theories, lifespan development, diversity and cultural issues, family systems, and how environmental factors affect human behavior. You need to know developmental milestones, understand cultural competence, recognize how oppression and discrimination impact clients, and apply person-in-environment thinking.

Assessment, Diagnosis, and Treatment Planning represents about 29% of the exam. That translates to approximately 44 questions. This domain is the heaviest on the clinical exam. You'll answer questions about conducting biopsychosocial assessments, performing mental status examinations, assessing risk, applying DSM-5-TR diagnostic criteria, developing treatment plans, and selecting appropriate interventions. Strong diagnostic skills matter here. You need to distinguish between similar diagnoses, recognize presenting symptoms, and understand when to refer or consult.

Psychotherapy, Clinical Interventions, and Case Management makes up roughly 27% of scored questions—about 41 questions. This domain tests your knowledge of therapeutic modalities, intervention techniques, crisis intervention, group and family therapy, and case management. You should know CBT, DBT, psychodynamic approaches, solution-focused therapy, motivational interviewing, and trauma-informed care. The questions ask which intervention fits which situation, how to handle resistance, when to terminate, and how to coordinate care.

Professional Values, Ethics, and Clinical Practice accounts for approximately 17% of the exam. That's about 26 questions. This domain covers the NASW Code of Ethics, confidentiality and privacy laws (including HIPAA), mandatory reporting, duty to warn, boundary issues, supervision, cultural competence in practice, and professional development. Ethics questions often present dilemmas where you must choose the most ethical course of action, sometimes between two options that both seem defensible.

These percentages are approximate and can vary slightly from one exam administration to another. The ASWB periodically updates content outlines and weightings based on practice analysis studies. Always check the current ASWB candidate handbook for the most recent information.

Here's what this distribution means for your study plan: You can't ignore any domain, but you should spend more time on Assessment/Diagnosis and Interventions/Case Management because they collectively represent over half the exam. If you're stronger in one area and weaker in another, adjust accordingly, but don't neglect the smaller domains. Ethics questions, while fewer in number, often separate passing from failing scores because they require nuanced judgment.

Score Requirements and Passing Standards

The ASWB uses scaled scoring, not percentage-based scoring. Your raw score (the number of questions you answer correctly out of 150 scored items) converts to a scaled score between 0 and 999. You need a scaled score of 400 to pass. This scaled approach allows the ASWB to account for variations in difficulty across different exam forms.

What does this mean practically? You don't need to answer every question correctly to pass. In fact, you can miss a significant number of questions and still achieve a passing score. The exact number varies based on the specific exam form's difficulty, but generally, answering around 93-106 questions correctly (roughly 62-70% of scored questions) puts you in passing range. Don't fixate on these numbers—they're estimates, not guarantees.

You'll receive your score immediately after completing the exam at the testing center. The computer calculates your results and displays them on screen. You'll also receive a printed score report before you leave the center. If you pass, the report confirms your passing score. If you don't pass, the report includes diagnostic information showing your performance in each content domain.

The score report doesn't tell you your exact raw score or which specific questions you missed. Instead, it shows how you performed in each domain using categories like "above the mean," "near the mean," or "below the mean" compared to other test-takers. This information guides your study focus if you need to retake the exam.

You can retake the exam if you don't pass, but you must wait 90 days between attempts for the first three attempts. After three failed attempts, you must wait six months before your next try. Each attempt requires a new application and fee. The ASWB doesn't limit the total number of attempts, but your state licensing board might impose restrictions.

Different states have different requirements beyond just passing the ASWB exam. Some require supervised clinical hours before you can sit for the exam. Others allow you to test before completing supervision. Some states accept only recent passing scores (within the past few years), while others accept older scores. Check with your specific state board to understand all requirements.

The pass rate for the ASWB Clinical exam hovers around 70-75% nationally. That means roughly one in four test-takers fails on their first attempt. Don't become part of that statistic because you didn't prepare adequately. The exam is passable, but it requires focused preparation.

Study Strategies and Test-Taking Tips

Walking into that testing center unprepared is like showing up to provide therapy without having reviewed your client's file. You might muddle through, but you won't perform at your best. Preparation isn't just about knowing the content—it's about knowing how to approach the exam itself, how to manage your time and your nerves, and how to think through questions the way the ASWB wants you to think.

Creating Your Study Plan

You need a study plan that fits your timeline, your learning style, and your current knowledge level. Three common timelines work for most test-takers: three months, two months, or one month. Choose based on how much time you have before your exam date and how much you already know.

The Three-Month Plan gives you the luxury of time. You can study at a comfortable pace without feeling rushed. Dedicate 10-15 hours per week to preparation. That's roughly 2-3 hours on weekdays and longer sessions on weekends, or whatever schedule fits your life.

Weeks 1-2: Complete a diagnostic practice exam and review all answers thoroughly. Identify your weak domains. Read through all study guide chapters, even the domains where you're strong. This creates a foundation and refreshes concepts you might have forgotten.

Weeks 3-5: Focus on your weakest domain. If Assessment and Diagnosis is your trouble spot, spend these three weeks there. Read the relevant chapters again, take notes, create flashcards, and work through all practice questions in that domain. Review the explanations for every question, right or wrong.

Weeks 6-8: Move to your second-weakest domain. Apply the same intensive study approach. By now, you should notice patterns in how questions are asked and what the ASWB emphasizes.

Weeks 9-10: Study your third-weakest domain. Even if this area feels comfortable, don't skip it. The ASWB might test aspects you haven't considered.

Week 11: Review your strongest domain and take the second full-length practice exam. Analyze your results. Have you improved in your weak areas? Are new gaps appearing?

Week 12: Final review of all domains, focusing on persistent weak spots. Take the third practice exam 3-4 days before your actual test. Spend the last days reviewing quick-reference materials, not learning new content.

The Two-Month Plan requires more intensive study—15-20 hours per week. The structure compresses but doesn't eliminate any steps.

Weeks 1-2: Diagnostic exam, identify weaknesses, and complete an initial read-through of all study materials.

Weeks 3-4: Intensive focus on weakest domain with all practice questions.

Weeks 5-6: Second-weakest domain with full practice question sets.

Week 7: Third-weakest domain and second practice exam.

Week 8: Review strongest domain, address any lingering gaps, and take the third practice exam. Final review in the last few days.

The One-Month Plan demands serious commitment—20-30 hours per week. This only works if you already have a solid foundation in clinical social work. If you're a recent graduate or haven't practiced in years, one month isn't enough.

Week 1: Diagnostic exam, identify critical weaknesses, and read through study materials focusing on weak areas.

Week 2: Intensive study of weakest domain plus all related practice questions.

Week 3: Study second-weakest domain, take second practice exam mid-week, adjust remaining study based on results.

Week 4: Review third-weakest domain, address any remaining gaps, take third practice exam early in the week, and spend final days on targeted review.

Regardless of your timeline, consistency matters more than marathon sessions. Studying two hours daily is more effective than cramming ten hours on Sunday. Your brain needs time to process and consolidate information.

Case Example 1: Robert chose the three-month plan but didn't stick to it. He studied intensively for two weeks, then stopped for a week because of work demands. This pattern repeated—bursts of study followed by gaps. When he took his exam, he'd forgotten material from his early study sessions. He passed, but admitted he would have scored higher with consistent effort. Regularity beats intensity.

Case Example 2: Lisa had only one month before her exam. She tried to cover everything equally, spending a few hours on each domain. She failed, scoring poorly across all areas. She hadn't given herself enough time to master any domain deeply. On her second attempt, she gave herself three months and followed the structured plan. She passed comfortably. Timeline matters, especially if your knowledge base has gaps.

Case Example 3: Ahmed used the two-month plan effectively. He worked full-time but protected his study time fiercely. He studied from 5:30 to 7:30 every morning before work, and four hours each Saturday. He tracked his progress weekly, adjusted when practice test results revealed unexpected weaknesses, and passed on his first attempt. His success came from protecting his study time and staying flexible within his plan.

Effective Question Analysis Techniques

The ASWB doesn't just test what you know—it tests how you think. Understanding how to analyze questions systematically improves your accuracy and speed.

Start by reading the question stem carefully. The stem is everything before the answer choices. It tells you what the question is really asking. Look for key words that define what you need to do: "What should the social worker do FIRST?" "Which response is MOST appropriate?" "What does this symptom presentation MOST likely indicate?"

Those qualifier words—first, most, best, least, primary—are critical. They tell you that multiple answers might be partially correct, but you're looking for the single best option according to the ASWB's standards. If a question asks what you should do first, all four answers might be things you'd eventually do, but only one represents the immediate priority.

Break down complex scenarios into components. Long question stems contain essential information and distracting details. Train yourself to identify what matters. If a question describes a 34-year-old married mother of two who works as a teacher and presents with depressed mood, loss of interest in activities, significant weight loss, sleep disturbance, and fatigue lasting three weeks, what's essential? The symptoms and duration matter for diagnosis. Her age might matter for developmental considerations. Her occupation and family status might be relevant for treatment planning, but they're secondary for a diagnostic question.

Look for what's being tested. Is this an ethics question? A diagnostic question? An intervention question? A question about professional boundaries? Knowing the category helps you frame your thinking. Ethics questions require you to apply NASW Code principles. Diagnostic questions need DSM-5-TR criteria. Intervention questions ask for evidence-based practice matching.

Consider the client's presenting problem and where they are in the helping process. A client in crisis needs crisis intervention, not long-term psychodynamic therapy. A client asking for help with a specific behavioral problem might benefit from CBT, not open-ended exploration of childhood experiences. Match the intervention to the situation.

Use the process of elimination actively. Read all four options before selecting your answer. Cross out options you know are wrong. If you can eliminate two choices, you've improved your odds significantly even if you need to guess between the remaining two.

Watch for absolute language in answer choices. Options that include words like "always," "never," "must," or "only" are often wrong. Social work practice rarely deals in absolutes. We work with context, individual circumstances, and professional judgment. An answer that says a social worker should "always" or "never" do something is usually too rigid to be correct.

Look for the social work response, not just the correct response. The ASWB tests social work practice, which means answers should reflect social work values: client self-determination, empowerment, strengths-based thinking, cultural competence, and person-in-environment perspective. If an answer choice sounds more like what a physician, psychologist, or case manager might do, it's probably not the best social work response.

Pay attention to ethical priorities. The NASW Code of Ethics establishes a hierarchy: clients' interests come first, then colleagues, then the profession, then society. When facing an ethical dilemma, ask yourself whose interests the question is asking you to prioritize. Usually, it's the client's interests, but sometimes questions test your understanding of when other considerations take precedence (like when safety issues require breaking confidentiality).

Managing Test Anxiety

Some anxiety is normal. A little nervousness can sharpen your focus. But excessive anxiety interferes with performance. You blank out on information you know, misread questions, or second-guess yourself into wrong answers.

Start managing anxiety weeks before the exam, not the night before. Build confidence through preparation. The better prepared you are, the less anxious you'll feel. Every practice question you answer correctly, every concept you master, reduces anxiety because it proves you can do this.

Practice under test-like conditions. Take your practice exams in quiet spaces, time yourself strictly, don't use notes or references, and sit for the full exam duration. This exposure helps your body and mind adapt to the testing experience. On exam day, the situation feels familiar rather than foreign.

Develop a pre-test routine. In the days before your exam, establish consistent sleep, eating, and exercise patterns. Don't radically change your routine the night before—if you normally drink coffee in the morning, do that on test day too. If you don't usually drink coffee, don't start on exam morning. Stick with what your body knows.

Use physical relaxation techniques. Deep breathing works because it activates your parasympathetic nervous system, which calms your body's stress response. Practice this: breathe in slowly through your nose for four counts, hold for four counts, exhale slowly through your mouth for four counts. Do this several times. You can use this technique during the exam if you feel anxiety rising.

Reframe negative thoughts. If you catch yourself thinking "I'm going to fail" or "I don't know anything," stop and reframe. Replace those thoughts with realistic, evidence-based ones: "I've prepared systematically" or "I've passed practice exams, so I can pass this one." Anxiety often comes from catastrophic thinking. Challenge those catastrophes with facts.

Manage physical symptoms. If your heart races, acknowledge it: "My heart is racing because I'm nervous, and that's okay. It doesn't mean anything is wrong." Don't fight the physical sensations—that makes them worse. Accept them, then redirect your attention to the task at hand.

On exam day, arrive early but not too early. Getting there 15-20 minutes before your appointment gives you time to check in without creating a long wait that builds anxiety. Bring your identification and authorization to test. Know what you can and cannot bring into the testing room.

If anxiety strikes during the exam, take a brief mental break. Close your eyes for 10 seconds, do a quick breathing exercise, then return to the question. You have time for these micro-breaks. Better to spend 30 seconds calming yourself than to miss the next five questions because you're spiraling.

Case Example 1: Sarah had significant test anxiety from past academic struggles. She began preparation three months out and incorporated anxiety management from day one. She practiced progressive muscle relaxation nightly, visualized herself successfully completing the exam, and took practice tests in the actual testing center (during open practice times for other exams). On test day, the environment felt familiar. Her anxiety stayed manageable, and she passed.

Case Example 2: Marcus ignored his anxiety during preparation, thinking it would resolve once he studied enough. He knew the material cold but panicked on exam day. His mind went blank on questions he could have answered easily. He failed by a small margin. Before his second attempt, he worked with a therapist on test anxiety, learned coping strategies, and practiced them during study sessions. His second attempt was successful.

Case Example 3: Jennifer's anxiety came from perfectionism. She'd agonize over each question, afraid of making mistakes. This slowed her down dramatically. She ran out of time and had to guess on the last 20 questions. She learned to set time limits per question during practice, force herself to move on even when uncertain, and accept that she didn't need perfection—just a passing score. Her second attempt, with better time management and reduced perfectionism, resulted in a pass.

Time Management Strategies

Four hours seems like plenty of time for 170 questions until you're sitting in that testing center and realize how quickly time passes. Effective time management keeps you from rushing at the end or obsessing so long over difficult questions that you never reach easier ones.

Calculate your pace. With 170 questions and 240 minutes, you have roughly 1.4 minutes per question. Round that to 90 seconds for easier math. Some questions take 30 seconds, others might take 2-3 minutes. The average should be around 90 seconds.

Create checkpoints. Plan to complete about 43 questions per hour. At the one-hour mark, you should be around question 43. At two hours, around question 86. At three hours, around question 129. This leaves you a buffer for the final 41 questions and review time if needed. If you're falling behind at a checkpoint, speed up. If you're ahead, you've built a cushion.

Don't get stuck. If you've spent two minutes on a question and still can't decide, make your best guess and move on. Mark it if the testing software allows, but don't let one difficult question derail your timing. You might miss that question, but you'll get to answer all the others. If you spend five minutes agonizing over it, you've stolen time from questions you might answer correctly.

Answer questions on your first read. Don't plan to skip questions and return to them unless absolutely necessary. Most testing software allows this, but the practice is inefficient. You'll spend time re-reading scenarios you've already read, and you'll create mental clutter by carrying unfinished questions in your working memory. Decide and move forward.

Watch the clock, but don't obsess. Check your progress at those hourly checkpoints, then trust your pace. Constant clock-watching creates anxiety and breaks your concentration. You've practiced pacing during your study sessions, so trust that training.

Budget more time for complex scenarios. A question presenting a detailed case vignette with multiple symptoms or ethical considerations deserves extra time. A straightforward factual question about DSM criteria or a developmental milestone takes less time. Learn to quickly categorize questions as you encounter them: "This is complex, I might need two minutes" or "This is straightforward, 45 seconds."

Use any extra time wisely. If you finish early, resist the urge to change answers wholesale. Research shows that your first instinct is often correct. Only change an answer if you spot a clear error in your reasoning or if you misread something the first time. Random second-guessing usually lowers scores.

How to Approach Scenario-Based Questions

Scenario-based questions are the heart of the ASWB Clinical exam. They present realistic practice situations and ask you to demonstrate clinical judgment. These questions test application, not just recall.

Read the scenario completely before looking at the question stem or answer choices. Don't jump ahead. The scenario provides context you need. Missing a detail can lead to the wrong answer.

Identify the client and the problem. Who is seeking help? What's the primary concern? A scenario might mention multiple people—a mother calling about her son's behavior, a couple in conflict, a client referred by his physician. Know who your client is and what they're asking for.

Note the setting and stage of intervention. Are you meeting this client for the first time? Is this an ongoing therapeutic relationship? Are you in crisis intervention mode or treatment planning mode? The stage of helping determines what's appropriate. You don't create a long-term treatment plan during an emergency, and you don't focus on crisis intervention when a client comes for their tenth session presenting a non-urgent concern.

Look for clinical indicators. Scenarios describing symptoms are asking you to recognize patterns. Count symptoms, note duration, assess severity, and consider differential diagnoses. If a scenario lists five symptoms consistent with major depression and two symptoms that might suggest bipolar disorder, the preponderance points toward depression unless other factors change the picture.

Consider developmental and cultural factors. A behavior concerning in one developmental stage might be normal in another. Cultural context affects symptom presentation, help-seeking behavior, and intervention appropriateness. If a scenario provides cultural information, it's there for a reason—use it.

Identify the specific question being asked. After reading the scenario, read the question stem carefully. Are you being asked to diagnose? Choose an intervention? Identify an ethical response? Make a referral? The question tells you what lens to use when evaluating the scenario.

Apply the best practice standard, not just acceptable practice. You might know three interventions that could work in a situation, but the ASWB wants the best one based on evidence, ethical guidelines, and professional standards. Look for the answer that best aligns with social work values and evidence-based practice.

Watch for "next step" questions. These often ask what the social worker should do first or next. Prioritize safety, ethical obligations, and immediate needs before long-term interventions. If a client expresses suicidal ideation, your next step is assessing imminent risk, not developing a treatment plan to address underlying depression.

Case Example 1: A scenario describes a 28-year-old client reporting sleep problems, decreased energy, difficulty concentrating, feelings of hopelessness, and loss of interest in activities she once enjoyed. These symptoms have been present for three weeks. Her appetite is unchanged. The question asks for the most likely diagnosis. Test-takers often overthink this, looking for what might make the scenario more complex. But the straightforward answer—Major Depressive Disorder—fits the presentation. The scenario gives you exactly what you need; don't add complications that aren't there.

Case Example 2: A scenario presents an ethical dilemma: Your client discloses that her husband, who is also your client (you see them separately), is having an affair. Your client asks if you knew about this. The question asks what you should do. This tests confidentiality boundaries. You cannot disclose information from one client to another, even if they're married. The correct response maintains both clients' confidentiality. Test-takers struggle with this because it feels unhelpful to the first client, but ethical obligations are clear.

Case Example 3: A question describes a client in his first session who appears disheveled, reports paranoid thoughts, demonstrates disorganized speech, and mentions he stopped taking his medications two weeks ago. The question asks what the social worker should do next. While a full psychosocial assessment is important, the immediate priority is addressing medication discontinuation and current psychiatric symptoms. The best answer involves coordinating with the client's psychiatrist or facilitating psychiatric evaluation, not beginning psychotherapy or discussing long-term goals.

Identifying Keywords and Eliminating Wrong Answers

Keywords direct your thinking. They specify what the question wants and what constraints apply. Missing a keyword leads to wrong answers even when you know the content.

"FIRST" and "NEXT" indicate sequence. These keywords ask about priorities and timing. Multiple actions might be appropriate, but only one comes first. Safety always comes first. Legal obligations (like mandated reporting) come before therapeutic goals. Assessment comes before intervention.

"MOST" and "BEST" indicate you're choosing the optimal option. All answers might be acceptable in some contexts, but one is superior for the specific situation presented. Look for the option that best aligns with evidence-based practice, professional ethics, and the client's presenting needs.

"EXCEPT" and "NOT" reverse the question. You're looking for the wrong answer or the exception to a rule. These questions trip up test-takers who read too quickly. Slow down, note the keyword, and look for the option that doesn't fit.

"ALWAYS" and "NEVER" in answer choices are red flags. Social work practice rarely deals in absolutes. If you see "The social worker should always..." or "The social worker must never..." be skeptical. These options are often incorrect because they ignore context and individual circumstances.

"PRIMARILY" and "MAINLY" ask for the predominant factor or response. Other factors might play a role, but one is primary. In diagnostic questions, this might mean identifying the most likely diagnosis when symptoms could fit multiple categories. In intervention questions, it means choosing the treatment approach that best addresses the primary presenting problem.

Now for elimination. You can't always spot the right answer immediately, but you can often spot wrong answers quickly.

Eliminate options that violate ethical principles. If an answer choice involves lying to a client, breaching confidentiality without legal justification, or imposing the social worker's values on a client, it's wrong. Cross it out.

Eliminate options that violate safety. If an answer ignores suicide risk, minimizes danger to others, or delays necessary emergency interventions, it's wrong. Safety trumps almost everything else.

Eliminate options outside the social worker's scope of practice. Social workers don't prescribe medications, perform psychological testing that requires psychologist credentials, or provide legal advice. If an answer has you doing something outside your professional role, eliminate it.

Eliminate options that skip necessary steps. If a question asks what to do in an initial session and an answer jumps to implementing a specific intervention without mentioning assessment, that's premature. Social workers assess before intervening.

Eliminate options that contradict information in the scenario. If the scenario states a client is uninsured and an answer choice assumes insurance coverage for recommendations, there's a disconnect. Stick with what the scenario tells you.

Eliminate options that reflect outdated practice. If you see terminology or approaches that are no longer current (older diagnostic terms, interventions that have been superseded by evidence-based practices), those are likely wrong. The ASWB tests current standards.

After elimination, you're often left with two plausible options. This is where careful reasoning matters. Compare them directly. Which one better addresses the specific question asked? Which one aligns more closely with social work values? Which one reflects more current evidence or practice standards?

Case Example 1: A question asks what a social worker should do first when a mandated client arrives for an initial appointment. Four options: A) Explain the limits of confidentiality, B) Conduct a full biopsychosocial assessment, C) Establish rapport and discuss the client's goals, D) Review the client's legal situation. "First" is your keyword. While all these actions are important, explaining confidentiality limits—especially with mandated clients who must understand what will be reported—comes before assessment or goal-setting. Option A is correct.

Case Example 2: A question describes symptoms and asks which diagnosis is MOST likely. The scenario fits criteria for both Adjustment Disorder and Major Depressive Disorder, but the symptoms are more severe and meet full criteria for MDD. The keyword "most" tells you to choose the best fit, not just an acceptable fit. Even though Adjustment Disorder is possible, MDD is the most likely diagnosis based on symptom severity and presentation.

Case Example 3: A question about intervention includes this option: "The social worker should always confront the client's defense mechanisms directly." The word "always" signals this is probably wrong. Direct confrontation isn't always therapeutic; it can rupture the therapeutic alliance, especially early in treatment or with fragile clients. This absolute language makes it the wrong choice, even if confrontation might sometimes be appropriate.

Pulling It Together

You now have a framework for approaching this exam. You know what the test looks like, how it's structured, what it tests, and how to prepare. You have strategies for managing your time, your anxiety, and the questions themselves. You know how to build a study plan that fits your timeline and how to adjust that plan based on your performance.

The ASWB Clinical exam tests whether you can apply social work knowledge, skills, and ethics in practice situations. It doesn't test trivia or obscure details. It tests judgment. Every question you work through in this book, every explanation you read, every mistake you analyze—all of it sharpens your clinical judgment.

Trust your preparation. You didn't choose social work because it was easy. You chose it because you want to help people navigate complex problems. The exam is just one more complex problem to navigate. You have the tools. Now use them.

Key Takeaways

1. Start with a diagnostic practice exam to identify your specific weak areas before creating your study plan.
2. Allocate study time proportionally to exam weighting—Assessment/Diagnosis and Interventions/Case Management represent over half the exam.
3. Consistency beats intensity in studying; regular short sessions work better than irregular marathon sessions.
4. Read question stems carefully and identify keywords (first, most, best, except) that direct your thinking.
5. Use systematic elimination to improve your odds; remove options that violate ethics, safety, or scope of practice.
6. Manage test anxiety starting weeks before the exam through preparation, practice under test conditions, and relaxation techniques.
7. Pace yourself at roughly 90 seconds per question and use hourly checkpoints to monitor progress.
8. Read complete scenarios before looking at questions; identify the client, problem, setting, and stage of intervention.
9. Choose the best social work response, not just a correct response—answers should reflect social work values and evidence-based practice.

10. You need approximately 62-70% correct to pass; perfection isn't required, solid preparation and good test-taking strategies are.

Chapter 1: Human Development Across the Lifespan

Human beings change from the moment of conception until death. As clinical social workers, you need to understand these changes—not as abstract concepts, but as living realities that shape every client who walks through your door. A 45-year-old woman struggling with depression brings her entire developmental history with her. The toddler who never learned to trust, the adolescent who couldn't separate, the young adult who avoided intimacy—all of these earlier selves live inside the person sitting across from you.

Development doesn't happen in a vacuum. It happens in families, in communities, in cultures that shape what we become. You can't separate a person's growth from the world they grew up in.

Developmental Theories

Erik Erikson's Psychosocial Stages

Erikson gave us eight stages of development, each with a crisis that must be resolved. These aren't just childhood issues—they span the entire life course. The quality of resolution at each stage affects all subsequent stages.

The first crisis happens in infancy: **trust versus mistrust** (birth to 18 months). An infant whose needs are met consistently learns that the world is safe. When caregivers are unreliable or rejecting, the infant learns mistrust. This basic orientation toward the world—safe or dangerous—colors everything that follows.

Consider Maria, a 32-year-old client who can't maintain relationships. In therapy, you discover her mother suffered from untreated postpartum depression. Maria spent her first year with a caregiver who was physically present but emotionally absent. The infant Maria couldn't understand depression—she only knew that crying didn't bring comfort. Now, the adult Maria expects abandonment and pushes people away before they can leave her.

Autonomy versus shame and doubt (18 months to 3 years) emerges when toddlers begin to assert independence. "No!" becomes their favorite word. Parents who support this growing autonomy—within safe limits—help children develop self-control and confidence. Overly critical or controlling parents create shame and doubt.

Initiative versus guilt (3 to 5 years) centers on purpose and direction. Preschoolers ask endless questions, make plans, and try new activities. When adults encourage this exploration, children develop initiative. When adults dismiss or ridicule their efforts, guilt takes root.

School-age children (6 to 11 years) face **industry versus inferiority**. Can I succeed at tasks that matter? Children compare themselves to peers. Those who experience success develop competence. Those who experience repeated failure develop feelings of inferiority that can last a lifetime.

Identity versus role confusion defines adolescence (12 to 18 years). Teenagers ask: Who am I? What do I believe? What will I become? This identity work happens through experimentation—with clothes, friends, ideas, values. Adolescents who navigate this successfully develop a coherent sense of self. Those who don't may drift or adopt identities without real commitment.

Young adulthood (19 to 40 years) brings **intimacy versus isolation**. Can I form close, committed relationships? This requires a solid identity—you need to know who you are before you can truly share yourself with another. People who fear losing themselves in relationships remain isolated.

Middle adulthood (40 to 65 years) centers on **generativity versus stagnation**. Am I contributing something of value? This might mean raising children, mentoring younger colleagues, creating art, or serving the community. People who can't find meaningful ways to contribute feel stagnant and unproductive.

Finally, late adulthood (65+ years) brings **integrity versus despair**. Looking back, was my life worthwhile? People who can accept their life—mistakes and all—achieve integrity. Those filled with regret experience despair.

Jean Piaget's Cognitive Development

Piaget showed us that children don't think like small adults—they have qualitatively different ways of understanding the world. These stages build on each other, and you can't skip steps.

The **sensorimotor stage** (birth to 2 years) defines infancy. Babies learn through their senses and actions. They develop **object permanence**—the understanding that objects continue to exist even when you can't see them. Before this develops (around 8-12 months), peek-a-boo is genuinely magical. The face that disappears has actually vanished from existence.

The **preoperational stage** (2 to 7 years) brings symbolic thought. Children can now use words and images to represent objects. But their thinking remains **egocentric**—they can't easily take another person's perspective. A four-year-old assumes everyone sees what she sees, knows what she knows.

A social worker evaluating a five-year-old might see this in action. The child says, "My daddy is mean." When asked why, she explains, "He won't let me have ice cream for breakfast." The child can't yet understand that her father's refusal reflects concern for her health, not meanness. Her thinking centers on her own immediate wants.

The **concrete operational stage** (7 to 11 years) brings logical thinking about concrete events. Children can now understand **conservation**—that quantity doesn't change when appearance changes. Pour water from a short, wide glass into a tall, narrow one, and the school-age child knows it's still the same amount of water. The preschooler thinks there's more because it looks higher.

The **formal operational stage** (12+ years) allows abstract thinking. Adolescents can think about possibilities, not just realities. They can reason about hypothetical situations, consider multiple perspectives, and think about thinking itself.

Lawrence Kohlberg's Moral Development

Kohlberg built on Piaget's work to describe how moral reasoning develops. He wasn't concerned with what people decide, but how they think about moral questions.

Preconventional morality (typical in young children) focuses on consequences. Right and wrong are defined by punishment and reward. "I shouldn't steal because I'll get in trouble." This isn't really morality—it's just avoiding punishment.

Conventional morality (typical in adolescents and adults) focuses on social rules and others' approval. "I shouldn't steal because stealing is against the law" or "because people would think badly of me." Right and wrong are defined by society's standards.

Postconventional morality (reached by some adults) recognizes that laws and social rules are human constructs. Moral principles may sometimes conflict with laws. A person at this level might say, "I shouldn't steal because it violates others' rights—but I would steal medicine to save a dying child because life is more sacred than property."

Most adults function at the conventional level. That's normal and healthy. You don't need postconventional reasoning to live an ethical life.

Infancy and Early Childhood

The first five years of life create the foundation for everything that follows. Brain development during this period is extraordinary—connections form at a rate that will never be matched again.

Infants are born ready to connect. They prefer faces to other visual stimuli. They can recognize their mother's voice within days. The infant brain is primed for relationship.

Attachment emerges from repeated interactions with caregivers. When a baby cries and someone responds—feeding her, changing her, soothing her—she learns that her signals have meaning and that people can be trusted to help. This becomes an **internal working model** of relationships.

Mary Ainsworth identified attachment patterns through the Strange Situation procedure. **Secure attachment** develops when caregivers are consistently responsive. These children use the caregiver as a secure base for exploration. When distressed, they seek comfort and are soothed.

Insecure-avoidant attachment develops when caregivers are consistently unresponsive or rejecting. These children learn that seeking comfort doesn't work, so they avoid the caregiver when distressed and suppress their emotions.

Insecure-ambivalent attachment develops with inconsistent caregiving. Sometimes the caregiver responds, sometimes not. These children are anxious and clingy. When distressed, they seek contact but aren't easily soothed—they've learned that comfort is unreliable.

Disorganized attachment develops when the caregiver is frightening or frightened. The child needs comfort from the very person who causes fear. This creates an unsolvable dilemma and often appears in homes with abuse or serious mental illness.

These patterns shape adult relationships. The securely attached infant becomes an adult who trusts others and seeks support when needed. The avoidant infant becomes an adult who dismisses emotional needs and maintains distance. The ambivalent infant becomes an adult who fears abandonment and seeks constant reassurance.

Early childhood brings rapid development in language, motor skills, and self-regulation. The toddler who had no impulse control gradually learns to wait, to share, to consider others. This happens through maturation, but also through countless small interactions with caregivers who set limits, explain feelings, and model self-control.

Play becomes the work of early childhood. Through play, children process experiences, practice skills, and learn social rules. A four-year-old who just visited the doctor plays "doctor" with her dolls—a way of mastering an experience that may have felt scary.

Adolescence and Identity Formation

Adolescence begins with puberty and ends when the person takes on adult roles. In modern society, this can span from age 11 to the late twenties.

Physical changes trigger psychological ones. The adolescent looks in the mirror and sees a stranger. Who is this person with the changing body, the unpredictable emotions, the sexual feelings?

Identity formation becomes the central task. Adolescents try on different selves like trying on clothes. This week's goth becomes next month's athlete. These experiments aren't confusion—they're the necessary work of identity development.

James Marcia described four identity statuses:

Identity diffusion means no exploration and no commitment. The adolescent hasn't seriously considered options and hasn't committed to any direction. "I don't know what I want to be, and I haven't really thought about it."

Identity foreclosure means commitment without exploration. The adolescent has adopted an identity—often from parents—without examining alternatives. "I'll be a doctor like my father. I never considered anything else."

Moratorium means active exploration without commitment. The adolescent is trying different options, questioning, experimenting. "I'm taking different classes, joining clubs, figuring out what fits."

Identity achievement means commitment after exploration. The adolescent has considered options and made genuine choices. "I've thought about different paths, and I've decided to pursue social work because it aligns with my values."

Healthy identity development requires both exploration and commitment. Parents who can tolerate uncertainty help adolescents explore. Those who demand premature closure create foreclosure.

Peer relationships gain enormous significance. The opinion of friends often matters more than parents' opinions—not because adolescents don't love their parents, but because peers help answer the question "Who am I among people like me?"

Consider Jason, a 16-year-old client referred for declining grades. He used to be studious, but now he skips homework to spend time with new friends. His parents see rebellion. You see identity work. Jason grew up in a family that valued academic achievement above all else. Now he's testing whether that fits who he wants to be. He needs to reject his parents' values temporarily to discover which ones he genuinely holds. This doesn't mean you ignore the failing grades—but you understand their meaning differently.

Risk-taking increases during adolescence, not because teenagers can't understand danger, but because they weigh rewards differently. The brain's reward system develops faster than the impulse control system. Social rewards—looking cool, impressing peers—activate the brain's pleasure centers intensely.

Adulthood and Aging

Young adulthood focuses on intimacy and achievement. People form committed relationships, establish careers, perhaps start families. These aren't just external events—they shape identity. The person you become through loving someone, raising children, building a career—this isn't the same person you were before.

Developmental theorists once thought development ended in young adulthood. We now know that's wrong. Development continues until death.

Daniel Levinson described adult development as alternating periods of stability and transition. Every 7-10 years, adults reevaluate their life structure. Is this still working? Does this still fit who I am?

The **midlife transition** (40-45 years) often brings questioning. You've lived long enough to see what's possible and what's not. Dreams you've carried since youth may now seem unreachable. This can trigger growth—a shift toward more authentic living—or crisis—desperate attempts to recapture youth.

Middle adulthood brings what Erikson called generativity—a concern for the next generation. This might mean raising children, but it extends beyond parenthood. It's about contributing, teaching, leaving something valuable behind.

Cognitive abilities change across adulthood. **Fluid intelligence**—the ability to solve novel problems and think quickly—peaks in the twenties and gradually declines. **Crystallized intelligence**—accumulated knowledge and wisdom—continues to grow into old age.

This means a 70-year-old may solve puzzles more slowly than a 20-year-old, but brings far more wisdom to complex human problems. As a clinical social worker, you'll often see this wisdom in older clients who understand themselves and others with a depth that younger clients haven't yet developed.

Late adulthood brings losses—physical decline, retirement, death of friends and partners. Depression isn't a normal part of aging, but grief is. You'll work with clients who are losing capacities they once took for granted. The man who defined himself through his work now faces retirement. The woman who prided herself on independence now needs help with basic tasks.

But late adulthood also brings gains. Many older adults report greater life satisfaction than middle-aged adults. They've learned what matters and what doesn't. They're less troubled by others' opinions. They appreciate simple pleasures more deeply.

Selective optimization with compensation describes how older adults maintain functioning. They select fewer activities (focusing on what matters most), optimize their performance in these areas (through practice and planning), and compensate for losses (using tools, asking for help).

Consider Eleanor, an 80-year-old client with arthritis who loved gardening. She can no longer kneel or dig. She might give up gardening entirely—or she might select (focus on container plants), optimize (choose plants that require less maintenance), and compensate (use raised beds and adaptive tools). This isn't just coping with loss—it's adaptive development.

Case Example: Marcus

Marcus is a 42-year-old African American man referred by his physician for depression. He reports low mood, poor sleep, and loss of interest in activities. His physician found no medical cause.

In your first session, Marcus seems reluctant. He says, "I don't really believe in therapy. My wife made me come." You recognize that many African American men have learned to distrust mental health services—for good historical reasons.

You take a developmental history. Marcus grew up in a single-parent home after his father left when he was eight. His mother worked two jobs. He learned early to be independent, to suppress emotional needs, to "be a man." This worked for years. He excelled in school, built a successful business, married, and had three children.

But now his oldest son is 16—the same age Marcus was when he took his first job to help his mother. His son shows no interest in work. He hangs out with friends Marcus considers "bad influences." Marcus tries to set limits, but his son rebels.

Marcus says, "I gave him everything I never had. Why isn't he grateful?"

You help Marcus see the developmental mismatch. Marcus had to grow up fast—his circumstances demanded it. His son has a different life. He has the luxury of adolescent exploration that Marcus never had. Marcus feels his son is wasting opportunities. His son feels controlled.

But there's more. Marcus is approaching midlife. He's achieved success by conventional standards, but at what cost? He worked constantly, rarely saw his children when they were young, has few friends. His wife complains that he's emotionally distant. He built the life he thought he should have—but does it fit who he is?

You work with Marcus on multiple levels. You help him understand his son's normal adolescent development. You help him examine his own midlife transition. You help him recognize how his childhood shaped both his strengths (resilience, work ethic) and his limitations (difficulty with intimacy, suppressed emotions).

Marcus's depression isn't just a symptom to eliminate—it's a signal that something needs to change. His old identity structure no longer fits. He needs to develop new ways of being—as a father, as a husband, as a man moving into the second half of life.

This takes months of work. Marcus starts spending time with his son—not lecturing, just being together. He joins a men's group at church. He and his wife start couple's therapy. His depression lifts, not because you eliminated symptoms, but because he's developing in new directions.

Practice Questions

1. A 15-year-old client tells you she doesn't know what she wants to study in college and hasn't thought much about it. According to Marcia's identity statuses, this represents:

A. Identity achievement
B. Identity foreclosure
C. Identity diffusion
D. Moratorium

2. According to Erikson, a 4-year-old child who is punished for asking questions and exploring may develop:

A. Mistrust
B. Shame and doubt
C. Guilt
D. Inferiority

3. A 70-year-old client maintains her independence by using a pill organizer, writing detailed lists, and asking her daughter to drive her to appointments. This illustrates:

A. Identity diffusion
B. Selective optimization with compensation
C. Concrete operational thinking
D. Role confusion

4. According to Piaget, a 3-year-old who believes her teddy bear is sad because it's sitting alone demonstrates:

A. Egocentrism
B. Conservation
C. Object permanence
D. Abstract reasoning

5. An infant whose mother is consistently unresponsive to crying is most likely to develop which attachment pattern?

A. Secure
B. Insecure-avoidant
C. Insecure-ambivalent
D. Disorganized

6. A client says, "I shouldn't cheat on my taxes because it's against the law and I could get in trouble." This represents which level of moral reasoning?

A. Preconventional
B. Conventional
C. Postconventional
D. Formal operational

7. According to Erikson, a 25-year-old who avoids committed relationships for fear of losing independence is struggling with:

A. Identity versus role confusion
B. Intimacy versus isolation
C. Generativity versus stagnation
D. Initiative versus guilt

8. A 9-year-old understands that water poured from a short, wide glass to a tall, narrow glass is the same amount. This demonstrates:

A. Egocentrism
B. Conservation
C. Object permanence
D. Symbolic thought

9. A 45-year-old client reports feeling like her life lacks meaning since her youngest child left for college. According to Erikson, she may be struggling with:

A. Intimacy versus isolation
B. Identity versus role confusion
C. Generativity versus stagnation
D. Integrity versus despair

10. According to Piaget, at what age do children typically develop object permanence?

A. 2-4 months
B. 8-12 months
C. 18-24 months
D. 3-4 years

11. A 17-year-old is actively exploring different religions, political views, and career options before making commitments. This represents:

A. Identity achievement
B. Identity foreclosure

C. Identity diffusion
D. Moratorium

12. An 8-month-old shows distress when his mother leaves the room but is quickly soothed when she returns. This most likely indicates:

A. Secure attachment
B. Insecure-avoidant attachment
C. Insecure-ambivalent attachment
D. Disorganized attachment

13. According to Erikson, the primary task of late adulthood is:

A. Intimacy versus isolation
B. Generativity versus stagnation
C. Integrity versus despair
D. Identity versus role confusion

14. A client says, "I believe in civil disobedience when laws are unjust, even though it means breaking the law." This represents which level of moral reasoning?

A. Preconventional
B. Conventional
C. Postconventional
D. Concrete operational

15. A 2-year-old insists on putting on her own shoes, even though it takes much longer. According to Erikson, parents who consistently do it for her may contribute to:

A. Mistrust
B. Shame and doubt
C. Guilt
D. Role confusion

16. According to Piaget, the ability to think about hypothetical situations and abstract concepts develops during:

A. Sensorimotor stage
B. Preoperational stage
C. Concrete operational stage
D. Formal operational stage

17. A 60-year-old finds satisfaction in mentoring young professionals at work. According to Erikson, this represents:

A. Identity achievement
B. Intimacy
C. Generativity
D. Integrity

18. An infant whose caregiver is sometimes responsive and sometimes not is most likely to develop which attachment pattern?

A. Secure
B. Insecure-avoidant
C. Insecure-ambivalent
D. Disorganized

19. A 5-year-old assumes that everyone knows what he knows and sees what he sees. This demonstrates:

A. Conservation
B. Egocentrism
C. Object permanence
D. Formal operational thinking

20. According to Erikson, a 10-year-old who experiences repeated academic failure may develop:

A. Mistrust
B. Shame and doubt
C. Guilt
D. Inferiority

21. A 30-year-old has followed his father's career path without considering alternatives. This represents:

A. Identity achievement
B. Identity foreclosure
C. Identity diffusion
D. Moratorium

22. Fluid intelligence typically:

A. Increases throughout adulthood
B. Peaks in young adulthood and gradually declines
C. Remains stable across the lifespan
D. Decreases in young adulthood and increases in late adulthood

23. A child who can think logically about concrete objects but struggles with abstract concepts is in Piaget's:

A. Sensorimotor stage
B. Preoperational stage
C. Concrete operational stage
D. Formal operational stage

24. According to Erikson, the primary developmental task of adolescence is:

A. Trust versus mistrust
B. Identity versus role confusion
C. Intimacy versus isolation
D. Initiative versus guilt

25. An infant whose parent is frightening or frightened is most likely to develop which attachment pattern?

A. Secure
B. Insecure-avoidant
C. Insecure-ambivalent
D. Disorganized

26. A client says, "I shouldn't lie because people would think badly of me." This represents which level of moral reasoning?

A. Preconventional
B. Conventional
C. Postconventional
D. Sensorimotor

27. According to Erikson, a 75-year-old who looks back on life with satisfaction and acceptance has achieved:

A. Generativity
B. Intimacy
C. Integrity
D. Identity

28. A 7-month-old continues to look for a toy after it's hidden under a blanket. This demonstrates:

A. Egocentrism
B. Conservation
C. Object permanence
D. Symbolic thought

29. According to Levinson, adults typically experience a major life reevaluation every:

A. 3-5 years
B. 7-10 years
C. 15-20 years
D. 25-30 years

30. A 14-year-old takes risks to impress peers, even though she understands the dangers. This is most likely because:

A. She lacks object permanence
B. She hasn't developed formal operational thinking

C. The brain's reward system develops faster than impulse control
D. She has identity diffusion

31. According to Erikson, a 35-year-old who has not formed intimate relationships may experience:

A. Role confusion
B. Isolation
C. Stagnation
D. Despair

32. Crystallized intelligence:

A. Decreases throughout adulthood
B. Peaks in young adulthood and declines
C. Continues to grow into old age
D. Remains stable across the lifespan

33. A 6-year-old compares her schoolwork to her classmates and feels inadequate. According to Erikson, repeated experiences like this could lead to:

A. Mistrust
B. Shame and doubt
C. Guilt
D. Inferiority

34. According to Piaget, a 4-year-old who uses a banana as a telephone is demonstrating:

A. Object permanence
B. Conservation
C. Symbolic thought
D. Abstract reasoning

35. A 50-year-old questions whether his career choice aligns with his values. This likely represents:

A. Identity diffusion
B. Midlife transition
C. Role confusion
D. Stagnation

36. A baby shows no distress when her mother leaves and ignores her when she returns. This most likely indicates:

A. Secure attachment
B. Insecure-avoidant attachment
C. Insecure-ambivalent attachment
D. Disorganized attachment

37. According to Kohlberg, which level of moral reasoning is most common in adults?

A. Preconventional
B. Conventional
C. Postconventional
D. All are equally common

38. A 3-year-old wants to help cook dinner but makes a mess. If parents respond with anger and criticism, Erikson would predict the child may develop:

A. Mistrust
B. Shame and doubt
C. Guilt
D. Inferiority

39. According to Erikson, identity formation primarily occurs during:

A. Early childhood
B. Middle childhood
C. Adolescence
D. Young adulthood

40. A 12-year-old can consider multiple solutions to a problem and think about future consequences. This indicates development of:

A. Preoperational thinking
B. Concrete operational thinking
C. Formal operational thinking
D. Postconventional thinking

41. Selective optimization with compensation in late adulthood involves:

A. Avoiding all challenging activities
B. Maintaining all previous activities without modification
C. Focusing on priorities and adapting strategies
D. Accepting decline without adjustment

42. An infant whose needs are consistently met is most likely to develop:

A. Autonomy
B. Trust
C. Initiative
D. Industry

43. According to Marcia, an adolescent who has committed to a career chosen by parents without exploring alternatives shows:

A. Identity achievement
B. Identity foreclosure

C. Identity diffusion
D. Moratorium

44. A 55-year-old finds meaning through volunteer work with youth. According to Erikson, this represents:

A. Identity
B. Intimacy
C. Generativity
D. Integrity

45. According to Piaget, understanding that 8+5 is the same as 5+8 requires:

A. Preoperational thinking
B. Concrete operational thinking
C. Formal operational thinking
D. Postconventional thinking

46. A client says, "I don't steal because stealing violates people's rights, regardless of the law." This represents which level of moral reasoning?

A. Preconventional
B. Conventional
C. Postconventional
D. Formal operational

47. According to Erikson, an infant whose caregiver is inconsistent may develop:

A. Autonomy
B. Mistrust
C. Shame
D. Guilt

48. Peer relationships become especially important during adolescence because they:

A. Replace family relationships
B. Help answer questions about identity
C. Indicate formal operational thinking
D. Demonstrate secure attachment

49. A 65-year-old maintains cognitive function by focusing on activities she does best and using memory aids for others. This demonstrates:

A. Identity diffusion
B. Selective optimization with compensation
C. Concrete operational thinking
D. Conventional moral reasoning

50. According to Erikson, looking back on life and feeling that it was wasted leads to:

A. Stagnation
B. Isolation
C. Despair
D. Inferiority

Answer Key with Detailed Explanations

1. C. Identity diffusion
This adolescent shows no commitment and hasn't engaged in exploration—the defining features of identity diffusion. She hasn't seriously considered her options (no exploration) and hasn't made any decisions (no commitment). Moratorium would involve active exploration. Identity achievement would require commitment after exploration. Identity foreclosure would mean commitment without exploration.

2. C. Guilt
The 4-year-old is in Erikson's initiative versus guilt stage. Children this age naturally ask questions and explore—this is healthy initiative. When adults punish or ridicule this behavior, children learn that their curiosity and ideas are bad, leading to guilt. Mistrust develops in infancy (0-18 months). Shame and doubt develop in toddlerhood (18 months-3 years). Inferiority develops in middle childhood (6-11 years).

3. B. Selective optimization with compensation
This client selects (chooses to maintain independence in specific areas), optimizes (uses tools and strategies to perform well), and compensates (asks for help where needed). This model describes successful aging—maintaining function by adapting strategies rather than giving up or refusing to modify approaches.

4. A. Egocentrism
Preschool children are egocentric—they attribute their own feelings and perspectives to others, including inanimate objects. The child assumes the teddy bear feels what she would feel in that situation. Conservation involves understanding that quantity doesn't change with appearance. Object permanence is understanding that objects exist when out of sight. Abstract reasoning develops in adolescence.

5. B. Insecure-avoidant
When caregivers are consistently unresponsive or rejecting, infants learn that seeking comfort doesn't work. They develop avoidant attachment—they don't seek proximity when distressed and show little emotion during separations or reunions. Secure attachment requires consistent responsiveness. Ambivalent attachment develops with inconsistent caregiving. Disorganized attachment occurs when the caregiver is frightening.

6. A. Preconventional
This reasoning focuses on personal consequences (getting in trouble), which defines preconventional morality. Conventional morality would focus on social rules or approval ("because it's wrong" or "because society condemns it"). Postconventional would focus on ethical principles beyond laws. Formal operational is a cognitive stage, not a moral reasoning level.

7. B. Intimacy versus isolation
Young adulthood (19-40 years) centers on intimacy versus isolation. Can I form close, committed relationships without losing myself? Fear of losing independence prevents intimacy and leads to isolation. Identity versus role confusion occurs in adolescence. Generativity versus stagnation occurs in middle adulthood. Initiative versus guilt occurs in early childhood.

8. B. Conservation
Conservation is understanding that quantity remains constant despite changes in appearance. This develops during concrete operational stage (7-11 years). Egocentrism is assuming others share your perspective. Object permanence is knowing objects exist when out of sight. Symbolic thought is using symbols to represent objects (develops earlier, in preoperational stage).

9. C. Generativity versus stagnation
Middle adulthood focuses on generativity—contributing to the next generation. When the vehicle for generativity (often parenting) ends, people may feel stagnant and without purpose. She needs to find new ways to contribute. Intimacy versus isolation occurs in young adulthood. Identity versus role confusion occurs in adolescence. Integrity versus despair occurs in late adulthood.

10. B. 8-12 months
Object permanence typically develops between 8-12 months. Before this, objects that disappear from view cease to exist in the infant's understanding. After this, infants will search for hidden objects. This is a major cognitive achievement of the sensorimotor stage.

11. D. Moratorium
Moratorium status involves active exploration without commitment. The adolescent is trying different options, questioning, experimenting—the healthy work of identity formation. Identity achievement would require commitment after exploration. Identity foreclosure would mean commitment without exploration. Identity diffusion would mean neither exploration nor commitment.

12. A. Secure attachment
Secure attachment is shown by using the caregiver as a secure base, showing distress at separation, and being quickly soothed upon reunion. Avoidant attachment shows little distress at separation and ignoring upon reunion. Ambivalent attachment shows extreme distress and difficulty being soothed. Disorganized attachment shows confused or contradictory behaviors.

13. C. Integrity versus despair
Late adulthood (65+ years) centers on reviewing life and achieving either integrity (acceptance) or despair (regret). Intimacy versus isolation occurs in young adulthood. Generativity versus stagnation occurs in middle adulthood. Identity versus role confusion occurs in adolescence.

14. C. Postconventional
Postconventional reasoning recognizes that moral principles may conflict with laws. The person appeals to principles (justice, human rights) that transcend legal rules. Preconventional focuses on consequences. Conventional focuses on following rules and social approval. Concrete operational is a cognitive stage, not a moral reasoning level.

15. B. Shame and doubt
Toddlerhood (18 months-3 years) focuses on autonomy versus shame and doubt. Toddlers need to practice independence. When adults don't allow this or criticize their efforts, children develop shame about their abilities and doubt about their competence. Mistrust develops in infancy. Guilt develops in early childhood. Role confusion develops in adolescence.

16. D. Formal operational stage
Formal operational thinking (beginning around age 12) allows abstract reasoning, hypothetical thinking, and logical reasoning about possibilities rather than just concrete realities. Sensorimotor involves learning through senses and actions. Preoperational involves symbolic thought but remains concrete. Concrete operational involves logical thinking about concrete objects and events.

17. C. Generativity
Generativity means contributing to the next generation—through mentoring, teaching, parenting, or creating something of lasting value. This is the primary task of middle adulthood (40-65 years). Identity achievement occurs in adolescence/young adulthood. Intimacy occurs in young adulthood. Integrity occurs in late adulthood.

18. C. Insecure-ambivalent
Inconsistent caregiving—sometimes responsive, sometimes not—creates insecure-ambivalent attachment. The infant can't predict whether needs will be met, leading to anxiety and clinginess. When distressed, the child seeks contact but isn't easily soothed. Secure attachment requires consistent responsiveness. Avoidant attachment develops with consistent unresponsiveness. Disorganized attachment occurs when the caregiver is frightening.

19. B. Egocentrism
Preschool children assume others share their knowledge and perspective—this is egocentrism. A child who knows something assumes everyone knows it. A child who sees something assumes everyone sees it. This gradually decreases as children develop the ability to take others' perspectives. Conservation involves understanding quantity constancy. Object permanence is knowing objects exist when unseen. Formal operational thinking involves abstract reasoning.

20. D. Inferiority
Middle childhood (6-11 years) focuses on industry versus inferiority. Children compare themselves to peers and evaluate their competence. Repeated failure leads to feelings of inferiority—"I'm not good at anything important." Mistrust develops in infancy. Shame and doubt develop in toddlerhood. Guilt develops in early childhood.

21. B. Identity foreclosure
Identity foreclosure means commitment without exploration. The person has adopted an identity (often from parents or culture) without considering alternatives. This may provide direction but lacks the authenticity of identity achievement, which requires genuine exploration and choice. Identity diffusion involves neither exploration nor commitment. Moratorium involves exploration without commitment.

22. B. Peaks in young adulthood and gradually declines
Fluid intelligence—the ability to solve novel problems, think quickly, and process new information—peaks in the twenties and gradually declines. This is normal aging, not pathology. Crystallized intelligence (accumulated knowledge and wisdom) continues to grow into old age, often compensating for declining fluid intelligence.

23. C. Concrete operational stage
Concrete operational thinking (7-11 years) allows logical reasoning about concrete objects and events but not abstract concepts. A child can solve math problems with real objects but struggles with algebraic variables. Sensorimotor involves learning through senses and actions. Preoperational involves symbolic thought but illogical thinking. Formal operational involves abstract reasoning.

24. B. Identity versus role confusion
Adolescence centers on identity formation. Who am I? What do I believe? What will I become? Successful resolution creates a coherent identity. Failure creates role confusion—uncertainty about self and direction. Trust versus mistrust occurs in infancy. Intimacy versus isolation occurs in young adulthood. Initiative versus guilt occurs in early childhood.

25. D. Disorganized
When the caregiver is the source of both fear and potential comfort, the infant faces an impossible situation. The person they need for safety is the person who frightens them. This creates disorganized attachment—confused, contradictory behaviors that reflect an unsolvable dilemma. This often occurs in homes with abuse, severe mental illness, or unresolved trauma in the caregiver.

26. B. Conventional
This reasoning focuses on social approval and what others think—characteristics of conventional morality. Right and wrong are defined by social standards and others' opinions. Preconventional would focus on punishment or reward. Postconventional would focus on ethical principles beyond social approval. Sensorimotor is a cognitive stage, not a moral reasoning level.

27. C. Integrity
Integrity means accepting your life—the good and bad, the successes and failures—as worthwhile. People who achieve integrity can look back without major regrets, accepting that they lived as well as they could given their circumstances. The alternative is despair—feeling that life was wasted and it's too late to change. Generativity occurs in middle adulthood. Intimacy occurs in young adulthood. Identity forms in adolescence.

28. C. Object permanence
Object permanence—understanding that objects continue to exist when out of sight—typically develops between 8-12 months. An infant who searches for a hidden toy demonstrates this understanding. Egocentrism is assuming others share your perspective. Conservation is understanding quantity constancy. Symbolic thought is using symbols to represent objects.

29. B. 7-10 years
Levinson found that adults experience major life structure evaluations approximately every 7-10 years. These transitions may be smooth or may feel like crises, but they involve questioning current

life structures and considering changes. The midlife transition (around 40-45) is one example, but transitions occur throughout adulthood.

30. C. The brain's reward system develops faster than impulse control
During adolescence, the brain's reward system (especially for social rewards) develops rapidly, while the prefrontal cortex (impulse control) develops more slowly. Adolescents understand risks but weight rewards differently—looking cool to peers activates reward centers intensely. This isn't poor judgment; it's normal brain development. Object permanence develops in infancy. Formal operational thinking develops in adolescence. Identity diffusion is about commitment and exploration, not risk-taking.

31. B. Isolation
Young adulthood focuses on intimacy versus isolation. Failure to form close, committed relationships leads to isolation—feeling alone and disconnected. This often stems from fear of losing oneself in relationships, which requires a solid identity first. Role confusion occurs in adolescence. Stagnation occurs in middle adulthood. Despair occurs in late adulthood.

32. C. Continues to grow into old age
Crystallized intelligence—accumulated knowledge, vocabulary, wisdom—continues to increase throughout adulthood and into old age. This often compensates for declining fluid intelligence. Older adults may solve new problems more slowly but bring more wisdom and experience to complex situations.

33. D. Inferiority
Middle childhood focuses on industry versus inferiority. Children naturally compare themselves to peers. Repeated experiences of inadequacy create feelings of inferiority—"I'm not as good as others." This can become a lasting sense of incompetence. Mistrust develops in infancy. Shame and doubt develop in toddlerhood. Guilt develops in early childhood.

34. C. Symbolic thought
Using one object to represent another (banana as telephone) demonstrates symbolic thought—a major achievement of the preoperational stage. Children can now use words, images, and objects to represent other things. Object permanence is knowing objects exist when unseen. Conservation is understanding quantity constancy. Abstract reasoning develops later.

35. B. Midlife transition
The midlife transition (typically 40-45 years) often involves questioning life choices. Have my decisions aligned with my true values? Is this the life I want? This can lead to growth and positive changes or to crisis and desperate attempts to recapture youth. Identity diffusion involves neither exploration nor commitment. Role confusion occurs in adolescence. Stagnation is about lack of contribution to the next generation.

36. B. Insecure-avoidant
Insecure-avoidant attachment is shown by little distress at separation and ignoring or avoiding the caregiver upon return. These infants have learned that the caregiver won't respond to their needs, so they suppress their attachment behaviors. Secure attachment shows distress and seeking comfort.

Ambivalent attachment shows extreme distress and difficulty being soothed. Disorganized shows confused behaviors.

37. B. Conventional
Most adults function at the conventional level of moral reasoning—basing moral judgments on social rules, laws, and others' approval. This is normal and healthy. Preconventional (focusing on consequences) is typical in children. Postconventional (reasoning from ethical principles that may conflict with laws) is reached by only some adults.

38. C. Guilt
Early childhood (3-5 years) focuses on initiative versus guilt. Children naturally take initiative—making plans, trying new things, helping. When adults punish or criticize these efforts, children learn that their ideas and actions are bad, leading to guilt. Mistrust develops in infancy. Shame and doubt develop in toddlerhood. Inferiority develops in middle childhood.

39. C. Adolescence
Identity formation is the primary task of adolescence (12-18 years). Teenagers ask: Who am I? What do I believe? What will I become? This work happens through experimentation and exploration. Early childhood focuses on initiative. Middle childhood focuses on industry. Young adulthood focuses on intimacy.

40. C. Formal operational thinking
Formal operational thinking (beginning around age 12) allows abstract reasoning, considering multiple possibilities, and thinking about future consequences. This is qualitatively different from concrete operational thinking, which is limited to logical reasoning about concrete objects and events. Preoperational thinking is illogical and egocentric. Postconventional refers to moral reasoning, not cognitive development.

41. C. Focusing on priorities and adapting strategies
Selective optimization with compensation means selecting what matters most (focus on priorities), optimizing performance in these areas (practice, plan), and compensating for losses (use tools, ask for help). This allows older adults to maintain functioning despite declining capacities. It's not about avoiding challenges or refusing to adapt.

42. B. Trust
Infancy (0-18 months) focuses on trust versus mistrust. When needs are consistently met, infants learn that the world is safe and people are reliable—this is basic trust. Autonomy develops in toddlerhood. Initiative develops in early childhood. Industry develops in middle childhood.

43. B. Identity foreclosure
Identity foreclosure means commitment without exploration. The adolescent has adopted an identity (from parents, culture) without considering alternatives. This provides direction but lacks the authenticity that comes from genuine exploration and choice. Identity achievement requires both exploration and commitment. Identity diffusion involves neither. Moratorium involves exploration without commitment.

44. C. Generativity
Generativity means contributing to the next generation and society. This can happen through parenting, mentoring, volunteering, creating, or any activity that leaves something valuable for those who follow. This is the primary task of middle adulthood. Identity forms in adolescence. Intimacy develops in young adulthood. Integrity develops in late adulthood.

45. B. Concrete operational thinking
Understanding mathematical operations and their reversibility (if 8+5=13, then 5+8=13) requires concrete operational thinking. This logical reasoning about concrete problems develops around age 7-11. Preoperational children can't grasp these relationships. Formal operational thinking involves abstract reasoning beyond concrete operations. Postconventional refers to moral reasoning.

46. C. Postconventional
Postconventional reasoning appeals to ethical principles (human rights, justice) that may transcend laws. The person recognizes that laws are human constructs and that moral principles may sometimes require violating laws. Preconventional focuses on personal consequences. Conventional focuses on rules and social approval. Formal operational refers to cognitive development.

47. B. Mistrust
Infancy focuses on trust versus mistrust. Inconsistent caregiving—sometimes responsive, sometimes not—teaches the infant that the world is unpredictable and people can't be relied upon. This creates basic mistrust. Autonomy develops in toddlerhood. Shame develops in toddlerhood. Guilt develops in early childhood.

48. B. Help answer questions about identity
Peers become especially important during adolescence because they help answer identity questions: Who am I among people like me? What do people like me value? Peer relationships don't replace family but serve different developmental functions. They're not primarily about cognitive development or attachment patterns.

49. B. Selective optimization with compensation
This client selects (focuses on what she does best), optimizes (continues practicing these skills), and compensates (uses memory aids for other tasks). This adaptive strategy allows older adults to maintain functioning despite age-related changes. Identity diffusion is about commitment and exploration. Concrete operational thinking is a childhood cognitive stage. Conventional moral reasoning is about social rules.

50. C. Despair
Late adulthood focuses on integrity versus despair. Integrity means accepting your life as worthwhile. Despair means feeling that life was wasted and it's too late for change—a profound regret. Stagnation (feeling unproductive) occurs in middle adulthood. Isolation (avoiding intimacy) occurs in young adulthood. Inferiority (feeling incompetent) develops in middle childhood.

Moving Forward

Understanding human development isn't about memorizing stages. It's about recognizing that the 40-year-old sitting across from you carries every year she's lived. The infant who wasn't comforted, the child who felt incompetent, the adolescent who couldn't form an identity—all of these earlier selves influence the adult seeking your help.

Development never stops. Your clients are still growing, still changing, still working on tasks that may have begun decades ago. The man who never developed trust in infancy can, with help, learn to trust now. The woman who foreclosed identity in adolescence can, in midlife, finally explore who she really is.

You're not just treating symptoms. You're supporting development at whatever stage your client has reached. That's the work.

Key Takeaways

- Development happens in stages, but each stage builds on earlier ones—unresolved issues from one stage affect all later stages
- Erikson's psychosocial stages span the entire lifespan, from trust versus mistrust in infancy to integrity versus despair in late adulthood
- Attachment patterns formed in infancy shape adult relationships—secure, avoidant, ambivalent, and disorganized patterns persist
- Piaget's cognitive stages show that children think qualitatively differently than adults—understanding this prevents unrealistic expectations
- Identity formation is the central task of adolescence, requiring both exploration and commitment to achieve genuine identity
- Adult development continues with regular transitions that require reevaluating life structures
- Moral reasoning develops from focusing on consequences to following social rules to reasoning from ethical principles
- Older adults adapt successfully through selective optimization with compensation—focusing on priorities and adapting strategies
- Every client brings their entire developmental history to therapy—effective treatment addresses both current issues and developmental foundations
- Development is never finished—people can work on tasks from earlier stages at any point in life

Chapter 2: Diversity, Social Justice, and Oppression

You can't do clinical social work without understanding power. Not just the power in your relationship with clients—though that matters too—but the power that shapes every client's life before they ever meet you. The power that determines who gets good schools and who doesn't. Who gets stopped by police and who doesn't. Who gets hired and who doesn't. Who gets believed and who doesn't.

Clinical work happens in a social context. Your client's depression isn't just about brain chemistry or family dynamics. It's about living in a world that may actively work against them. The anxiety you're treating may be a reasonable response to real danger. The "paranoia" may be justified vigilance.

Cultural Competence and Humility

For years, we talked about cultural competence—learning about different cultures so you could work effectively with diverse clients. The idea was good. The execution often wasn't. Social workers studied lists: Asians value family. Latinos value respect. Native Americans value spirituality. These generalizations helped no one and sometimes hurt.

Real competence starts with humility. Cultural humility means recognizing that you can never fully understand another person's cultural experience. You can learn. You can listen. But you'll always be an outsider to experiences you haven't lived.

Cultural humility has three components:

First, **lifelong learning and self-reflection**. You examine your own cultural identity, biases, and assumptions. You recognize that learning about other cultures never ends. Each client teaches you something new.

Second, **addressing power imbalances**. You acknowledge the power you hold as a therapist and work to minimize its harmful effects. You recognize that institutional power affects the therapeutic relationship.

Third, **institutional accountability**. You examine how your agency's policies and practices affect diverse clients. You work to change systems, not just help individuals adapt to unfair systems.

Cultural humility means you don't assume. A client from Mexico may have completely different experiences than a client from El Salvador, even though both are "Latino." A Black client from Nigeria has different experiences than a Black client whose family has been in the U.S. for generations. A gay man in his twenties grew up in a different world than a gay man in his seventies.

You ask. You listen. You accept correction. When you make assumptions—and you will—you apologize and adjust.

Race, Ethnicity, and Immigration

Race is a social construct, not a biological reality. There's more genetic variation within racial groups than between them. But race is real in its effects. The social meaning attached to skin color shapes lives profoundly.

Racism isn't just individual prejudice. It's a system that advantages some groups and disadvantages others. You can be "not racist" personally while participating in racist systems. When your agency requires documentation that undocumented immigrants can't provide, that's institutional racism—regardless of anyone's intentions.

Racial trauma describes the cumulative effects of racism on mental health. This includes:

- Direct experiences of discrimination and violence
- Vicarious trauma from witnessing racism against others
- Anticipatory anxiety about future racism
- Intergenerational transmission of trauma

A Black client's hypervigilance isn't paranoia—it's adaptive. A Latino client's mistrust of authorities isn't resistance—it's learned from experience. An Asian client's academic pressure isn't just "tiger parenting"—it may reflect awareness that they face higher standards to achieve the same outcomes.

Microaggressions—brief, everyday slights that communicate hostile or derogatory messages—accumulate. "You're so articulate" said to a Black professional. "Where are you really from?" asked of an Asian American. "You don't look Jewish." Each incident seems small. The cumulative effect is enormous.

Immigration adds layers of complexity. Immigrants may experience:

- **Acculturative stress** from navigating two cultures
- **Loss and grief** for their country of origin
- **Family separation** across borders or generations
- **Documentation status anxiety** and fear of deportation
- **Discrimination** as both immigrants and racial minorities

Children of immigrants often become cultural brokers—translating language and culture for parents. This can create role reversals where children carry adult responsibilities. The stress of living between cultures, never fully belonging to either, shapes development.

Case Example: Aisha

Aisha is a 28-year-old Black woman referred by her physician for "noncompliance" with diabetes management. The referral note says she "refuses to follow medical advice" and "doesn't take her condition seriously."

In your first session, Aisha seems wary. She answers questions briefly. You recognize that she has good reasons to mistrust helping professionals—they've often failed Black women.

You start differently. You acknowledge the referral: "Your doctor is concerned about your diabetes management. But I'm more interested in hearing your perspective. What's this been like for you?"

Aisha relaxes slightly. She explains that she can't afford the recommended foods. The doctor suggested fresh vegetables and lean proteins—but she lives in a food desert where the nearest grocery store is an hour away by bus. The corner store has processed foods and little produce.

The doctor recommended exercise—but Aisha works two jobs to support her three children. She leaves before dawn and returns after dark. Her neighborhood isn't safe for evening walks. The gym membership the doctor suggested costs more than she spends on food weekly.

The doctor told her to "reduce stress"—but Aisha's rent just increased. Her oldest son was stopped by police three times last month for "looking suspicious" in his own neighborhood. Her daughter's school called her a "problem child" for defending herself against racist comments.

The doctor never asked about any of this. He just labeled her noncompliant.

You help Aisha identify realistic strategies within her actual life constraints. You connect her with food assistance programs and community resources. You write a letter to her doctor explaining the social determinants of health affecting her diabetes management.

But you also validate her reality: "Your doctor saw noncompliance. I see a woman managing impossible circumstances with limited resources. The problem isn't that you don't care about your health. The problem is that the medical system doesn't account for the reality of your life."

This is clinical social work informed by awareness of racism and social inequality. You don't just help Aisha adjust to an unfair system—you advocate for systemic change while supporting her immediate needs.

LGBTQ+ Populations

Sexual orientation and gender identity shape development and mental health in specific ways. LGBTQ+ individuals face unique stressors that affect clinical presentation.

Minority stress theory explains elevated mental health problems in LGBTQ+ populations. This stress comes from:

- **External stressors**: Discrimination, violence, rejection, legal inequalities
- **Internalized stigma**: Negative beliefs about oneself based on societal messages
- **Concealment**: Energy spent hiding identity and monitoring behavior
- **Anticipation of rejection**: Hypervigilance for potential discrimination

Coming out isn't a single event—it's a lifelong process. Each new situation requires a decision: Do I disclose? Is it safe? What will I lose or gain?

Family rejection has severe consequences. LGBTQ+ youth who experience family rejection are:

- 8 times more likely to attempt suicide
- 6 times more likely to report high levels of depression
- 3 times more likely to use illegal drugs
- 3 times more likely to engage in unprotected sex

But family acceptance dramatically improves outcomes. Even small actions matter: using correct names and pronouns, expressing affection, supporting gender expression, standing up for the young person.

Transgender and gender non-conforming individuals face additional stressors. **Gender dysphoria**—distress from the mismatch between gender identity and assigned sex—can be severe. But it's not mental illness. The distress comes from:

- Body characteristics that don't match identity
- Social misgendering and use of wrong pronouns
- Legal barriers to changing documentation
- Lack of access to medical transition if desired
- Violence and discrimination

Treatment focuses on supporting the person's identity, not changing it. This might include:

- Social transition (name, pronouns, presentation)
- Medical transition (hormones, surgery) if desired
- Family therapy to support acceptance
- Advocacy for safe environments
- Connection with affirming communities

Older LGBTQ+ adults face unique challenges. Many came of age before Stonewall, when homosexuality was classified as mental illness and could result in imprisonment. They experienced profound oppression and may mistrust helping professionals. Many remained closeted and now face aging without partners or children. Some move back into the closet in senior housing where they fear discrimination.

Disability and Accessibility

Disability affects one in four adults in the United States. Yet clinical social work training often neglects disability issues. The **medical model** views disability as a problem located in the individual that needs to be fixed or cured. The **social model** recognizes that disability results from the interaction between individual differences and social barriers.

A person who uses a wheelchair isn't disabled by their body—they're disabled by stairs without ramps, buses without lifts, buildings without accessible bathrooms. Remove the barriers, and the disability often disappears.

Ableism—discrimination against people with disabilities—pervades society and mental health services. It appears in:

- Physical inaccessibility of buildings and offices
- Information not provided in accessible formats
- Assumptions about quality of life and capacity
- Infantilization and paternalism
- Inspiration porn—treating people with disabilities as inspirational simply for living their lives

People with disabilities face specific mental health risks:

- Higher rates of trauma from medical procedures and bullying
- Social isolation from exclusion and inaccessibility
- Poverty from employment discrimination and additional costs
- Loss and grief related to disability or degenerative conditions
- Internalized ableism from societal messages

Invisible disabilities—chronic pain, mental illness, chronic fatigue, autoimmune conditions—create additional challenges. People face skepticism, accusations of faking, pressure to "push through" and prove their disability. The effort of appearing "normal" is exhausting.

Intersectionality matters profoundly. Being disabled and Black, disabled and poor, disabled and LGBTQ+—each intersection creates unique experiences. A wheelchair user who is also undocumented faces barriers that someone with citizenship doesn't.

Clinical work requires:

- **Physical accessibility**: Ramps, accessible bathrooms, service animals welcome
- **Communicative accessibility**: Materials in multiple formats, sign language interpreters
- **Attitudinal accessibility**: Respect for autonomy, presumption of competence
- **Flexibility**: Accommodating fatigue, pain, medical appointments
- **Knowledge**: Understanding how disability affects the presenting problem

Socioeconomic Factors

Poverty kills. It shortens lives, causes illness, and creates trauma. Yet we often treat poverty as a personal failing rather than a structural condition.

Economic inequality has grown dramatically. The richest 1% now own more wealth than the bottom 90% combined. This isn't just statistics—it's your clients' reality.

Poverty creates chronic stress. The stress of not knowing if you can pay rent. The stress of choosing between medication and food. The stress of working multiple jobs and still falling behind. This chronic stress affects brain development in children and mental health in adults.

The **allostatic load** describes cumulative wear and tear from chronic stress. Poor individuals have higher allostatic load, leading to earlier aging and more health problems.

Food insecurity affects one in eight Americans. This doesn't just mean hunger—it means:

- Constant worry about food running out
- Sacrificing nutrition for calories (processed foods are cheap)
- Skipping meals to feed children
- Emergency room visits for nutrition-related problems

Housing instability creates profound insecurity. Eviction isn't just losing housing—it's trauma. Children who experience eviction are more likely to experience hunger, illness, and school difficulties. Their mothers are more likely to experience depression.

Homelessness destroys health. Sleep deprivation, exposure to weather, violence, lack of hygiene facilities—these create both physical and mental health crises. Yet services often require documentation or sobriety that homeless individuals can't provide.

Work affects health. Low-wage workers often face:

- Irregular schedules that prevent planning
- No sick leave or health insurance
- Physically demanding or dangerous conditions
- Exposure to toxic substances
- Workplace discrimination

The working poor—people employed full-time but still in poverty—face particular stress. They work hard but can't get ahead. The American myth that hard work guarantees success fails them daily.

Education stratifies opportunity. Poor children attend underfunded schools with fewer resources. They're more likely to be suspended or expelled. They're less likely to attend college. This isn't about ability—it's about access.

Case Example: The Martinez Family

The Martinez family comes to therapy because 10-year-old Miguel is "acting out" at school. His teacher reports that he's aggressive, defiant, and often falls asleep in class.

Your assessment reveals a family under enormous stress. Both parents work—the father in construction, the mother cleaning houses. They work opposite shifts so someone can always be with the children. They rarely see each other.

The family lives in a two-bedroom apartment with Miguel, his two younger siblings, and his grandmother. Miguel shares a bedroom with his siblings. He has no quiet place to do homework. The apartment has mold that triggers his asthma, but they can't afford to move.

Miguel's father was injured at work three months ago. Worker's compensation is disputed. The family fell behind on bills. They've been eating rice and beans almost exclusively. Miguel is hungry.

The school sent Miguel to the principal for falling asleep. No one asked why. At home, he cares for his siblings while his parents work. He often doesn't sleep until his parents return near midnight. He wakes early to get his siblings ready for school.

The school labeled Miguel's behavior a problem. You see a child carrying adult responsibilities while dealing with hunger, inadequate sleep, and housing stress.

You work on multiple levels:

- Connect the family with food assistance and medical care
- Advocate with the school for understanding and support
- Help the family identify stress reduction strategies
- Support Miguel's need to be a child, not a parent
- Work with parents on distributing responsibilities differently
- Address the trauma of poverty and instability

This is clinical social work grounded in understanding that individual problems often reflect social conditions. You can't treat Miguel's "behavior problem" without addressing his family's poverty.

Oppression and Liberation

Oppression operates on multiple levels:

Individual level: Internalized oppression occurs when people believe negative messages about their group. A woman believes women are naturally worse at math. A poor person believes poverty reflects personal failure. A person with a disability believes they're a burden.

Interpersonal level: Discrimination, microaggressions, and prejudice in relationships. A qualified candidate not hired due to accent. A couple harassed for holding hands. A student's intelligence questioned due to race.

Institutional level: Policies and practices that disadvantage certain groups. Schools that suspend Black students at higher rates for identical behaviors. Banks that deny mortgages in certain neighborhoods. Immigration policies that separate families.

Cultural level: Societal norms and values that privilege some groups. Beauty standards based on white features. Success defined by accumulation of wealth. Health defined as absence of disability.

Liberation requires working at all levels. You help clients challenge internalized oppression. You address interpersonal discrimination. You advocate for institutional change. You work to shift cultural narratives.

Empowerment in clinical practice means:

- Recognizing clients' strengths and resilience
- Understanding survival strategies as adaptive, not pathological
- Supporting client autonomy and self-determination
- Connecting personal struggles to social conditions
- Facilitating collective action and community connection
- Advocating for systemic change

You don't just help individuals cope with oppression—you work to dismantle it.

Practice Questions

1. Cultural humility differs from cultural competence primarily by emphasizing:

A. Learning facts about different cultures
B. Achieving expertise in cultural practices
C. Lifelong learning and self-reflection
D. Mastering communication techniques

2. A Black client describes feeling constantly watched in stores. The social worker should recognize this as:

A. Paranoid thinking requiring assessment
B. A reasonable response to racial profiling
C. Projection of internal anxiety
D. Evidence of persecution delusions

3. Microaggressions are best described as:

A. Minor conflicts that don't significantly impact mental health
B. Brief, everyday slights that communicate derogatory messages
C. Unintentional comments that should be ignored
D. Direct expressions of prejudice and hatred

4. According to minority stress theory, LGBTQ+ individuals experience elevated mental health problems primarily due to:

A. Internal psychological deficits
B. Family dysfunction and poor parenting
C. Chronic stress from stigma and discrimination
D. Confusion about identity

5. The social model of disability emphasizes:

A. Medical treatment to cure disabilities
B. Individual limitations and deficits
C. Social barriers that create disability
D. Psychological adjustment to limitations

6. Racial trauma can best be understood as:

A. Individual oversensitivity to racial issues
B. Cumulative psychological impact of racism
C. Paranoid interpretation of neutral events
D. Anger management problems

7. A transgender client reports distress about their body and social misgendering. This describes:

A. Body dysmorphic disorder
B. Delusional disorder
C. Gender dysphoria
D. Narcissistic personality disorder

8. Acculturative stress refers to:

A. Pressure to completely abandon one's culture
B. Stress from navigating multiple cultural contexts
C. Inability to adapt to any culture
D. Rejection of both original and new cultures

9. Children of immigrants who translate and mediate between cultures often experience:

A. Enhanced self-esteem and competence
B. Role reversal and premature responsibility
C. Delayed cognitive development
D. Improved family relationships

10. Institutional racism differs from individual prejudice by:

A. Being less harmful to affected individuals
B. Operating through organizational policies and practices
C. Being intentional and conscious
D. Only affecting employment and housing

11. A social worker working with an older gay client should understand that this client likely:

A. Never experienced significant discrimination
B. Came of age when homosexuality was criminalized
C. Has always been open about sexual orientation
D. Has the same experiences as younger gay clients

12. Allostatic load describes:

A. The weight of social responsibilities
B. Cumulative wear from chronic stress
C. Genetic predisposition to illness
D. Normal aging processes

13. Food insecurity is best defined as:

A. Complete absence of food
B. Consistent uncertainty about food access
C. Preference for processed foods
D. Occasional hunger between meals

14. A client from El Salvador and a client from Mexico are both Latino but may have:

A. Identical cultural experiences and values
B. Very different histories and experiences
C. The same immigration experiences
D. Interchangeable cultural identities

15. Internalized oppression occurs when:

A. People fight against discrimination
B. People believe negative messages about their group
C. People experience external discrimination
D. People reject their cultural identity

16. A wheelchair user reports that inaccessible buildings prevent them from accessing services. The social worker should recognize this as:

A. The client's personal problem to solve
B. A social barrier requiring advocacy
C. Unrealistic expectations
D. Resistance to treatment

17. Family acceptance of LGBTQ+ youth:

A. Has minimal impact on mental health outcomes
B. Dramatically improves mental health and reduces risk
C. Should wait until adulthood
D. Is less important than peer acceptance

18. A poor client working two jobs misses appointments. The social worker should consider:

A. The client isn't motivated for treatment
B. Practical barriers to accessing services
C. The client has poor time management
D. The need for consequences for missed sessions

19. Inspiration porn refers to:

A. Treating people with disabilities as inspirational simply for living
B. Appropriate recognition of disability achievements
C. Sexual exploitation of people with disabilities
D. Motivational stories about overcoming challenges

20. Eviction affects children's development by:

A. Building resilience and coping skills
B. Creating trauma and instability
C. Having minimal long-term impact
D. Teaching important life lessons

21. Cultural brokers in immigrant families:

A. Help families navigate systems effectively
B. Always benefit from this role
C. Should be encouraged for all children
D. Experience no negative effects

22. A Native American client describes historical trauma affecting their family. The social worker should understand this as:

A. An excuse for current problems
B. Intergenerational transmission of trauma from colonization
C. Individual family dysfunction
D. Resistance to moving forward

23. Ableism in mental health settings most commonly appears through:

A. Providing accommodations for disabilities
B. Physical and communicative inaccessibility
C. Treating all clients equally
D. Requiring medical documentation

24. A Latina client experiences discrimination at work but doesn't report it. This might reflect:

A. Acceptance of mistreatment
B. Realistic fear of retaliation and job loss
C. Low self-esteem requiring treatment
D. Cultural values against confrontation

25. The concept of intersectionality recognizes that:

A. All forms of oppression are identical
B. Multiple identities create unique experiences
C. Only one identity matters at a time
D. Some identities cancel out others

26. A client says they don't "see color" and treat everyone the same. The social worker should recognize this as:

A. An ideal approach to diversity
B. Color-blindness that ignores racial realities
C. Evidence of cultural competence
D. The goal of anti-racist practice

27. Undocumented immigrants may avoid mental health services due to:

A. Lack of mental health problems
B. Cultural stigma only
C. Fear of deportation and family separation
D. Preference for traditional healing

28. A client with chronic pain reports that others accuse them of faking. This reflects:

A. Accurate perception of malingering
B. Discrimination against invisible disabilities
C. The client's need for attention
D. Normal skepticism about pain

29. Economic inequality affects mental health primarily through:

A. Individual choice and responsibility
B. Chronic stress and limited resources
C. Genetic factors in poor populations
D. Cultural values about success

30. A Muslim client reports increased anxiety after 9/11. The social worker should consider:

A. Generalized anxiety disorder
B. Religious issues requiring spiritual counseling
C. Impact of discrimination and hate crimes
D. Paranoid ideation

31. Gentrification affects communities of color by:

A. Improving neighborhoods for all residents
B. Displacing long-term residents and destroying community
C. Creating equal opportunities for everyone
D. Having no mental health impact

32. A deaf client requests a sign language interpreter. The social worker should:

A. Suggest the client learn to lip read
B. Provide written notes instead
C. Provide a qualified interpreter
D. Work with family members as interpreters

33. Environmental racism refers to:

A. Individual prejudice about the environment
B. Disproportionate exposure of communities of color to environmental hazards
C. Cultural differences in environmental values
D. Equal distribution of environmental problems

34. A client with a disability says they don't want to be "fixed." The social worker should:

A. Explain the benefits of treatment
B. Respect their perspective and autonomy
C. Consider this resistance to change
D. Refer to medical providers

35. Passing privilege refers to:

A. Academic success
B. Ability to be perceived as part of a dominant group
C. Gaining acceptance through hard work
D. Receiving special treatment

36. A refugee client describes nightmares about violence in their home country. This most likely represents:

A. Pre-migration trauma requiring treatment
B. Adjustment disorder to new country
C. Exaggeration to gain sympathy
D. Cultural expression of distress

37. Code-switching describes:

A. Changing communication styles across contexts
B. Dishonesty about identity
C. Confusion about cultural identity
D. Rejection of one's culture

38. A low-income client can't afford copays for therapy. The social worker should:

A. Refuse services until payment is arranged
B. Explore sliding scale fees and free resources
C. Provide less frequent sessions
D. Suggest the client get a better job

39. Heteronormativity creates stress for LGBTQ+ individuals by:

A. Providing clear social expectations
B. Assuming heterosexuality as default and normal
C. Encouraging family formation
D. Having no significant impact

40. A client with limited English proficiency brings a child to interpret. The social worker should:

A. Allow this for convenience
B. Provide a professional interpreter
C. Use simple English and speak slowly
D. Communicate through written notes

41. The school-to-prison pipeline disproportionately affects:

A. All students equally
B. Students of color and students with disabilities
C. Students who break rules
D. Students from wealthy families

42. A social worker makes an assumption about a client's culture and the client corrects them. The social worker should:

A. Defend their knowledge
B. Apologize and thank the client
C. Change the subject
D. Explain their training

43. Sanctuary trauma describes:

A. Trauma occurring in safe spaces
B. Harm caused by helping systems meant to provide safety
C. Religious trauma
D. Childhood trauma in the home

44. A client identifies as gender fluid. The social worker should:

A. Encourage the client to choose one gender
B. Assess for identity confusion
C. Respect and use the client's identity and pronouns
D. Explain biological sex differences

45. Redlining historically prevented:

A. School segregation
B. Black families from accessing mortgages in certain areas
C. Employment discrimination
D. Voting rights restrictions

46. A client experiences both racism and sexism. The social worker should understand that:

A. These experiences are separate and unrelated
B. One identity is more important than the other
C. The combination creates unique experiences
D. The client should focus on one issue at a time

47. Medical mistrust in Black communities reflects:

A. Ignorance about health benefits
B. Historical exploitation and unethical research
C. Cultural resistance to Western medicine
D. Personal paranoia

48. A social worker's agency requires documentation that undocumented clients cannot provide. This represents:

A. Necessary administrative procedures
B. Institutional racism creating barriers
C. Protection against fraud
D. Standard clinical practice

49. Chosen family for LGBTQ+ individuals:

A. Replaces biological family
B. Provides support when biological family rejects
C. Is less important than biological family
D. Indicates failure to reconcile with family

50. A client living in poverty reports feeling hopeless about the future. The social worker should:

A. Treat this as depression requiring medication
B. Recognize realistic response to structural barriers
C. Focus on positive thinking
D. Challenge cognitive distortions

Answer Key with Detailed Explanations

1. C. Lifelong learning and self-reflection
Cultural humility emphasizes ongoing learning, self-examination of biases, and recognition that you can never fully understand another's cultural experience. Unlike cultural competence (which suggests achievable expertise), cultural humility acknowledges the limitations of your understanding and the need for continuous growth. It focuses on the relationship and power dynamics, not just acquiring cultural knowledge.

2. B. A reasonable response to racial profiling
Black individuals frequently experience being followed in stores, having their purchases scrutinized, and being treated as potential thieves—this is racial profiling, not paranoia. The social worker must

recognize this as a realistic response to actual discrimination, not a symptom of mental illness. Pathologizing normal reactions to racism causes further harm and misses the real issue.

3. B. Brief, everyday slights that communicate derogatory messages
Microaggressions are subtle, often unintentional expressions of prejudice that accumulate over time. Examples include "You're so articulate" (implying surprise that a person of color speaks well) or "Where are you really from?" (implying someone isn't truly American). While individual incidents may seem minor, the cumulative effect significantly impacts mental health.

4. C. Chronic stress from stigma and discrimination
Minority stress theory explains that LGBTQ+ individuals experience chronic stress from external discrimination, internalized stigma, concealment efforts, and anticipation of rejection. This chronic stress—not anything inherent to being LGBTQ+—accounts for elevated rates of depression, anxiety, and suicidality. The problem is societal oppression, not LGBTQ+ identity itself.

5. C. Social barriers that create disability
The social model recognizes that disability results from barriers in the environment, not just individual impairments. A wheelchair user isn't disabled by their body but by stairs without ramps, inaccessible transportation, and discriminatory attitudes. This model shifts focus from "fixing" individuals to removing barriers and creating accessible environments.

6. B. Cumulative psychological impact of racism
Racial trauma describes the mental health impact of experiencing, witnessing, or anticipating racism. This includes direct discrimination, vicarious trauma from seeing violence against people who share your identity, and the stress of constant vigilance. It's a legitimate trauma response, not oversensitivity or misinterpretation.

7. C. Gender dysphoria
Gender dysphoria describes distress from the mismatch between gender identity and assigned sex. This might include distress about body characteristics, being misgendered, or social treatment. The distress—not being transgender—is the clinical issue. Treatment supports the person's identity through social and potentially medical transition, not attempts to change their identity.

8. B. Stress from navigating multiple cultural contexts
Acculturative stress emerges from living between cultures—maintaining connection to heritage culture while adapting to a new culture. This might include language barriers, conflicting values, discrimination, and loss of social status. The stress comes from navigating these tensions, not from immigration itself.

9. B. Role reversal and premature responsibility
When children interpret, translate documents, and negotiate systems for parents, they take on adult responsibilities prematurely. This role reversal can create stress, parentification, and loss of childhood. While these children may develop skills, the burden often comes at a developmental cost.

10. B. Operating through organizational policies and practices
Institutional racism operates through policies, practices, and norms that disadvantage certain racial groups—often without conscious intent. Examples include school discipline policies that

disproportionately affect Black students, hiring practices that screen out ethnic names, or health systems that provide lower quality care to minorities. It's systemic, not just individual prejudice.

11. B. Came of age when homosexuality was criminalized
Older LGBTQ+ adults often came of age when homosexuality was classified as mental illness, was criminalized, and could result in loss of employment, housing, or children. Many experienced profound oppression and may mistrust helping professionals. Understanding this history is essential to working effectively with older LGBTQ+ clients.

12. B. Cumulative wear from chronic stress
Allostatic load describes the cumulative biological burden from chronic stress—the wear and tear on body systems from repeatedly activating stress responses. Poor individuals experience higher allostatic load due to chronic financial stress, discrimination, dangerous environments, and limited resources. This accelerates aging and increases disease risk.

13. B. Consistent uncertainty about food access
Food insecurity means worrying whether food will run out before you can buy more, not having money for nutritious food, skipping meals to feed children, or relying on emergency food. It's chronic uncertainty about food access, not just occasional hunger. This creates constant stress and affects both physical and mental health.

14. B. Very different histories and experiences
Latino/Hispanic is an umbrella term encompassing people from many countries with distinct histories, cultures, and experiences. Someone from El Salvador who fled civil war has different experiences than someone from Mexico with multi-generational U.S. presence. Cultural humility means not assuming shared experiences based on broad categories.

15. B. People believe negative messages about their group
Internalized oppression occurs when people accept and believe society's negative messages about their group. A woman believes women are naturally worse at math. A poor person believes poverty reflects personal failure. This internalization of oppressive beliefs causes shame, low self-esteem, and self-limiting behaviors.

16. B. A social barrier requiring advocacy
Inaccessible buildings are environmental barriers that disable people—not personal problems for individuals to solve alone. The social worker should recognize this as requiring systemic advocacy and change, not just helping the client adapt. This reflects the social model of disability, which locates disability in social barriers, not individual limitations.

17. B. Dramatically improves mental health and reduces risk
Family acceptance of LGBTQ+ youth dramatically reduces suicide risk, depression, and substance use while improving self-esteem and overall health. Even small gestures matter—using correct names and pronouns, expressing affection, and advocating for the young person. Conversely, family rejection has devastating consequences for mental health and well-being.

18. B. Practical barriers to accessing services
Poor clients often face enormous barriers to accessing services—inflexible work schedules, lack of

transportation, childcare needs, and inability to afford time off work. Missed appointments often reflect these structural barriers, not lack of motivation. Social workers must adapt services to accommodate these realities rather than blaming clients.

19. A. Treating people with disabilities as inspirational simply for living
Inspiration porn treats people with disabilities as inspirational simply for doing ordinary activities—going to school, having a job, living their lives. This objectifies people with disabilities and reinforces the assumption that their lives must be tragic or that they're somehow special for existing. It's patronizing, not respectful.

20. B. Creating trauma and instability
Eviction creates profound trauma and instability for children. They may experience school disruption, loss of belongings and community, hunger, and homelessness. Children who experience eviction have higher rates of depression, anxiety, and health problems. Eviction isn't a learning experience—it's a traumatic event with lasting consequences.

21. A. Help families navigate systems effectively
While cultural brokers help families navigate systems and provide valuable services, this role often comes with costs. Children may experience role reversal, premature responsibility, exposure to adult concerns, and loss of childhood. The benefits don't eliminate the burdens of carrying adult responsibilities as a child.

22. B. Intergenerational transmission of trauma from colonization
Historical trauma describes the cumulative emotional and psychological wounding across generations from massive group trauma—including colonization, genocide, forced removal, and cultural destruction experienced by Native Americans. This trauma is transmitted across generations through biological, psychological, and social mechanisms. It's a legitimate clinical concept, not an excuse.

23. B. Physical and communicative inaccessibility
Ableism in mental health settings commonly appears through inaccessible buildings, lack of materials in accessible formats, no sign language interpreters, and assumptions about capacity and quality of life. These barriers communicate that people with disabilities aren't valued or expected. Accessibility isn't special treatment—it's civil rights.

24. B. Realistic fear of retaliation and job loss
People of color often don't report discrimination because retaliation is real. They may be labeled "difficult," passed over for promotion, or fired for pretextual reasons. For someone living paycheck to paycheck, losing a job means losing housing and food security. Not reporting discrimination often reflects realistic assessment of risks, not acceptance or low self-esteem.

25. B. Multiple identities create unique experiences
Intersectionality recognizes that people hold multiple identities (race, class, gender, sexuality, disability, etc.) that interact to create unique experiences. A Black lesbian faces different experiences than a white lesbian or a Black heterosexual man. You can't understand someone's experience by examining one identity in isolation—the intersections matter.

26. B. Color-blindness that ignores racial realities
"Not seeing color" sounds egalitarian but actually ignores the reality that race shapes life experiences profoundly. Color-blindness prevents recognition of racism and its effects. It's a form of denial that allows racial inequities to persist while claiming equality. Genuine anti-racism requires seeing and acknowledging racial realities, not pretending they don't exist.

27. C. Fear of deportation and family separation
Undocumented immigrants often avoid services—including mental health care—due to realistic fear that seeking help could lead to detention, deportation, and family separation. Recent policies have increased this fear. Social workers must understand these barriers and create safe, confidential spaces while advocating against policies that prevent people from accessing needed care.

28. B. Discrimination against invisible disabilities
People with chronic pain, chronic fatigue, autoimmune conditions, and other invisible disabilities frequently face skepticism and accusations of faking. Because the disability isn't visible, others assume it doesn't exist. This discrimination creates additional stress beyond the disability itself and prevents people from accessing needed accommodations and support.

29. B. Chronic stress and limited resources
Economic inequality affects mental health through chronic stress (worrying about money, food, housing), limited access to resources (healthcare, healthy food, safe housing), and experiences of discrimination and shame. Poverty isn't a personal failing—it's a structural condition that creates toxic stress affecting brain development, physical health, and mental health.

30. C. Impact of discrimination and hate crimes
Muslim Americans experienced dramatic increases in discrimination, hate crimes, and surveillance after 9/11. Anxiety in this context reflects realistic response to increased danger and hostility, not generalized anxiety disorder. The social worker must recognize how social and political events affect clients' mental health and validate these realistic concerns.

31. B. Displacing long-term residents and destroying community
Gentrification displaces long-term residents who can no longer afford rising rents, destroys social networks and community connections, and erases cultural spaces and institutions. While it may improve infrastructure, the benefits go to new residents while original residents are pushed out. This displacement causes trauma, loss, and mental health problems.

32. C. Provide a qualified interpreter
Providing a qualified sign language interpreter is a civil rights requirement under the ADA, not an optional accommodation. Written notes don't provide equal access—sign language has different grammar and structure than English. Family members shouldn't interpret for clinical sessions due to confidentiality concerns and the burden it places on family dynamics.

33. B. Disproportionate exposure of communities of color to environmental hazards
Environmental racism describes the pattern of communities of color and poor communities being disproportionately exposed to environmental hazards—toxic waste sites, air pollution, water

contamination, and industrial facilities. This isn't coincidence—it reflects historical discrimination in housing, zoning, and enforcement. These environmental hazards cause serious health problems.

34. B. Respect their perspective and autonomy
Many people with disabilities reject the medical model that views them as needing to be "fixed." They see disability as part of their identity, not a problem to eliminate. Social workers must respect this perspective and client autonomy. Treatment should focus on the client's goals—which might be accommodations and barrier removal, not changing their body or identity.

35. B. Ability to be perceived as part of a dominant group
Passing privilege refers to being able to be perceived as part of a more privileged group—a light-skinned person of color passing as white, a bisexual person in a heterosexual relationship being assumed straight, or someone with an invisible disability not being identified as disabled. This can provide safety but also requires concealment and creates stress.

36. A. Pre-migration trauma requiring treatment
Refugees often experienced violence, persecution, loss, and trauma before migration. These experiences cause PTSD, depression, and other mental health problems. The trauma occurred before arrival and requires culturally appropriate trauma treatment. This isn't adjustment disorder or cultural expression—it's response to genuine trauma.

37. A. Changing communication styles across contexts
Code-switching means adapting language, behavior, and presentation to different contexts—speaking differently at work than with family, or changing behavior in white spaces versus spaces with people of color. This isn't dishonesty—it's a survival strategy in contexts where authentic self-expression might lead to discrimination or danger. The need to code-switch creates stress.

38. B. Explore sliding scale fees and free resources
When clients can't afford copays, social workers must find solutions—sliding scale fees, pro bono services, community resources, or advocacy for policy changes. Refusing services or suggesting clients "get a better job" ignores structural barriers and abandons clients who need help. Economic barriers shouldn't prevent access to needed mental health services.

39. B. Assuming heterosexuality as default and normal
Heteronormativity is the assumption that heterosexuality is normal, natural, and universal—reflected in questions about opposite-sex partners, forms that only allow male/female spouse options, and children's books showing only heterosexual families. This creates stress for LGBTQ+ individuals who must constantly correct assumptions, come out repeatedly, and exist in spaces that don't acknowledge their reality.

40. B. Provide a professional interpreter
Children should never be used as interpreters for clinical sessions. This places inappropriate burdens on children, exposes them to adult content, compromises confidentiality, and creates role reversal. Professional interpreters are required to ensure effective communication and maintain appropriate clinical boundaries. This is both ethical practice and often a legal requirement.

41. B. Students of color and students with disabilities
The school-to-prison pipeline describes how students—particularly students of color and students with disabilities—are pushed out of schools and into the criminal justice system through harsh discipline, police presence in schools, and zero-tolerance policies. Black students are suspended and expelled at dramatically higher rates than white students for identical behaviors.

42. B. Apologize and thank the client
When a client corrects your cultural assumptions, apologize for the error, thank them for the correction, and adjust your understanding. Don't defend your knowledge or training—accept that the client is the expert on their own experience. This demonstrates cultural humility and builds trust. Making mistakes is inevitable; how you respond to correction matters.

43. B. Harm caused by helping systems meant to provide safety
Sanctuary trauma describes harm caused by systems meant to help—child welfare agencies that separate families, mental health systems that force treatment, shelters with dehumanizing rules. People seeking safety encounter new trauma from the systems meant to protect them. This recognition helps explain why people avoid services and mistrust helpers.

44. C. Respect and use the client's identity and pronouns
Gender fluid individuals experience gender as changing over time or across contexts. Social workers must respect this identity, use the client's pronouns (which may change), and avoid pathologizing gender diversity. This isn't confusion—it's how the client experiences gender. Treatment addresses the client's goals, not changing their identity to fit binary expectations.

45. B. Black families from accessing mortgages in certain areas
Redlining was the systematic denial of mortgages and insurance to Black families in certain neighborhoods, marked in red on maps. This prevented Black families from building wealth through homeownership and created segregated neighborhoods. The effects persist today in wealth gaps, segregated schools, and neighborhood quality disparities. This is structural racism, not ancient history.

46. C. The combination creates unique experiences
Intersectionality recognizes that experiencing both racism and sexism creates unique experiences that aren't just additive—they're multiplicative. A Black woman faces experiences that neither white women nor Black men face. The intersections of identities create distinct experiences of discrimination, resilience, and identity that must be understood in their complexity.

47. B. Historical exploitation and unethical research
Medical mistrust in Black communities reflects historical reality—the Tuskegee syphilis study, forced sterilization, Henrietta Lacks' cells taken without consent, and ongoing disparities in care quality. This isn't paranoia or ignorance—it's rational response to historical exploitation and ongoing discrimination in healthcare. Social workers must acknowledge this history and build trust.

48. B. Institutional racism creating barriers
When agency policies require documentation that certain groups can't provide, this creates discriminatory barriers regardless of intent. Undocumented immigrants, homeless individuals, and others may lack required documents. These policies exclude vulnerable populations from services.

This is institutional racism—policies that create racial disparities in access, even without discriminatory intent.

49. B. Provides support when biological family rejects
Chosen family—friends and community members who provide family-like support—becomes especially important for LGBTQ+ individuals whose biological families reject them. This isn't replacing family or indicating failure—it's creating support systems when biological family fails to provide acceptance. Chosen family can be as meaningful and important as biological family.

50. B. Recognize realistic response to structural barriers
When someone living in poverty feels hopeless about the future, this may reflect realistic assessment of structural barriers, not just depression requiring medication. Economic mobility has decreased. Poverty is increasingly difficult to escape. Recognizing this reality doesn't mean ignoring treatable depression, but it means understanding hopelessness in context and addressing both individual symptoms and structural barriers.

Reflection on Practice

Social justice work in clinical practice isn't optional—it's central to competent care. You can't separate individual problems from social contexts. The woman with depression may need therapy, but she also needs affordable housing. The adolescent with anxiety may need coping skills, but he also needs safety from police harassment.

This doesn't mean you abandon clinical skills. You still assess, diagnose, and treat. But you do so with awareness that symptoms often reflect social conditions. You work at multiple levels—supporting individual clients, advocating for policy changes, and working to dismantle oppressive systems.

The work is difficult. You'll face your own biases. You'll make mistakes. You'll work in systems that perpetuate the problems you're trying to solve. Cultural humility means staying engaged despite these challenges—learning, reflecting, and working for change.

Your clients are the experts on their experiences. Listen to them. Believe them. Let them teach you. This is where real understanding begins.

Essential Points to Remember

- Cultural humility requires lifelong learning, self-reflection, and recognition that you can never fully understand another's cultural experience
- Racism, sexism, homophobia, and other forms of oppression create real trauma and mental health consequences—not individual oversensitivity
- The social model of disability locates problems in social barriers, not individual limitations—focus on removing barriers, not fixing people
- Minority stress explains elevated mental health problems in marginalized groups through chronic stress from discrimination, not inherent deficits

- Intersectionality recognizes that multiple identities create unique experiences that can't be understood by examining one identity alone
- Microaggressions accumulate over time to create significant mental health impact, even when individual incidents seem minor
- Economic inequality creates toxic stress through poverty, food insecurity, housing instability, and chronic worry about survival
- Family acceptance dramatically improves outcomes for LGBTQ+ youth, while rejection increases suicide risk and mental health problems
- Historical trauma from colonization, slavery, and genocide transmits across generations and affects current mental health in affected communities
- Institutional racism operates through policies and practices that create disparities, regardless of individual intent or conscious prejudice
- Clinical symptoms often reflect realistic responses to oppression and structural barriers, not just individual pathology requiring treatment
- Effective practice requires working at multiple levels—individual support, advocacy for policy change, and efforts to dismantle oppressive systems

Chapter 3: Family Systems and Dynamics

Families create us. The patterns you learned in your first relationships—how to connect, how to fight, how to need, how to separate—these patterns shape every relationship that follows. You can't understand a client without understanding their family. And you can't understand a family without seeing it as a system.

A system is more than the sum of its parts. A family isn't just individual people living together. It's a network of relationships with patterns, rules, and structures that organize behavior. Change one part of the system, and ripples spread throughout.

Family Structure and Roles

Every family has structure—the organization of relationships, power, and boundaries. Structure isn't good or bad in itself. What matters is whether the structure supports healthy development and adaptation.

Subsystems are smaller units within the family. The most common subsystems are:

The **parental subsystem** includes adults responsible for caregiving and decision-making. In two-parent families, this means the parents work together. In single-parent families, one person carries this role. In extended family households, grandparents or other relatives may be part of this subsystem.

The **sibling subsystem** includes children learning to relate to peers. This is where children practice negotiation, cooperation, and conflict resolution. Birth order affects experiences within this subsystem—oldest children often take leadership roles, youngest children may be protected or dismissed.

The **spousal subsystem** includes the intimate partnership between adults. This subsystem needs privacy and boundaries separate from parenting. When these boundaries blur—when children become confidants for adult issues—problems emerge.

Boundaries define who participates in what and how. Clear boundaries are firm but flexible. They protect subsystems while allowing appropriate interaction.

Rigid boundaries create isolation. Family members are disengaged—they barely know what's happening in each other's lives. An adolescent could be struggling with depression, and parents might not notice. Rigid boundaries prevent needed support and connection.

Diffuse boundaries create enmeshment. Everyone knows everything about everyone. There's no privacy, no separateness. A mother might read her daughter's diary, insisting "we don't have secrets." Diffuse boundaries prevent healthy individuation.

Roles are patterns of behavior expected from family members. Some roles support healthy functioning—the caretaker who ensures everyone's needs are met, the mediator who helps resolve conflicts. Other roles develop in response to dysfunction.

The **hero child** achieves and performs to make the family look good. This child excels in school, sports, or other visible areas. The family points to this child as proof that everything is fine—even when it isn't. The hero child carries enormous pressure to maintain this image.

The **scapegoat** gets blamed for family problems. This child acts out, gets in trouble, and draws negative attention. The family can point to this child as the problem—avoiding examination of deeper issues. The scapegoat actually serves a function, allowing the family to avoid addressing real problems.

The **lost child** disappears into the background. This child doesn't cause trouble or demand attention. The family may barely notice this child, who learns to meet their own needs and expect nothing from others. This child often appears "fine" but experiences profound loneliness.

The **mascot** uses humor and entertainment to relieve family tension. When conflict emerges, the mascot cracks jokes or acts silly. The family laughs, tension decreases temporarily, but real issues remain unaddressed. The mascot learns to suppress their own needs to manage others' emotions.

These roles aren't chosen consciously. They develop in response to family needs and dynamics. Understanding roles helps explain behavior that might otherwise seem puzzling.

Case Example: The Chen Family

The Chen family seeks therapy because 14-year-old Amy has been caught shoplifting. The parents describe Amy as "our problem child" who has always been difficult. They contrast her with her older brother David, who excels academically and causes no trouble.

In family sessions, you observe the pattern. Amy acts sullen and defiant. David sits quietly, the model child. When you ask the parents about their relationship, they become uncomfortable. Mother changes the subject to Amy's behavior. Father agrees that Amy is the issue they need to fix.

You recognize Amy as the scapegoat. As long as everyone focuses on Amy's misbehavior, no one examines the parents' failing marriage or David's crushing anxiety hidden behind perfect performance. Amy's shoplifting serves a function—it keeps the family focused on her instead of more threatening issues.

You also notice boundaries. David has become a parental child—he mediates between his parents, comforts his mother, and takes responsibility for Amy. The spousal subsystem has dissolved, with mother using David as her emotional confidant. Amy is both scapegoated and parentified—she's blamed for problems while also being expected to care for her mother's emotional needs.

Treatment requires shifting the focus. You work with the parents on their relationship and appropriate boundaries. You help David step back from the parental role and focus on his own development. You help Amy separate her behavior from her role as family problem. As the family structure changes, Amy's acting out decreases—it's no longer needed.

Attachment Theory

Attachment is the emotional bond between a child and caregiver. This bond provides security, shapes the child's internal working model of relationships, and affects development across the lifespan.

John Bowlby developed attachment theory, and Mary Ainsworth identified attachment patterns through research. But attachment isn't just theory—it's lived reality for every person who walks into your office.

Secure attachment develops when caregivers respond consistently to the child's needs. The child learns: I can count on people to help me. My needs matter. The world is safe enough to explore because I have a secure base to return to.

Securely attached children use their caregiver as a secure base. They explore their environment, checking back periodically. When distressed, they seek comfort and are soothed. As adults, they trust others, seek support when needed, and form healthy intimate relationships.

Insecure-avoidant attachment develops when caregivers are consistently unresponsive or rejecting. The child learns: Seeking help doesn't work. I must handle things alone. Needing others leads to rejection.

Avoidantly attached children don't seek comfort when distressed. They appear independent—but it's not healthy independence. It's adaptation to a world where needs go unmet. As adults, they dismiss emotional needs, maintain distance in relationships, and feel uncomfortable with intimacy.

Insecure-ambivalent attachment develops with inconsistent caregiving. Sometimes the caregiver responds, sometimes not. The child learns: I can't predict whether my needs will be met. I must escalate to get attention. Relationships are unreliable.

Ambivalently attached children are anxious and clingy. When distressed, they seek contact but aren't easily soothed—they've learned that comfort is unpredictable. As adults, they fear abandonment, seek constant reassurance, and struggle with anxiety in relationships.

Disorganized attachment develops when the caregiver is frightening or frightened. The child needs comfort from the very person who causes fear. This creates an unsolvable dilemma.

Children with disorganized attachment show confused, contradictory behaviors. They might approach the caregiver while looking away, or freeze in the caregiver's presence. As adults, they struggle with profound relationship difficulties, often repeating patterns of trauma in their intimate partnerships.

Attachment patterns persist into adulthood, but they can change. You don't ask clients about their attachment history directly—you observe it in their relationships, including the therapeutic relationship.

The therapeutic relationship can provide a corrective emotional experience. An avoidantly attached client who has never trusted anyone slowly learns that you're consistent and reliable. An ambivalently attached client who fears abandonment experiences you maintaining boundaries while remaining engaged. The relationship itself becomes healing.

Internal working models can be revised. The adult who learned in infancy that people can't be trusted can learn—through new relationship experiences—that some people are trustworthy. This doesn't erase early experiences, but it creates new possibilities.

Attachment affects parenting. Parents tend to raise children with the attachment pattern they experienced—unless they've examined and worked through their own attachment history. An avoidantly attached parent may have difficulty responding to a child's emotional needs. An ambivalently attached parent may become anxious and overprotective.

Family Life Cycle

Families develop through predictable stages, each with specific tasks and challenges. The **family life cycle** helps you understand normal transitions and anticipate difficulties.

Couple formation begins when two people commit to a partnership. The task is developing a shared life while maintaining individual identities. Couples must negotiate:

- How to manage money
- How to divide household labor
- How much time to spend together versus apart
- How to relate to extended families
- Whether and when to have children

Conflict during this stage often centers on these negotiations. The couple is creating new patterns, not just combining existing ones.

Families with young children face demands of caregiving while maintaining the couple relationship. New parents experience sleep deprivation, loss of spontaneity, and identity shifts. The parental subsystem must form without eliminating the spousal subsystem—couples who lose their partnership in the process of becoming parents struggle.

Extended family relationships shift. New grandparents have opinions about parenting. Boundaries need renegotiation. Cultural expectations about grandparent involvement vary widely—what feels supportive to one family feels intrusive to another.

Families with adolescents must allow increasing independence while maintaining connection. Parents shift from direct control to influence. Adolescents need freedom to explore identity while still having parental support and structure.

This stage often revives parents' own adolescent issues. A father who rebelled against strict parents may be overly permissive. A mother who became pregnant as a teenager may become overly restrictive. Unresolved issues from parents' own adolescence affect how they respond to their teenager.

Launching children requires parents to let go while remaining available. Young adults need to separate and establish independence. Parents must develop new roles and rediscover their couple relationship—or create new identities if single.

Empty nest isn't necessarily crisis. Many parents report increased satisfaction once children launch. But parents whose identity centers entirely on parenting may struggle. Couples who maintained connection adapt more easily than couples who stayed together "for the children."

Families in later life face aging, grandparenting, and often caregiving. Adult children may need to care for aging parents—a role reversal that creates stress for everyone. Decisions about living arrangements, medical care, and end-of-life planning require family negotiation.

Death of a spouse or partner is often the most difficult transition. The surviving partner must reconstruct identity and life without their longtime companion. Adult children must support grieving parents while managing their own grief.

Non-traditional family life cycles follow different patterns. Single parents face all developmental tasks while carrying sole responsibility. Stepfamilies must integrate members with different histories and loyalties. Same-sex couples navigate stages without the cultural scripts available to heterosexual couples.

The key isn't following a prescribed path—it's successfully navigating transitions. Families get stuck when they can't adapt to new developmental demands.

Intergenerational Patterns

What happens in one generation affects the next—and the next. **Intergenerational transmission** describes how patterns, roles, and trauma pass through families across time.

Murray Bowen's **family systems theory** emphasizes these patterns. Differentiation of self—the ability to maintain your own identity while remaining emotionally connected to family—varies across generations. Low differentiation in one generation predicts low differentiation in the next.

Triangulation occurs when two people pull in a third to reduce anxiety between them. A couple in conflict focuses on a child's behavior instead of addressing their relationship. The child's misbehavior reduces tension between the parents—temporarily. But it prevents the couple from resolving their issues and burdens the child with regulating the parents' relationship.

Triangles are extremely stable. The child who reduces parental tension through misbehavior may continue this pattern into adulthood—acting out whenever stress emerges. The pattern outlives its original function.

Genograms map family patterns across generations. You draw a family tree including:

- Family structure (who is in the family, relationships)
- Critical events (deaths, divorces, migrations)
- Patterns (substance use, mental illness, violence)
- Relationship quality (close, distant, conflictual)

Patterns emerge visually. You might see depression in every generation of women. Substance use problems in men across three generations. Conflictual mother-daughter relationships repeating. Oldest children carrying family responsibility.

These patterns aren't destiny. Awareness creates the possibility of change. A client who sees three generations of problematic drinking can consciously choose a different path. A mother who recognizes she's repeating her own mother's harsh criticism can work to parent differently.

Legacies and loyalty bind families across generations. Children feel obligated to carry out parents' unfulfilled dreams, to maintain family traditions, to avoid surpassing parents' achievements. These invisible loyalties shape choices in powerful ways.

A daughter might sabotage her own success to avoid surpassing her mother who sacrificed her career for family. A son might choose a profession his father wanted instead of following his own interests. These aren't conscious decisions—they're expressions of family loyalty operating below awareness.

Family secrets create particular problems. The secret everyone knows but no one discusses—the father's alcoholism, the mother's mental illness, the grandfather's abuse—shapes behavior while remaining unspoken. Children sense the secret, fill in gaps with imagination, and often blame themselves.

Bringing secrets into open discussion reduces their power. This doesn't mean forcing disclosure—it means creating space where truth can be spoken if family members choose.

Trauma transmission occurs across generations. Children of Holocaust survivors, descendants of enslaved people, Native Americans whose grandparents attended boarding schools—all may experience effects of trauma they didn't directly experience.

Transmission happens through multiple pathways:

- **Parenting affected by trauma**: A parent with PTSD may be overprotective or emotionally distant
- **Narrative transmission**: Stories told (or not told) about family history shape identity
- **Epigenetic changes**: Trauma may alter gene expression in ways that affect offspring
- **Attachment disruption**: Traumatized parents may struggle to provide secure attachment

Understanding intergenerational trauma helps you recognize that a client's struggles may have roots extending far beyond their individual experiences.

Case Example: The Johnson Family

Robert, a 35-year-old Black man, enters therapy for anger problems. His partner threatens to leave unless he gets help. Robert describes explosive rage over minor frustrations—his partner forgetting to buy milk, a coworker arriving late to a meeting.

You create a genogram with Robert. Patterns emerge immediately. Robert's father was violent—he beat Robert's mother and the children. Robert swore he would never be like his father. Yet here he is, struggling with rage.

Robert's grandfather was also violent. He grew up in the Jim Crow South, experiencing constant degradation and threat. He couldn't express anger toward white people without risking death, so rage got displaced onto his family. Robert's father experienced the same pattern—anger at racism with nowhere safe to direct it, resulting in violence at home.

Robert is carrying three generations of rage at injustice and violence. His individual anger has historical roots. He experiences contemporary racism—being followed in stores, stopped by police, passed over for promotion—and his rage connects to generations of similar experiences.

Treatment addresses multiple levels. Robert learns skills for managing anger in the moment. But you also help him understand his rage in historical context. The anger isn't just about milk or meetings—it's about injustice, past and present.

Robert works to break the cycle. He processes his own experiences of racism and trauma. He grieves what his father and grandfather endured. He learns to express anger without violence. He's creating a new pattern for his own children—one where anger can be felt and expressed safely.

Practice Questions

1. In family systems theory, a triangle occurs when:

A. Three people form a close relationship
B. Two people pull in a third to reduce anxiety
C. Parents disagree about discipline
D. Extended family interferes in nuclear family

2. A child who appears independent and doesn't seek comfort when distressed most likely has which attachment pattern?

A. Secure
B. Insecure-avoidant
C. Insecure-ambivalent
D. Disorganized

3. The "hero child" in a dysfunctional family:

A. Is genuinely well-adjusted and successful
B. Achieves to make the family look good despite dysfunction
C. Takes responsibility for family problems
D. Uses humor to deflect tension

4. Clear boundaries in families are:

A. Rigid and inflexible
B. Nonexistent to promote closeness

C. Firm but flexible
D. Constantly changing

5. Enmeshment in families is characterized by:

A. Appropriate privacy and individuation
B. Isolation and disconnection
C. Diffuse boundaries and lack of separateness
D. Clear generational hierarchies

6. An adult who fears abandonment and seeks constant reassurance in relationships likely experienced:

A. Secure attachment
B. Insecure-avoidant attachment
C. Insecure-ambivalent attachment
D. Disorganized attachment

7. The family life cycle stage when parents must shift from control to influence is:

A. Families with young children
B. Families with adolescents
C. Launching children
D. Families in later life

8. A genogram is primarily used to:

A. Diagnose mental illness
B. Map family patterns across generations
C. Determine custody arrangements
D. Assess individual functioning

9. Parentification occurs when:

A. Parents become overly strict
B. A child takes on parental responsibilities
C. Parents divorce and remarry
D. Extended family provides childcare

10. Disorganized attachment typically develops when:

A. Caregivers are consistently unresponsive
B. Caregiving is inconsistent
C. The caregiver is frightening or frightened
D. Multiple caregivers are involved

11. The scapegoat in a family system:

A. Actually causes all family problems
B. Gets blamed for family problems, serving a function

C. Is the youngest child
D. Refuses to participate in family dysfunction

12. Differentiation of self refers to:

A. Becoming completely independent from family
B. Maintaining identity while staying emotionally connected
C. Separating from family completely
D. Avoiding all family contact

13. A couple who avoids addressing relationship problems by focusing on their child's behavior demonstrates:

A. Good parenting
B. Triangulation
C. Clear boundaries
D. Differentiation

14. The spousal subsystem requires:

A. Complete transparency with children
B. Privacy and boundaries separate from parenting
C. Involvement of extended family
D. Children's participation in decision-making

15. Internal working models of relationships are formed primarily during:

A. Adolescence
B. Young adulthood
C. Infancy and early childhood
D. Middle age

16. A family where everyone knows everything about everyone and there's no privacy demonstrates:

A. Secure attachment
B. Clear boundaries
C. Enmeshment
D. Differentiation

17. The "lost child" in a dysfunctional family:

A. Gets the most attention
B. Disappears into the background
C. Acts out to express family pain
D. Takes care of everyone else

18. Intergenerational trauma transmission occurs through:

A. Genetic factors only
B. Storytelling only
C. Multiple pathways including parenting, narrative, and biology
D. Direct experience only

19. A child who shows contradictory behaviors—approaching the caregiver while looking away—likely has:

A. Secure attachment
B. Insecure-avoidant attachment
C. Insecure-ambivalent attachment
D. Disorganized attachment

20. Family secrets affect children by:

A. Protecting them from difficult information
B. Creating anxiety and often self-blame
C. Having no significant impact
D. Building family cohesion

21. The empty nest stage is:

A. Always a crisis for parents
B. Easier for couples who maintained connection
C. Typically the most difficult life stage
D. Only difficult for mothers

22. Rigid boundaries in families lead to:

A. Enmeshment
B. Healthy independence
C. Isolation and disengagement
D. Strong family bonds

23. A child who uses humor to relieve family tension is the:

A. Hero
B. Scapegoat
C. Lost child
D. Mascot

24. Attachment patterns:

A. Never change after childhood
B. Can be revised through new relationship experiences
C. Are determined solely by genetics
D. Don't affect adult relationships

25. The primary task of couple formation is:

A. Having children
B. Developing shared life while maintaining individual identities
C. Separating completely from families of origin
D. Establishing financial security

26. Bowen's concept of triangulation describes:

A. Healthy three-person relationships
B. Pulling in a third person to reduce two-person anxiety
C. Three generations living together
D. Sibling rivalry

27. A parent who becomes overly restrictive with their teenager because they became pregnant as an adolescent demonstrates:

A. Good judgment based on experience
B. Unresolved issues from their own adolescence affecting parenting
C. Appropriate protective parenting
D. Secure attachment

28. The therapeutic relationship can:

A. Replace family relationships
B. Provide a corrective emotional experience
C. Cure attachment disorders completely
D. Eliminate all relationship problems

29. Families with young children must:

A. Eliminate the couple relationship
B. Focus exclusively on children
C. Maintain parental subsystem without eliminating spousal subsystem
D. Include children in all decisions

30. Invisible loyalties in families:

A. Don't significantly affect behavior
B. Shape choices in powerful but unconscious ways
C. Only affect children
D. Always involve positive obligations

31. A consistently responsive caregiver facilitates:

A. Insecure-avoidant attachment
B. Insecure-ambivalent attachment
C. Secure attachment
D. Disorganized attachment

32. Oldest children who take on family leadership roles in the sibling subsystem:

A. Always become parentified
B. Experience normative birth order effects
C. Will definitely develop problems
D. Should be prevented from leading

33. Cultural expectations about grandparent involvement:

A. Are universal across cultures
B. Vary widely across cultural groups
C. Don't affect family functioning
D. Should always favor minimal involvement

34. An avoidantly attached adult typically:

A. Seeks support readily
B. Fears abandonment
C. Dismisses emotional needs and maintains distance
D. Shows contradictory relationship behaviors

35. The family life cycle concept:

A. Prescribes one correct path
B. Helps understand normal transitions and anticipate difficulties
C. Only applies to traditional nuclear families
D. Ignores cultural variations

36. Parentified children:

A. Benefit from increased responsibility
B. Carry adult burdens that interfere with development
C. Always become well-adjusted adults
D. Are found only in single-parent families

37. A family stuck at a life cycle transition:

A. Will naturally unstick over time
B. Can't adapt to new developmental demands
C. Is functioning optimally
D. Doesn't need professional help

38. The concept of subsystems in family therapy emphasizes:

A. Individual functioning only
B. Smaller units within the family with different functions
C. Nuclear family over extended family
D. Parents over children

39. Depression appearing in multiple generations of women in a family:

A. Proves genetic causation
B. Is coincidental
C. Represents an intergenerational pattern worth examining
D. Can't be changed

40. A client who sabotages success to avoid surpassing a parent demonstrates:

A. Lack of ability
B. Poor motivation
C. Invisible family loyalty
D. Healthy modesty

41. Same-sex couples navigating family life cycle stages:

A. Follow identical patterns to heterosexual couples
B. Navigate without available cultural scripts
C. Experience no unique challenges
D. Can't successfully raise children

42. Stepfamilies face the unique challenge of:

A. No challenges beyond nuclear families
B. Integrating members with different histories and loyalties
C. Always failing to bond
D. Excluding biological parents

43. Bringing family secrets into open discussion:

A. Always causes harm
B. Should be forced on unwilling family members
C. Can reduce their power when family chooses disclosure
D. Is never appropriate

44. A child who becomes a parental child:

A. Benefits from maturity and responsibility
B. Mediates parents and carries inappropriate burdens
C. Is fulfilling a healthy family role
D. Will definitely become a good parent

45. Families in later life face:

A. No significant developmental tasks
B. Aging, grandparenting, and often caregiving role reversals
C. Easier transitions than earlier stages
D. Only positive changes

46. A child who appears anxious, clingy, and is difficult to sooth when distressed likely has:

A. Secure attachment
B. Insecure-avoidant attachment
C. Insecure-ambivalent attachment
D. Disorganized attachment

47. Epigenetic changes related to trauma:

A. Don't affect offspring
B. May alter gene expression in ways that affect offspring
C. Only occur with direct trauma exposure
D. Are completely reversible

48. The "mascot" role in a dysfunctional family:

A. Successfully resolves family problems
B. Uses humor to manage tension while real issues remain unaddressed
C. Is the healthiest family role
D. Only occurs in large families

49. Launching children successfully requires parents to:

A. Cut off all contact
B. Maintain complete control
C. Let go while remaining available
D. Focus entirely on grandchildren

50. An infant with a frightening caregiver faces:

A. Normal developmental challenges
B. An unsolvable dilemma needing comfort from source of fear
C. No particular attachment difficulties
D. Automatic secure attachment

Answer Key with Detailed Explanations

1. B. Two people pull in a third to reduce anxiety
Triangulation occurs when two people experiencing anxiety or conflict pull in a third person to reduce tension between them. For example, parents in conflict focus on a child's behavior instead of addressing their relationship problems. The triangle reduces immediate anxiety but prevents resolution of the underlying issue and burdens the third person with managing others' relationships.

2. B. Insecure-avoidant
Children with insecure-avoidant attachment learned that seeking comfort doesn't work—caregivers were consistently unresponsive or rejecting. They appear independent and don't seek comfort when distressed, but this isn't healthy independence—it's adaptation to unavailable caregivers. They've learned to suppress attachment needs because expressing them led to rejection.

3. B. Achieves to make the family look good despite dysfunction
The hero child excels and achieves to create the appearance that the family is functioning well, even

when significant problems exist. This child carries enormous pressure to maintain the image of family success and often struggles with perfectionism, fear of failure, and difficulty acknowledging their own needs. Achievement serves the family's need to appear functional.

4. C. Firm but flexible
Clear boundaries are firm enough to protect subsystems and define roles, but flexible enough to allow appropriate interaction and adaptation to changing needs. They're not rigid (which creates isolation) or diffuse (which creates enmeshment). Clear boundaries allow both connection and appropriate separateness.

5. C. Diffuse boundaries and lack of separateness
Enmeshment occurs when boundaries are diffuse—family members are overly involved in each other's lives with little privacy or individual identity. Everyone knows everything about everyone. There's no appropriate separateness. This prevents healthy individuation and makes it difficult for family members to develop autonomous identities.

6. C. Insecure-ambivalent attachment
Adults with insecure-ambivalent attachment patterns experienced inconsistent caregiving as children—sometimes the caregiver responded, sometimes not. They learned that relationships are unpredictable. As adults, they fear abandonment, seek constant reassurance, experience relationship anxiety, and have difficulty trusting that others will be there for them.

7. B. Families with adolescents
Families with adolescents must navigate the shift from parental control to parental influence. Adolescents need increasing autonomy to develop identity, while still requiring parental guidance and support. Parents must allow exploration and independence while maintaining connection and appropriate boundaries—a delicate balance that challenges many families.

8. B. Map family patterns across generations
Genograms are visual maps of family structure, relationships, and patterns across multiple generations. They help identify recurring patterns (substance use, mental illness, relationship dynamics), critical events (deaths, divorces, migrations), and family roles. Patterns that might not be obvious in verbal history often become clear when mapped visually.

9. B. A child takes on parental responsibilities
Parentification occurs when a child carries adult responsibilities—emotionally caring for parents, managing household tasks, or parenting younger siblings. This role reversal interferes with normal child development. The child's needs go unmet while they meet others' needs. This can create competence but at the cost of childhood and age-appropriate development.

10. C. The caregiver is frightening or frightened
Disorganized attachment develops when the caregiver is both the source of fear and the potential source of comfort—an unsolvable dilemma for the infant. This typically occurs with abuse, severe mental illness, or unresolved trauma in the caregiver. The infant needs comfort from the very person who frightens them, creating confused, contradictory attachment behaviors.

11. B. Gets blamed for family problems, serving a function
The scapegoat is blamed for family problems, but this serves a function—allowing the family to avoid examining deeper issues. The scapegoat's misbehavior becomes the focus, preventing attention to parents' marital problems, substance use, or other dysfunction. The scapegoat isn't causing problems—they're expressing family dysfunction and providing a distraction from real issues.

12. B. Maintaining identity while staying emotionally connected
Differentiation of self means maintaining your own identity, values, and functioning while remaining emotionally connected to family. It's not about cutting off or becoming independent—it's about being yourself within relationships. People with good differentiation can be close to family without losing themselves or having their functioning disrupted by family anxiety.

13. B. Triangulation
When a couple avoids addressing their relationship problems by focusing on a child's behavior, they're triangulating the child. The child's issues reduce tension between the parents temporarily, but prevent resolution of the couple's problems. The child becomes the identified patient when the real problem is the couple's relationship.

14. B. Privacy and boundaries separate from parenting
The spousal subsystem—the intimate partnership between adults—requires privacy and boundaries separate from the parental role. Couples need time, conversation, and intimacy that doesn't include children. When these boundaries disappear, the couple relationship suffers, which ultimately affects the entire family system.

15. C. Infancy and early childhood
Internal working models of relationships—expectations about whether people are trustworthy, whether needs will be met, whether you're worthy of love—are formed primarily through early attachment experiences in infancy and childhood. These models shape all subsequent relationships, though they can be revised through later relationship experiences.

16. C. Enmeshment
Enmeshment describes families with diffuse boundaries where everyone knows everything about everyone and there's no privacy or appropriate separateness. Family members are overly involved in each other's lives. This prevents healthy individuation and creates anxiety because personal experiences and feelings immediately become family issues.

17. B. Disappears into the background
The lost child avoids attention, doesn't make demands, and disappears into the background. The family may barely notice this child, who appears "fine" and self-sufficient. But the lost child experiences profound loneliness and learns that their needs don't matter. They cope by becoming invisible and expecting nothing from others.

18. C. Multiple pathways including parenting, narrative, and biology
Intergenerational trauma transmission occurs through multiple mechanisms: parenting affected by trauma, narratives told about family history, possibly epigenetic changes affecting gene expression,

attachment disruptions, and modeled coping strategies. It's not just one pathway—trauma affects the next generation through complex interactions of biological, psychological, and social factors.

19. D. Disorganized attachment
Contradictory behaviors—approaching while looking away, freezing in the caregiver's presence, seeking contact but appearing fearful—characterize disorganized attachment. These confused behaviors reflect the child's impossible situation: needing comfort from the person who frightens them. The child has no organized strategy for getting needs met safely.

20. B. Creating anxiety and often self-blame
Family secrets—things everyone knows but no one discusses—create anxiety and confusion for children. Children sense the secret, try to make sense of gaps in information, and often blame themselves for family tension. Secrets prevent children from understanding their reality and frequently lead to shame and self-blame for problems they didn't cause.

21. B. Easier for couples who maintained connection
The empty nest stage isn't automatically a crisis. Many parents report increased satisfaction once children launch. Couples who maintained their relationship throughout parenting typically adapt well—they rediscover each other. Couples who stayed together "for the children" or lost their connection while parenting struggle more with this transition.

22. C. Isolation and disengagement
Rigid boundaries create isolation and disengagement. Family members barely know what's happening in each other's lives. There's little emotional connection or support. A child could be struggling significantly and parents might not notice. Rigid boundaries prevent the connection and support that families need to function well.

23. D. Mascot
The mascot uses humor and entertainment to relieve family tension. When conflict emerges or anxiety rises, the mascot cracks jokes, acts silly, or distracts everyone. The family laughs, tension decreases temporarily, but real issues remain unaddressed. The mascot learns to suppress their own needs to manage others' emotions through humor.

24. B. Can be revised through new relationship experiences
While attachment patterns formed in childhood tend to persist, they can change through new relationship experiences, including therapy. The therapeutic relationship can provide a corrective emotional experience—an avoidantly attached person learning to trust, an ambivalently attached person experiencing consistency. Internal working models can be revised, though this requires time and repeated positive experiences.

25. B. Developing shared life while maintaining individual identities
The primary task of couple formation is creating a shared life—negotiating how to live together, manage money, relate to families of origin, and make decisions—while maintaining individual identities. Couples must find balance between "we" and "I," creating partnership without losing self. This foundation affects all subsequent family development.

26. B. Pulling in a third person to reduce two-person anxiety
Triangulation describes pulling a third person into a two-person relationship to reduce anxiety. Parents in conflict focus on a child. Two coworkers in tension complain to a third. The triangle reduces immediate anxiety but prevents resolution between the original two people and burdens the third person with managing others' relationships.

27. B. Unresolved issues from their own adolescence affecting parenting
Parents' unresolved adolescent issues often resurface when their children reach adolescence. A parent who became pregnant as a teenager may become overly restrictive—not because it's what their adolescent needs, but because the parent's own anxiety and unresolved issues drive the behavior. Effective parenting requires working through your own developmental issues.

28. B. Provide a corrective emotional experience
The therapeutic relationship can provide a corrective emotional experience—a consistent, trustworthy relationship different from early attachment experiences. This doesn't cure attachment difficulties instantly or completely, but it can begin to revise internal working models. The relationship itself becomes part of the healing process.

29. C. Maintain parental subsystem without eliminating spousal subsystem
Families with young children must maintain the parental subsystem (caregiving and decision-making) while preserving the spousal subsystem (intimate partnership). Parents who lose their couple relationship in the process of parenting often struggle. The couple relationship actually supports good parenting—it doesn't compete with it.

30. B. Shape choices in powerful but unconscious ways
Invisible loyalties are obligations to family that operate below conscious awareness but powerfully shape choices. A daughter might sabotage success to avoid surpassing her mother. A son might choose his father's career despite different interests. These aren't conscious decisions—they're expressions of family loyalty and unconscious beliefs about what family membership requires.

31. C. Secure attachment
Consistent, responsive caregiving facilitates secure attachment. The infant learns that needs will be met, people are trustworthy, and the world is safe enough to explore. This creates an internal working model of self as worthy and others as reliable, which supports healthy development and relationships throughout life.

32. B. Experience normative birth order effects
Oldest children often naturally take leadership roles in the sibling subsystem—this is a normative birth order effect, not necessarily pathological. Problems arise when this becomes parentification—when the oldest child carries actual parental responsibilities. Leadership among siblings is normal; parenting siblings while parents are present is problematic.

33. B. Vary widely across cultural groups
Cultural expectations about grandparent involvement vary dramatically. In some cultures, grandparents are expected to be highly involved in child-rearing. In others, nuclear family autonomy

is valued. What feels supportive in one culture feels intrusive in another. Social workers must understand cultural context rather than imposing their own cultural expectations.

34. C. Dismisses emotional needs and maintains distance
Avoidantly attached adults dismiss emotional needs, maintain distance in relationships, and feel uncomfortable with intimacy. They learned in infancy that seeking closeness led to rejection, so they suppress attachment needs and present as independent. This isn't healthy autonomy—it's adaptation to early experiences of unavailability.

35. B. Helps understand normal transitions and anticipate difficulties
The family life cycle concept helps social workers understand normal developmental transitions and anticipate predictable difficulties. It's not a prescription for one correct path—families follow different patterns. But understanding common stages helps identify when families are stuck and what developmental tasks they're navigating.

36. B. Carry adult burdens that interfere with development
Parentified children carry adult emotional or practical responsibilities that interfere with normal development. While they may appear competent and mature, they're missing childhood experiences and having their own needs go unmet. This can create skills but at significant developmental cost, often leading to adult difficulties with boundaries and self-care.

37. B. Can't adapt to new developmental demands
Families get stuck at life cycle transitions when they can't adapt to new developmental demands. Parents can't let adolescents individuate. Couples can't adjust to empty nest. Families can't incorporate new members. Being stuck isn't a choice—it reflects difficulty navigating change. Professional help can facilitate the necessary adaptations.

38. B. Smaller units within the family with different functions
Subsystems are smaller units within the family (parental, sibling, spousal) that serve different functions. Each subsystem has appropriate boundaries and roles. The parental subsystem handles caregiving and decisions. The sibling subsystem allows children to practice peer relationships. The spousal subsystem maintains the couple relationship. Healthy families have clear, functional subsystems.

39. C. Represents an intergenerational pattern worth examining
Depression appearing across generations represents an intergenerational pattern that warrants examination. This might involve genetic factors, learned coping patterns, trauma transmission, or family dynamics that create risk. Recognizing the pattern doesn't determine whether it's primarily biological or environmental—it highlights the need to understand family context and create opportunities for change.

40. C. Invisible family loyalty
Sabotaging success to avoid surpassing a parent reflects invisible family loyalty—an unconscious belief that family membership requires not exceeding parents' achievements. This isn't about ability or motivation—it's about loyalty operating below awareness. Making these loyalties conscious creates the possibility of choosing whether to honor them.

41. B. Navigate without available cultural scripts
Same-sex couples navigate family life cycle stages without the readily available cultural scripts that heterosexual couples have. They must create their own paths through couple formation, decisions about children, relationships with families of origin, and later life transitions. This isn't inherently problematic, but it requires more conscious negotiation without cultural templates.

42. B. Integrating members with different histories and loyalties
Stepfamilies face the unique challenge of integrating members who come with different histories, loyalties, and expectations. Children have loyalties to both biological parents. Adults bring parenting styles from previous relationships. Families must negotiate new structures while honoring existing bonds—a complex process requiring patience and flexibility.

43. C. Can reduce their power when family chooses disclosure
Bringing family secrets into open discussion can reduce their power—but this works when family members choose disclosure, not when it's forced. Making the unspoken spoken allows family members to understand reality, reduces shame and self-blame, and creates possibility for change. But timing and readiness matter—forced disclosure can cause harm.

44. B. Mediates parents and carries inappropriate burdens
A parental child mediates between parents, provides emotional support to adults, and carries responsibilities beyond their developmental capacity. This creates premature maturity and apparent competence, but the child's own needs go unmet. The role interferes with normal development and often creates adult difficulties with boundaries, self-care, and relationships.

45. B. Aging, grandparenting, and often caregiving role reversals
Families in later life face aging, grandparenting, role reversals when adult children care for aging parents, decisions about living arrangements, and often end-of-life planning. These transitions require significant adaptation. They're not inherently negative, but they involve loss, change, and negotiation of new family roles and structures.

46. C. Insecure-ambivalent attachment (continued)
Children with insecure-ambivalent attachment are anxious, clingy, and difficult to soothe when distressed because they experienced inconsistent caregiving. They can't predict whether needs will be met, so they remain anxious and escalate to get attention. When comfort comes, they struggle to trust it because past experience taught them it's unreliable. This pattern often continues into adult relationships characterized by fear of abandonment and need for constant reassurance.

47. B. May alter gene expression in ways that affect offspring
Epigenetic changes related to trauma may alter gene expression in ways that affect offspring, even without direct trauma exposure. Trauma can modify how genes are expressed—turning some on or off—and these modifications may be passed to the next generation. This doesn't mean trauma damage is permanent or unchangeable, but it helps explain how trauma effects can appear in people who didn't directly experience the original trauma.

48. B. Uses humor to manage tension while real issues remain unaddressed
The mascot uses humor and playfulness to manage family tension and anxiety. When conflict

emerges, the mascot makes everyone laugh, temporarily reducing stress. But this prevents the family from addressing real problems. The mascot learns to suppress their own needs and feelings to manage others' emotions, often becoming the family entertainer while their own struggles go unnoticed.

49. C. Let go while remaining available
Successfully launching children requires parents to let go of control and daily involvement while remaining available for support and connection. Young adults need freedom to make their own decisions and mistakes, but they also need to know parents are there if needed. This balance—releasing without abandoning—allows healthy separation and ongoing relationship.

50. B. An unsolvable dilemma needing comfort from source of fear
An infant with a frightening caregiver faces an impossible situation—they need comfort and safety from the very person who frightens them. The caregiver is both the source of fear and the only potential source of comfort. This creates disorganized attachment because the infant has no organized strategy for getting needs met safely. The approach-avoidance conflict produces confused, contradictory behaviors.

Understanding What Holds Families Together

Family systems don't exist in isolation. They're embedded in communities, cultures, and historical moments that shape what's possible and what's expected. The family struggling in your office carries not just their individual histories, but generations of patterns, cultural legacies, and social forces beyond their control.

You can't fix families by treating individuals. The depressed mother, the acting-out adolescent, the distant father—these aren't separate problems. They're parts of a system that maintains equilibrium, even when that equilibrium is painful. Change one part, and the whole system responds.

Your work involves seeing patterns others can't see. The family points to one person as the problem. You recognize that person as the symptom bearer—the one expressing what the whole family experiences. You help families see their own patterns, understand their own structures, and choose different ways of being together.

This isn't about blame. The parents who create insecure attachment often experienced it themselves. The family maintaining dysfunctional patterns isn't choosing dysfunction—they're doing the best they can with the models they inherited. Your job is creating space for new possibilities, for patterns to shift, for families to reorganize in healthier ways.

Families are resilient. Even families with severe dysfunction have strengths. The parentified child develops competence. The scapegoat develops independence. The enmeshed family knows how to connect. Your work involves helping families build on strengths while changing patterns that no longer serve them.

Core Principles for Your Practice

- Family systems operate as organized wholes—changing one part affects all other parts through interconnected relationships

- Attachment patterns formed in infancy shape relationship expectations throughout life, but these patterns can be revised through new experiences
- Family roles develop in response to system needs and serve functions, even when those roles are dysfunctional or harmful
- Boundaries define who participates in what and how—clear boundaries allow both connection and appropriate separateness
- Intergenerational patterns transmit across generations through multiple pathways including parenting, narrative, and possibly biology
- Family life cycle stages bring predictable transitions and challenges that require adaptation and reorganization
- Triangulation reduces immediate anxiety but prevents resolution of underlying issues and burdens the third person
- Enmeshment prevents healthy individuation while rigid boundaries create isolation—both extremes interfere with development
- Family secrets create anxiety and confusion, often leading to self-blame for problems children didn't cause
- The therapeutic relationship itself can provide corrective emotional experiences that begin to revise internal working models
- Cultural context shapes family structures, roles, and expectations—what's normative in one culture may be problematic in another
- Families get stuck when they can't adapt to new developmental demands—professional help facilitates necessary adaptations

Chapter 4: Environmental and Social Factors

Every client lives in multiple systems. The individual sits within a family, which exists within a community, embedded in social structures, shaped by culture and history. You can't understand the person without understanding these contexts. The woman's depression isn't just about her brain chemistry—it's about the neighborhood where she lives, the job she can't find, the services she can't access.

Social workers have always understood this. While other professions focus narrowly on the individual, social work maintains a dual focus—person and environment. You work with individuals, but you see the systems shaping their lives.

Social Systems Theory

General systems theory provides a framework for understanding how parts interact to create wholes. A system is a set of elements in relationship, where the whole is greater than the sum of its parts.

Key concepts apply across all systems:

Boundaries define what's inside and outside the system. A family has boundaries—who's in, who's out. A community has boundaries—geographic, cultural, social. Boundaries can be open (allowing exchange with environment), closed (limiting exchange), or somewhere between.

Input and output describe what enters and leaves the system. A family receives input (money, food, information, social support) and produces output (contributions to community, next generation, cultural practices). Problems arise when input is inadequate or output is blocked.

Feedback loops are circular processes where output affects future input. **Negative feedback** maintains stability—like a thermostat keeping temperature constant. **Positive feedback** amplifies change—like a microphone creating increasingly loud feedback. Both are necessary, but problems arise when systems get stuck in one type.

Homeostasis is the tendency of systems to maintain equilibrium. Families develop patterns that maintain stability, even when those patterns are dysfunctional. An alcoholic family organizes around drinking. When the alcoholic gets sober, the system destabilizes. Other members may unconsciously work to restore the familiar pattern because change feels dangerous.

Equifinality means different paths can lead to the same outcome. Two children in poverty—one becomes depressed, one becomes resilient. The same starting point produces different results based on intervening factors. This gives hope—if multiple paths lead to problems, multiple paths also lead to solutions.

Multifinality means the same starting point leads to different outcomes. Not everyone who experiences trauma develops PTSD. Not every child in poverty struggles academically. Understanding what creates different trajectories helps you identify protective factors and intervention points.

Ecological systems theory, developed by Urie Bronfenbrenner, maps how environmental systems affect development:

The **microsystem** includes immediate environments—family, school, peer group, neighborhood. These are direct, daily interactions that most immediately affect the person.

The **mesosystem** includes connections between microsystems—the relationship between family and school, between peers and family. A child whose parents know their teachers has stronger support than a child with no connection between home and school.

The **exosystem** includes settings that affect the person indirectly—a parent's workplace, community services, local government. A parent losing a job affects the child, even though the child isn't directly involved in the workplace.

The **macrosystem** includes broad cultural values, laws, and social conditions. Economic systems, cultural beliefs, political structures—these shape everything below them.

The **chronosystem** adds time—historical events, life transitions, developmental stages. The same person at different times, or different cohorts at the same age, have different experiences based on historical context.

Case Example: Marcus (Ecological Perspective)

Marcus is a 10-year-old African American boy referred for behavioral problems at school. Using an ecological lens reveals multiple system levels:

Microsystem: Marcus lives with his mother and younger sister in a one-bedroom apartment. His mother works two jobs—retail during the day, cleaning offices at night. She's rarely home. Marcus spends after-school hours caring for his sister. At school, Marcus has few friends and conflicts with teachers who perceive him as "disrespectful."

Mesosystem: There's no connection between home and school. Marcus's mother can't attend conferences—she'd lose pay. Teachers have tried calling, but mother works when school calls. The school sees an uninvolved parent. The mother sees a school that doesn't understand her reality.

Exosystem: Mother's employer offers no sick leave or schedule flexibility. The family lost housing assistance due to administrative error and is appealing. The local community center closed due to budget cuts—Marcus used to go there after school.

Macrosystem: Economic inequality means mother's wages don't cover basic needs despite full-time work. Racism affects how Marcus is perceived at school—behaviors that would be seen as "spirited" in white children are seen as "aggressive" in him. Educational funding formulas mean Marcus's school has fewer resources than suburban schools.

Chronosystem: Mother recently left an abusive relationship. The family moved, disrupting Marcus's schooling and friendships. Developmental timing matters—Marcus is approaching adolescence, when peer relationships become critical, but he's isolated.

The school labeled Marcus the problem. An ecological view reveals a child managing impossible circumstances within systems that fail him at multiple levels. Intervention requires working across systems—not just treating Marcus individually.

You help the school understand Marcus's caregiving responsibilities and trauma history. You connect mother with legal aid for the housing appeal. You advocate for policy changes allowing flexible parent-teacher communication. You find a new after-school program and help Marcus access it. You work with Marcus individually on coping skills and friendship building.

This is social work—simultaneous attention to individual and environment, recognizing that both must change.

Person-in-Environment Perspective

The **person-in-environment (PIE) perspective** is social work's signature contribution. Other professions see individuals. Social work sees individuals in context.

This perspective recognizes that problems arise at the interface between person and environment. A person with a mobility disability isn't inherently limited—they're disabled by stairs without ramps, buses without lifts, attitudes that assume inability. Change the environment, and the disability often disappears.

Assessment using PIE considers:

Personal factors: Age, developmental stage, cognitive abilities, mental health, physical health, personality, coping skills, strengths, vulnerabilities.

Environmental factors: Family, community, culture, economic resources, social support, physical environment, access to services, experiences of discrimination.

Transactions: How person and environment affect each other. A depressed person withdraws, reducing social support, increasing depression. An anxious parent hovers, preventing child's independence, increasing both anxiety and dependence.

The PIE perspective prevents victim-blaming. When a client "fails" to improve, you don't just look at their motivation or effort. You examine environmental barriers. Can they afford treatment? Is transportation available? Do they have childcare? Is the intervention culturally appropriate? Does bias affect how they're treated?

You also avoid environmental determinism—the idea that environment completely determines outcomes. People have agency. They make choices within constraints. Your work involves expanding choices by changing both person and environment.

Goodness of fit describes the match between person and environment. Problems arise from poor fit, not just individual pathology or environmental deficits. A highly active child in a rigid classroom—

poor fit. An introverted adult in a job requiring constant social interaction—poor fit. The same person in a different environment might thrive.

Intervention can change the person (building skills, changing thoughts), change the environment (modifying classrooms, finding better job fit), or improve the transaction (helping person and environment adapt to each other).

Community Resources and Support Systems

Communities provide resources that buffer stress and support well-being. But access to resources is distributed unequally.

Social capital describes the value of social networks and connections. People with high social capital know people who can help—someone who knows about job openings, someone who can provide a reference, someone with a car when transportation is needed.

Poor communities often have strong internal social capital but limited bridging capital—connections to people with different resources and opportunities. Everyone knows each other, helps each other, but no one has connections to resources beyond the community.

Formal supports are organized services—mental health centers, medical clinics, schools, social service agencies. These provide professional help but often have barriers:

- Location difficult to reach without transportation
- Hours incompatible with work schedules
- Eligibility requirements that exclude those in greatest need
- Cultural insensitivity driving people away
- Waitlists that delay help until crisis escalates

Informal supports include family, friends, neighbors, faith communities, mutual aid groups. These provide immediate, accessible help but can be overwhelmed when needs are extensive or persistent.

Your role involves:

Resource assessment: What resources exist? What gaps remain? What barriers prevent access?

Connection: Helping clients navigate systems, access resources, overcome barriers.

Advocacy: Working to create resources, remove barriers, change policies that prevent access.

Capacity building: Helping communities develop resources and strengthen networks.

Mutual aid and self-help groups provide unique benefits. People with shared experiences offer understanding that professionals can't match. A parent who lost a child to suicide understands grief in ways a therapist without that experience doesn't. These groups provide support, information, hope, and practical strategies.

You refer clients to groups, help them start groups, and partner with groups to expand services. You recognize that professional help isn't always the most powerful intervention—sometimes it's connection with others who truly understand.

Faith communities provide support for many clients. Religious beliefs offer meaning, community, and coping strategies. You don't need to share clients' faith, but you must respect it and help them access faith-based support when desired.

Some clients experience conflict between faith and other identities—LGBTQ+ individuals in non-affirming religious communities, women in patriarchal religious structures. You help clients navigate these tensions, find affirming communities, or integrate conflicting aspects of identity.

Impact of Trauma and Adversity

Trauma and chronic adversity affect development, health, and functioning in profound ways. The **Adverse Childhood Experiences (ACE) Study** documented connections between childhood adversity and adult health.

ACEs include:

- Physical, emotional, or sexual abuse
- Physical or emotional neglect
- Household substance abuse
- Household mental illness
- Domestic violence
- Parental separation or divorce
- Incarcerated household member

The study found dose-response relationships—more ACEs predict worse outcomes. People with 4+ ACEs compared to those with none:

- 4-12 times higher risk for alcoholism, drug abuse, depression, suicide attempt
- 2-4 times higher risk for smoking, poor self-rated health, sexually transmitted disease
- 1.4-1.6 times higher risk for physical inactivity and severe obesity

These aren't moral failures or poor choices—they're adaptations to trauma. Substance use numbs pain. Smoking regulates stress. Sexual behavior seeks connection or reenacts trauma. Obesity may provide protective weight or result from stress-driven eating.

Toxic stress describes chronic activation of stress response systems without adequate support to buffer effects. Normal stress activates responses briefly, then returns to baseline. Toxic stress keeps systems activated, causing wear and tear on developing brains and bodies.

Children experiencing toxic stress show:

- Hypervigilance and exaggerated startle response
- Difficulty concentrating and learning
- Problems with emotional regulation
- Aggressive or withdrawn behavior
- Physical health problems including frequent illness

Adults with childhood toxic stress experience:

- Higher rates of mental illness
- Chronic health conditions including heart disease, diabetes, autoimmune disorders
- Difficulties in relationships and parenting
- Economic struggles and employment problems

These effects aren't inevitable. **Protective factors** buffer stress and promote resilience:

Individual factors: Easy temperament, intelligence, problem-solving skills, sense of purpose, positive self-concept.

Relationship factors: At least one stable, caring adult relationship; positive peer relationships; connection to prosocial adults.

Community factors: Access to quality education, safe neighborhoods, economic opportunity, mental health and medical services.

Cultural factors: Strong cultural identity, spiritual beliefs, cultural practices that provide meaning and connection.

Your assessment identifies both risk and protective factors. Intervention builds on strengths while addressing risks.

Trauma-informed care recognizes the widespread impact of trauma and integrates this understanding into all aspects of service:

Realize the widespread impact of trauma and potential paths for recovery.

Recognize signs and symptoms of trauma in clients, families, and staff.

Respond by integrating trauma knowledge into policies, procedures, and practices.

Resist re-traumatization by avoiding practices that recreate trauma dynamics.

This means:

- Prioritizing physical and emotional safety
- Building trust through transparency and consistency

- Supporting client choice and control
- Recognizing that symptoms are adaptations, not pathology
- Understanding that "difficult" behavior often reflects trauma responses
- Addressing power imbalances in the helping relationship

Complex trauma results from prolonged, repeated trauma, usually interpersonal and often beginning in childhood. Unlike single-incident trauma, complex trauma affects core developmental processes:

- Attachment and relationships
- Sense of self and identity
- Emotional regulation
- Behavioral control
- Cognition and learning
- Physical health

Traditional PTSD treatment may be insufficient for complex trauma. Treatment must address not just traumatic memories but fundamental difficulties with relationships, self-regulation, and identity.

Historical and collective trauma affects entire communities across generations. Native Americans dealing with effects of genocide and forced assimilation. African Americans carrying trauma of slavery and ongoing racism. Holocaust survivors and descendants. Refugees from war and persecution.

This trauma isn't just individual—it's embedded in communities, transmitted across generations, and maintained by ongoing oppression. Healing requires both individual and collective approaches.

Case Example: Sarah

Sarah, a 28-year-old white woman, enters therapy for depression and relationship problems. She reports chronic emptiness, unstable relationships, and self-harm through cutting.

Initial assessment reveals extensive childhood trauma. Sarah's father was alcoholic and violent. Her mother was depressed and emotionally unavailable. Sarah experienced physical abuse, witnessed domestic violence, and had her emotional needs consistently ignored—ACE score of 5.

Sarah learned early that the world is dangerous and people can't be trusted. She developed hypervigilance, scanning for threat. She learned to suppress her needs because expressing them led to punishment. She used cutting to regulate overwhelming emotions—pain she could control when everything else felt chaotic.

Adult Sarah struggles with relationships. She's drawn to chaotic, unstable partners—familiar territory. When relationships feel close, she sabotages them—closeness triggers fear. She alternates between clinging desperately and pushing people away.

Work is difficult. She's intelligent and capable, but authority figures trigger her. She perceives criticism where none exists. She quits jobs before she can be fired—abandoning before being abandoned.

Your treatment is trauma-informed. You prioritize safety—in the therapeutic relationship, in Sarah's life. You work slowly, building trust through consistency and transparency. You explain what you're doing and why, giving Sarah control and choice.

You help Sarah understand her symptoms as adaptations. Hypervigilance kept her safe in childhood. Emotional suppression prevented punishment. Cutting regulated feelings when no one helped her learn regulation. Self-sabotage prevented deeper disappointment. These strategies made sense given her childhood—they just don't serve her now.

You work on multiple levels:

Individual: Processing trauma, building emotion regulation skills, challenging negative self-beliefs.

Relational: Using the therapeutic relationship to provide new experiences of safety and trust.

Environmental: Connecting Sarah with support groups, helping her find employment that doesn't trigger authority issues.

Systemic: Advocating for trauma-informed practices in the mental health system.

Recovery takes years. Sarah gradually learns that some people can be trusted. She develops skills for managing emotions without self-harm. She begins to believe she's worthy of care. The work is slow, with setbacks, but Sarah is building a life not determined by trauma.

Practice Questions

1. According to ecological systems theory, a parent's workplace belongs to which system?

A. Microsystem
B. Mesosystem
C. Exosystem
D. Macrosystem

2. Homeostasis in family systems refers to:

A. Healthy functioning
B. Tendency to maintain equilibrium even when dysfunctional
C. Progressive change over time
D. Open communication

3. A child with an ACE score of 4 or higher has:

A. No increased health risks
B. Slightly elevated risk for some problems
C. Significantly elevated risk for multiple health and mental health problems
D. Guaranteed poor outcomes

4. The person-in-environment perspective recognizes that problems arise:

A. Solely from individual pathology
B. Solely from environmental deficits
C. At the interface between person and environment
D. Randomly without clear causes

5. Social capital refers to:

A. Financial resources
B. Educational achievement
C. Value of social networks and connections
D. Government benefits

6. Toxic stress differs from normal stress by:

A. Being more intense
B. Chronic activation without adequate buffering
C. Affecting only children
D. Having no long-term effects

7. According to trauma-informed care, "difficult" client behavior should be understood as:

A. Manipulation requiring firm limits
B. Attention-seeking requiring ignoring
C. Trauma responses requiring understanding
D. Personality defects requiring confrontation

8. Equifinality means:

A. All outcomes are equally likely
B. Different paths can lead to the same outcome
C. The same path always produces the same outcome
D. Outcomes are predetermined

9. Bridging social capital refers to:

A. Connections within one's own community
B. Connections to people with different resources and opportunities
C. Professional relationships only
D. Family relationships

10. Complex trauma differs from single-incident trauma by:

A. Being less severe
B. Affecting only adults
C. Resulting from prolonged, repeated trauma affecting core development
D. Being easier to treat

11. The mesosystem includes:

A. Immediate environments like family and school
B. Connections between microsystems
C. Broad cultural values
D. Historical events

12. Protective factors:

A. Eliminate all risk
B. Buffer stress and promote resilience
C. Only involve individual characteristics
D. Are unnecessary if risks are low

13. Goodness of fit refers to:

A. Physical health
B. Match between person and environment
C. Family relationships
D. Educational achievement

14. Negative feedback in systems:

A. Causes problems
B. Maintains stability
C. Amplifies change
D. Should be eliminated

15. Historical trauma:

A. Affects only those who directly experienced it
B. Ends when the original trauma ends
C. Affects entire communities across generations
D. Has no current relevance

16. The macrosystem includes:

A. Individual family dynamics
B. School and neighborhood
C. Broad cultural values, laws, and social conditions
D. Peer relationships

17. Mutual aid groups provide unique benefits because:

A. They're led by professionals
B. Members share experiences and understand each other
C. They're free
D. They require no commitment

18. When a family maintains dysfunction to preserve familiar patterns, this demonstrates:

A. Homeostasis
B. Positive feedback
C. Equifinality
D. Multifinality

19. A client who experienced childhood neglect now struggles with relationships, emotion regulation, and identity. This pattern suggests:

A. Simple PTSD
B. Complex trauma
C. Adjustment disorder
D. Normal development

20. Formal supports include:

A. Family and friends
B. Faith communities
C. Organized services like mental health centers
D. Informal neighbor networks

21. Positive feedback loops:

A. Maintain stability
B. Amplify change
C. Are always beneficial
D. Prevent all problems

22. The chronosystem adds which dimension to ecological theory?

A. Space
B. Relationships
C. Time
D. Culture

23. A person with mobility disability encountering inaccessible buildings demonstrates:

A. Personal pathology
B. Problems arising from person-environment transactions
C. Individual limitation only
D. Untreatable condition

24. ACEs predict adult health problems through:

A. Genetic transmission only
B. Direct physical damage only
C. Toxic stress affecting developing brains and bodies
D. Coincidence

25. Trauma-informed care prioritizes:

A. Rapid symptom reduction
B. Confronting avoidance
C. Physical and emotional safety
D. Medication management

26. Poor communities often have:

A. No social capital
B. Strong internal capital but limited bridging capital
C. Equal resources to wealthy communities
D. No protective factors

27. Multifinality means:

A. Multiple problems require multiple treatments
B. The same starting point leads to different outcomes
C. All paths lead to the same place
D. Families have multiple functions

28. Self-harm in trauma survivors often functions as:

A. Attention-seeking behavior
B. Manipulation of others
C. Emotion regulation when other skills weren't learned
D. Evidence of personality disorder

29. The exosystem affects individuals:

A. Through direct daily interaction
B. Indirectly through settings they're not directly involved in
C. Not at all
D. Only in childhood

30. Barriers to accessing formal supports include:

A. Location and transportation only
B. Cost only
C. Multiple factors including location, hours, eligibility, cultural sensitivity
D. No significant barriers exist

31. When assessing using PIE, you consider:

A. Personal factors only
B. Environmental factors only
C. Personal, environmental, and transactional factors
D. Diagnosis only

32. Children experiencing toxic stress show:

A. Normal development
B. Hypervigilance, concentration difficulties, emotional dysregulation
C. Enhanced coping abilities
D. No observable effects

33. Systems with closed boundaries:

A. Function optimally
B. Limit exchange with environment
C. Promote growth
D. Are always pathological

34. A client's substance use following childhood trauma should be understood as:

A. Moral failure
B. Poor choice
C. Adaptation to regulate pain and stress
D. Unrelated to trauma

35. Faith communities provide:

A. Professional mental health services
B. Meaning, community, and support for many clients
C. Replacement for therapy
D. No relevant support

36. The dose-response relationship in ACE research means:

A. All ACEs have equal impact
B. One ACE is as harmful as many
C. More ACEs predict worse outcomes
D. ACEs don't actually affect health

37. Environmental determinism:

A. Accurately explains all behavior
B. Inappropriately assumes environment completely determines outcomes
C. Recognizes human agency
D. Is the basis of PIE perspective

38. Input and output in systems describe:

A. Computer functions only
B. What enters and leaves the system
C. Individual thoughts
D. Family rules

39. Hypervigilance in trauma survivors:

A. Is paranoia requiring medication
B. Was adaptive in dangerous environments
C. Should be immediately eliminated
D. Has no function

40. Community capacity building involves:

A. Providing all services professionally
B. Helping communities develop resources and strengthen networks
C. Removing informal supports
D. Replacing mutual aid with professional services

41. A highly active child struggling in a rigid classroom demonstrates:

A. ADHD requiring medication
B. Poor fit between person and environment
C. Bad parenting
D. Hopeless situation

42. Collective trauma:

A. Affects only individuals
B. Isn't scientifically valid
C. Affects entire communities across generations
D. Ends immediately after traumatic events

43. Systems theory suggests that changing one part of a system:

A. Has no effect on other parts
B. Affects all parts through interconnection
C. Only affects directly connected parts
D. Is impossible

44. Adults with childhood toxic stress experience:

A. No lasting effects
B. Higher rates of mental illness and chronic health conditions
C. Enhanced coping abilities
D. The same outcomes as those without toxic stress

45. The microsystem includes:

A. Cultural values
B. Historical events
C. Immediate environments like family and school
D. Indirect influences

46. Re-traumatization in service settings occurs when:

A. Trauma is discussed
B. Practices recreate trauma dynamics like powerlessness
C. Clients receive services
D. Providers show empathy

47. An intervention changing both person and environment demonstrates:

A. Confusion about focus
B. PIE perspective in action
C. Impossibility
D. Poor clinical judgment

48. Informal supports can be:

A. Completely replaced by formal services
B. Overwhelmed when needs are extensive
C. Ignored in treatment planning
D. Used without consideration of limitations

49. The relationship between ACEs and adult health:

A. Is coincidental
B. Operates through toxic stress affecting development
C. Is exaggerated
D. Only affects mental health

50. Recognizing client agency within environmental constraints involves:

A. Blaming victims
B. Ignoring environment
C. Seeing people as passive
D. Acknowledging both choices and limitations

Answer Key with Detailed Explanations

1. C. Exosystem

A parent's workplace belongs to the exosystem—settings that affect the child indirectly. The child doesn't directly participate in the workplace, but parental work schedules, stress, income, and flexibility all affect the child. Job loss, promotion, workplace stress—all these exosystem factors ripple into the child's microsystem.

2. B. Tendency to maintain equilibrium even when dysfunctional
Homeostasis describes systems' tendency to maintain stability and equilibrium, even when current patterns are dysfunctional. A family organizes around alcoholism—when the alcoholic gets sober, the system destabilizes and members may unconsciously work to restore familiar patterns. Homeostasis isn't inherently healthy or unhealthy—it's just the system's tendency toward stability.

3. C. Significantly elevated risk for multiple health and mental health problems
ACE research shows dose-response relationships—more adverse experiences predict worse outcomes. People with 4+ ACEs have 4-12 times higher risk for alcoholism, drug abuse, depression, and suicide attempt compared to those with no ACEs. But this is risk, not destiny—protective factors matter, and outcomes vary based on many factors beyond ACE count.

4. C. At the interface between person and environment
The person-in-environment perspective recognizes that problems arise from transactions between person and environment, not solely from individual pathology or environmental deficits. A person with a disability isn't inherently limited—they're disabled by environmental barriers. Change either the person (building skills) or environment (removing barriers), and the problem may resolve.

5. C. Value of social networks and connections
Social capital describes the value of relationships and networks. People with high social capital know people who can provide help, information, opportunities, and resources. Poor communities may have strong internal social capital (everyone helps each other) but limited bridging capital (connections to people with different resources and opportunities).

6. B. Chronic activation without adequate buffering
Toxic stress involves chronic activation of stress response systems without adequate adult support to buffer effects. Normal stress activates systems briefly, then returns to baseline. Toxic stress keeps systems activated, causing wear and tear on developing brains and bodies. The key difference is chronicity and lack of buffering, not intensity alone.

7. C. Trauma responses requiring understanding
Trauma-informed care recognizes that "difficult" behaviors—aggression, withdrawal, noncompliance, dissociation—often reflect trauma responses, not manipulation or personality defects. These behaviors made sense in traumatic contexts and served protective functions. Understanding this prevents re-traumatization through punitive responses and guides interventions that address underlying trauma.

8. B. Different paths can lead to the same outcome
Equifinality means multiple paths can reach the same destination. Two children experience poverty—one becomes depressed, one becomes resilient. Different intervening factors create different outcomes from similar starting points. This concept provides hope—if multiple paths lead to problems, multiple paths also lead to solutions.

9. B. Connections to people with different resources and opportunities
Bridging social capital refers to connections across different social groups—relationships with people who have different resources, information, and opportunities than your immediate community. This

differs from bonding social capital (connections within your group). Poor communities may have strong bonding capital but limited bridging capital to access broader opportunities.

10. C. Resulting from prolonged, repeated trauma affecting core development
Complex trauma results from prolonged, repeated trauma—usually interpersonal and often beginning in childhood. Unlike single-incident trauma, complex trauma affects fundamental developmental processes: attachment, self-concept, emotional regulation, behavioral control, cognition. Traditional PTSD treatment addressing single traumatic memories may be insufficient—complex trauma requires addressing core developmental disruptions.

11. B. Connections between microsystems
The mesosystem includes connections between microsystems—relationships between family and school, peers and family, neighborhood and religious community. A child whose parents know teachers has mesosystem support. Disconnection between microsystems (parents can't attend school events, no communication between home and school) weakens the mesosystem.

12. B. Buffer stress and promote resilience
Protective factors buffer the impact of stress and adversity, promoting resilience despite risk. They don't eliminate risk or guarantee good outcomes, but they reduce the likelihood of problems. Protective factors operate at individual (temperament, intelligence), relationship (stable caring adult), community (quality education, safety), and cultural (strong identity, spiritual beliefs) levels.

13. B. Match between person and environment
Goodness of fit describes how well person and environment match. A highly active child in a rigid classroom—poor fit. An introverted adult in a job requiring constant social interaction—poor fit. The same person in a different environment might thrive. Problems often reflect poor fit, not inherent pathology. Intervention can change person, environment, or both to improve fit.

14. B. Maintains stability
Negative feedback maintains system stability—like a thermostat keeping temperature constant. When temperature rises, cooling activates; when it falls, heating activates. In families, negative feedback might look like: conflict emerges, someone makes a joke, tension reduces, equilibrium restores. This maintains stability, which isn't inherently good or bad.

15. C. Affects entire communities across generations
Historical and collective trauma affects entire communities and transmits across generations. Native Americans dealing with genocide effects, African Americans carrying slavery trauma, Holocaust descendants—the trauma isn't just individual. It's embedded in communities, transmitted through multiple pathways, and often maintained by ongoing oppression. Healing requires both individual and collective approaches.

16. C. Broad cultural values, laws, and social conditions
The macrosystem includes broad cultural values, economic systems, political structures, laws, and social conditions that shape everything below. Cultural beliefs about family, economic inequality, racism, gender norms—these macrosystem factors influence all other systems without directly interacting with the individual.

17. B. Members share experiences and understand each other
Mutual aid and self-help groups provide unique benefits because members share experiences. A parent who lost a child to suicide understands grief in ways a therapist without that experience can't. Shared experience creates credibility, hope (someone like me recovered), practical strategies, and deep understanding. This isn't replacement for professional help, but it's powerful support.

18. A. Homeostasis
When families maintain dysfunctional patterns to preserve familiar equilibrium, this demonstrates homeostasis—the system's tendency toward stability. Change feels dangerous even when current patterns are harmful. Family members may unconsciously sabotage positive changes to restore familiar patterns. Understanding homeostasis helps explain why change is difficult even when everyone wants it.

19. B. Complex trauma
Difficulties with relationships, emotion regulation, and identity following childhood neglect suggest complex trauma. This isn't simple PTSD (which focuses on traumatic memories). Complex trauma affects core developmental processes. Prolonged, repeated interpersonal trauma during critical developmental periods disrupts fundamental capacities for connection, self-regulation, and coherent identity.

20. C. Organized services like mental health centers
Formal supports are organized, professional services—mental health centers, medical clinics, social service agencies, schools. These provide professional help but often have barriers: location, hours, eligibility requirements, waitlists, cultural insensitivity. Informal supports (family, friends, neighbors) provide immediate help but can be overwhelmed by extensive needs.

21. B. Amplify change
Positive feedback loops amplify change—like a microphone creating increasingly loud feedback. In families, this might look like: parent anxiety increases, child becomes anxious, parent gets more anxious, child gets worse, parent panics. The cycle escalates. Positive feedback isn't good or bad—it just describes amplification. Both negative (stabilizing) and positive (amplifying) feedback are necessary; problems arise when stuck in either.

22. C. Time
The chronosystem adds the dimension of time to ecological theory. This includes historical events, life transitions, developmental timing, cohort effects. The same person at different ages, or different cohorts at the same age, have different experiences. A child experiencing parental divorce at age 5 has different impacts than the same divorce at age 15.

23. B. Problems arising from person-environment transactions
A person with mobility disability encountering inaccessible buildings demonstrates how problems arise from person-environment transactions. The disability isn't inherent limitation—it's created by environmental barriers. Change the environment (add ramps, elevators, accessible transportation), and the disability often disappears. This is the essence of the PIE perspective.

24. C. Toxic stress affecting developing brains and bodies
ACEs predict adult health problems through toxic stress pathways. Chronic stress without buffering affects developing brains and bodies—stress hormones, inflammatory processes, brain structure changes. Children adapt to dangerous environments in ways that protect short-term survival but create long-term health risks. Substance use, smoking, obesity—these are adaptations to regulate stress, not moral failures.

25. C. Physical and emotional safety
Trauma-informed care prioritizes physical and emotional safety above all else. Survivors experienced profound lack of safety—creating safety now is foundational. This means predictable environments, transparent processes, client choice and control, absence of re-traumatization. Without safety, other interventions can't succeed and may cause harm.

26. B. Strong internal capital but limited bridging capital
Poor communities often have strong internal social capital—neighbors help each other, everyone knows everyone, people share resources. But they may lack bridging capital—connections to people with different resources and opportunities. Everyone helps, but no one has access to jobs, education, or resources beyond the community. Building bridging capital expands opportunities.

27. B. The same starting point leads to different outcomes
Multifinality means the same starting point produces different outcomes. Not everyone who experiences trauma develops PTSD. Not all children in poverty struggle academically. Intervening factors—protective relationships, individual strengths, access to resources—create different trajectories. Understanding multifinality helps identify what creates resilience versus problems.

28. C. Emotion regulation when other skills weren't learned
Self-harm in trauma survivors often functions as emotion regulation. When overwhelming feelings arise and no one taught regulatory skills, people find their own methods. Cutting, burning, hitting—these create pain that's controllable when emotions feel uncontrollable. Understanding the function prevents judgment and guides intervention toward building alternative regulatory skills.

29. B. Indirectly through settings they're not directly involved in
The exosystem affects individuals indirectly through settings they don't directly participate in. A child isn't involved in a parent's workplace, but workplace policies (flexibility, leave, stress, wages) affect the child. Community decisions about services, local government actions—these exosystem factors shape lives indirectly.

30. C. Multiple factors including location, hours, eligibility, cultural sensitivity
Barriers to formal supports are multiple and interconnected: location difficult to reach without transportation, hours incompatible with work schedules, eligibility requirements excluding those in greatest need, waiting lists delaying help, cultural insensitivity driving people away, language barriers, documentation requirements. Effective intervention requires addressing all these barriers, not just one.

31. C. Personal, environmental, and transactional factors
PIE assessment considers personal factors (age, abilities, mental health, strengths), environmental factors (family, community, resources, discrimination), and transactions (how person and environment

affect each other). All three are necessary—focusing only on person or only on environment misses the complete picture and limits intervention effectiveness.

32. B. Hypervigilance, concentration difficulties, emotional dysregulation
Children experiencing toxic stress show hypervigilance (constantly scanning for threat), concentration and learning difficulties (can't focus when brain is in threat mode), emotional dysregulation (can't manage feelings without adult help that wasn't provided), and behavioral problems (aggression or withdrawal). These are adaptations to danger, not inherent deficits.

33. B. Limit exchange with environment
Systems with closed boundaries limit exchange with the environment—little input from outside, little output to the world. Families with closed boundaries are isolated, don't access community resources, don't participate in broader systems. This isn't always pathological (temporary closing during crisis might be protective), but chronic closed boundaries prevent adaptation and growth.

34. C. Adaptation to regulate pain and stress
Substance use following childhood trauma should be understood as adaptation—an attempt to regulate pain and stress when healthier regulatory skills weren't learned. People aren't weak or making poor choices—they're using available methods to manage overwhelming internal experiences. Understanding this prevents moral judgment and guides intervention toward building alternative coping strategies.

35. B. Meaning, community, and support for many clients
Faith communities provide meaning, belonging, community, support, and coping strategies for many clients. Religious beliefs help people make sense of suffering, find purpose, and maintain hope. You don't need to share clients' faith, but you must respect it, help them access faith-based support when desired, and recognize faith as a potential strength and resource.

36. C. More ACEs predict worse outcomes
The dose-response relationship in ACE research means more adverse experiences predict increasingly worse outcomes. One ACE increases risk moderately. Four or more ACEs dramatically increase risk across multiple domains. This isn't deterministic—protective factors matter—but it demonstrates that cumulative adversity has cumulative effects.

37. B. Inappropriately assumes environment completely determines outcomes
Environmental determinism inappropriately assumes that environment completely determines outcomes, denying human agency and choice. The PIE perspective recognizes that environment profoundly shapes possibilities, but people make choices within constraints. Social workers work to expand choices by changing environments while recognizing that people maintain agency even in oppressive conditions.

38. B. What enters and leaves the system
Input and output describe what enters and leaves a system. Families receive input (money, food, social support, information) and produce output (contributions to community, next generation, cultural transmission). Problems arise when input is inadequate (insufficient resources) or output is blocked (isolation preventing contribution).

39. B. Was adaptive in dangerous environments
Hypervigilance in trauma survivors was adaptive in dangerous environments—constantly scanning for threat prevented harm. It's not paranoia or pathology—it's a protective strategy that made sense given circumstances. The problem is that hypervigilance continues even in safe environments. Treatment helps people recognize safety cues and calibrate threat responses appropriately.

40. B. Helping communities develop resources and strengthen networks
Community capacity building involves helping communities develop their own resources, strengthen social networks, and increase ability to address problems collectively. This isn't about professionals providing all services—it's about supporting communities to help themselves, building on existing strengths, and creating sustainable local resources.

41. B. Poor fit between person and environment
A highly active child struggling in a rigid classroom demonstrates poor fit between person and environment. The child's activity level isn't inherently pathological—it just doesn't match environmental demands. The same child in a different setting (activity-based learning, frequent movement breaks, outdoor time) might thrive. Intervention can modify the child, the environment, or both to improve fit.

42. C. Affects entire communities across generations
Collective trauma affects entire communities and transmits across generations through multiple pathways: disrupted parenting, cultural narratives, possibly epigenetic changes, ongoing oppression maintaining trauma effects. This isn't individual PTSD multiplied—it's trauma embedded in community structures, relationships, and cultural identity. Healing requires both individual and collective approaches.

43. B. Affects all parts through interconnection
Systems theory recognizes that changing one part of a system affects all parts through interconnection. A child gets better in therapy, but the family system organized around the child's problems destabilizes. A parent stops drinking, and the family must reorganize. Understanding systems helps predict these ripple effects and work with the whole system, not just the identified patient.

44. B. Higher rates of mental illness and chronic health conditions
Adults with childhood toxic stress experience significantly higher rates of mental illness (depression, anxiety, PTSD, substance use) and chronic health conditions (heart disease, diabetes, autoimmune disorders, cancer). This operates through biological pathways—chronic stress affects developing brains and bodies—and behavioral pathways—adaptive strategies like substance use create health risks.

45. C. Immediate environments like family and school
The microsystem includes immediate environments where the person directly participates—family, school, peer group, neighborhood, workplace. These are daily, direct interactions that most immediately affect development and functioning. The quality of microsystems significantly predicts outcomes.

46. B. Practices recreate trauma dynamics like powerlessness
Re-traumatization occurs when service practices recreate trauma dynamics—powerlessness (no choice or control), violation of boundaries, broken trust, physical/emotional harm. Examples: forced treatment, restraints, punitive responses to trauma symptoms, staff abuse. Trauma-informed care specifically works to avoid re-traumatization by prioritizing safety, choice, and trustworthiness.

47. B. PIE perspective in action
Interventions changing both person and environment demonstrate the PIE perspective in practice. You might help a client build coping skills (person) while also advocating for workplace accommodations (environment). You teach parenting strategies (person) while connecting family to food assistance (environment). Effective practice often requires multi-level intervention.

48. B. Overwhelmed when needs are extensive
Informal supports (family, friends, neighbors) provide immediate, accessible help, but they can become overwhelmed when needs are extensive, persistent, or specialized. A friend can provide support during acute crisis but may not sustain help for chronic mental illness. Effective practice recognizes both the value and limitations of informal supports, building on strengths while adding formal support when needed.

49. B. Operates through toxic stress affecting development
The relationship between ACEs and adult health operates primarily through toxic stress pathways affecting child development. Chronic stress without buffering affects developing brains (structure, function, stress response systems) and bodies (inflammatory processes, immune function). Children adapt in ways that protect immediate survival but create long-term health vulnerabilities.

50. D. Acknowledging both choices and limitations
Recognizing client agency within environmental constraints means acknowledging that people make choices, but choices happen within limits created by social structures, resources, and power dynamics. This avoids both victim-blaming (ignoring constraints) and environmental determinism (denying agency). Social workers expand choices by changing environments while respecting that clients make their own decisions.

Putting It All Together

Social work happens where person meets environment. You can't separate them. The client's depression isn't just about neurotransmitters or childhood experiences—it's about the job they can't find, the neighborhood where they live, the services they can't access, the discrimination they face daily.

Your assessment maps multiple system levels. You see the individual, the family, the community, the broader social structures. You recognize that problems at one level create problems at others. A parent's unemployment (exosystem) affects family stress (microsystem) affects child development (individual).

Your intervention works across levels. You help individuals build skills, change thoughts, process trauma. You help families reorganize patterns and improve communication. You connect people to resources and remove barriers to access. You advocate for policy changes and work to dismantle oppressive systems.

This is complex work. You need individual clinical skills and systems change skills. You need to sit with a trauma survivor in profound pain and also testify at a city council meeting about housing policy. Both matter. Both are social work.

The person-in-environment perspective prevents you from blaming individuals for problems created by social conditions. But it also prevents you from seeing people as passive victims. People have agency. They make choices, resist oppression, create meaning, and build lives within constraints. Your job is expanding those possibilities.

Core Understanding for Practice

- Ecological systems theory maps how environmental systems at multiple levels affect individual development and functioning
- Person-in-environment perspective locates problems at the interface between individuals and contexts, not solely in either
- Social systems operate through feedback loops, boundaries, and homeostasis that maintain patterns even when dysfunctional
- Adverse childhood experiences create toxic stress that affects development through biological and behavioral pathways
- Protective factors at individual, relationship, community, and cultural levels buffer stress and promote resilience despite adversity
- Community resources include both formal services and informal supports, each with strengths and limitations
- Trauma-informed care recognizes widespread trauma impact and prioritizes safety, choice, and avoiding re-traumatization
- Complex trauma from prolonged interpersonal harm affects core developmental capacities beyond traumatic memories
- Historical and collective trauma affects entire communities across generations through multiple transmission pathways
- Effective intervention requires working across system levels—individual, family, community, and policy—simultaneously
- Goodness of fit between person and environment predicts functioning better than examining either in isolation
- Social capital—particularly bridging capital connecting people across different groups—provides access to opportunities and resources

Chapter 5: Clinical Assessment Methods

Assessment is detective work. You gather clues—what the client says, how they say it, what they don't say. You observe body language, thought patterns, emotional responses. You ask questions that open doors to understanding. Every piece of information fits into a larger picture of who this person is, what they're experiencing, and what they need.

But assessment isn't just information gathering. It's the beginning of treatment. The questions you ask communicate what matters. The way you listen builds trust. Clients often say that the first session—when someone finally heard their full story—was healing in itself.

Good assessment is both art and science. You need technical knowledge of diagnostic criteria, risk factors, and assessment tools. You also need the ability to create safety, to read between the lines, to understand what the client is trying to tell you even when they can't find the words.

Biopsychosocial Assessment

The biopsychosocial model recognizes that human problems arise from the interaction of biological, psychological, and social factors. You can't understand depression by looking at neurotransmitters alone, or at negative thoughts alone, or at life stressors alone. You need all three.

Biological factors include genetics, medical conditions, medications, substance use, brain chemistry, hormones, nutrition, sleep, and physical health. A client's anxiety might be triggered by hyperthyroidism. Depression might worsen with chronic pain. Cognitive problems might stem from medication side effects.

You ask about medical history—current conditions, past illnesses, surgeries, injuries. You ask about medications—prescribed, over-the-counter, supplements. Many clients don't realize that blood pressure medication can cause depression, that steroids can trigger mania, that even common cold medicines can interact with psychiatric medications.

Family medical and psychiatric history matters. Mental illness runs in families—not because of weak character, but because of genetics and learned patterns. A client with three generations of depression has different risk factors than someone with no family history.

Sleep and appetite changes often signal mental health problems. Depression disrupts sleep—either insomnia or hypersomnia. Anxiety keeps people awake. Mania eliminates the need for sleep. Changes in eating—increased or decreased—accompany many disorders.

Psychological factors include thoughts, emotions, behaviors, coping strategies, personality traits, self-concept, and past experiences. You assess how the client thinks about themselves, others, and the world. You notice patterns—all-or-nothing thinking, catastrophizing, personalization.

You ask about trauma history—childhood abuse, neglect, violence, losses. You ask carefully, respecting the client's pace. Some clients are ready to discuss trauma immediately. Others need time to build trust. Pushing too hard too soon can re-traumatize.

Coping strategies reveal a lot. How does the client handle stress? Some exercise, talk to friends, use humor. Others drink, isolate, or self-harm. All coping strategies serve a function—even destructive ones. Understanding the function helps you find healthier alternatives.

Social factors include relationships, work, education, housing, finances, culture, religion, community, and social support. A client's depression might be triggered by job loss. Anxiety might worsen with housing instability. Psychosis might be misunderstood as demonic possession in some cultural contexts.

You assess current living situation—who lives with the client, what's the quality of relationships, is the home safe? You ask about work or school—is it a source of satisfaction or stress? You explore financial stability—can basic needs be met?

Social support is protective. Clients with strong support systems generally do better than isolated clients. But support quality matters more than quantity. One genuine, reliable friend beats a dozen superficial connections.

Cultural and religious beliefs shape how people understand and express distress. Some cultures somatize emotional pain—experiencing depression as physical symptoms. Some see mental illness as spiritual crisis. You respect these beliefs while providing effective treatment.

Integration is where assessment becomes powerful. You don't just collect information in three categories. You see how factors interact. A client with genetic vulnerability to depression (biological) develops negative thinking patterns after childhood abuse (psychological) and becomes socially isolated after losing a job (social). All three factors maintain the depression.

Case Example: Maria's Depression

Maria, a 45-year-old Latina woman, presents with depression. A purely biological view might focus on medication. A purely psychological view might focus on cognitive distortions. But the biopsychosocial assessment reveals complexity.

Biological: Maria has hypothyroidism, poorly controlled. Thyroid dysfunction commonly causes depression. She's also perimenopausal—hormonal changes affect mood. She sleeps four hours nightly and survives on coffee and sugar. Her mother and sister both have depression.

Psychological: Maria experienced emotional neglect as a child. Her parents worked constantly, leaving her to raise younger siblings. She learned that her needs don't matter, that she must care for everyone else. She believes she's selfish if she prioritizes herself. When overwhelmed, she withdraws and stops eating.

Social: Maria works two jobs to support her three children and sends money to her parents in Mexico. She has no time for friends or activities she enjoys. She stopped attending church—her primary source of support—because she works Sundays. Her children's father provides no support. She feels trapped and hopeless.

Treatment addresses all three levels. You refer Maria to her physician for thyroid management. You help her challenge beliefs about selfishness and develop self-care skills. You connect her with financial assistance and help her find a Spanish-speaking support group. You work with her to gradually reduce work hours and reconnect with church community.

Three months later, Maria's depression has significantly improved. Was it the thyroid medication? The therapy? The social support? The answer is yes—all of them working together.

Mental Status Examination

The Mental Status Examination (MSE) is a systematic assessment of current psychological functioning. It's like a snapshot of the client's mental state at the time of the interview. The MSE has specific components, each revealing different aspects of functioning.

Appearance describes how the client looks. You note grooming, hygiene, clothing appropriateness, physical health indicators. Poor grooming might suggest depression, self-neglect, or cognitive impairment. Bizarre dress might suggest mania or psychosis. Multiple layers of clothing in summer might suggest homelessness or paranoia.

But you interpret carefully. Disheveled appearance might simply mean the client rushed from work. Eccentric clothing might be cultural or personal style. You look for patterns and changes, not just single observations.

Behavior includes motor activity, eye contact, and interaction style. Is the client agitated or lethargic? Making appropriate eye contact or avoiding it? Cooperative or hostile? You note psychomotor retardation (slowed movements) in depression, agitation in anxiety, and purposeless movement in mania.

Cultural factors affect behavior. Direct eye contact is respectful in some cultures, disrespectful in others. What looks like avoidance might be cultural appropriateness.

Speech describes how the client talks—rate, volume, tone, amount. Pressured speech (rapid, difficult to interrupt) suggests mania. Slow, monotone speech suggests depression. Loud, rapid speech might indicate anxiety or anger. Minimal speech might suggest depression, psychosis, or cultural reserve.

Mood and affect are related but different. **Mood** is what the client reports—"I feel depressed," "I'm anxious." **Affect** is what you observe—the emotional expression you see.

You describe affect quality (happy, sad, angry, anxious), range (broad, restricted, flat), appropriateness (congruent or incongruent with content), and stability (stable or labile). Flat affect—showing no emotion—might indicate depression or schizophrenia. Labile affect—rapidly shifting emotions—might suggest borderline personality disorder or neurological problems.

Incongruent affect raises concerns. A client smiling while describing trauma suggests dissociation or psychosis. Laughing while discussing death might indicate inappropriate affect seen in schizophrenia.

Thought process describes how the client thinks—the flow and form of thoughts. Logical, linear thinking is normal. Tangential thinking goes off-topic. Circumstantial thinking eventually reaches the point but takes a winding path. Loose associations jump between unrelated ideas.

Flight of ideas—rapidly jumping between loosely connected thoughts—suggests mania. Thought blocking—sudden stops mid-sentence—suggests schizophrenia. Perseveration—repeating the same response—suggests cognitive impairment or psychosis.

Thought content describes what the client thinks about. You assess for delusions (fixed false beliefs), obsessions (intrusive, unwanted thoughts), suicidal or homicidal ideation, and preoccupations.

Delusions come in types: persecutory (people are out to get me), grandiose (I have special powers), referential (TV is sending me messages), somatic (my organs are rotting). You assess conviction—does the client firmly believe despite evidence to the contrary?

Perception describes unusual sensory experiences. Hallucinations are perceptions without stimuli—hearing voices no one else hears, seeing things others don't see. Illusions are misperceptions of real stimuli—seeing a coat rack as a person.

Auditory hallucinations are most common in schizophrenia. Command hallucinations—voices telling the client what to do—raise safety concerns, especially if commanding harm. Visual hallucinations might suggest medical conditions, substance use, or certain mental illnesses.

Cognition includes orientation, attention, concentration, and memory. You assess orientation to person (knows who they are), place (knows where they are), time (knows the date), and situation (understands why they're here).

Disorientation suggests delirium, dementia, severe psychosis, or dissociation. You test attention and concentration—can the client focus on questions? Can they do simple calculations? Memory assessment includes immediate (repeat three words), recent (recall those words later), and remote (significant life events).

Insight and judgment assess self-awareness and decision-making. Insight is understanding one's condition. Does the client recognize they have a problem? Do they understand how it affects their life? Poor insight is common in psychosis, mania, and some personality disorders.

Judgment is decision-making ability. You assess through questions about hypothetical situations: "What would you do if you found a stamped, addressed envelope on the ground?" Poor judgment suggests impulsivity, cognitive impairment, or active symptoms.

Case Example: James's MSE

James, a 32-year-old man, presents to the emergency room after his family called police reporting bizarre behavior.

Appearance: Disheveled, wearing shorts and T-shirt in winter, multiple layers of aluminum foil visible under clothing. Poor hygiene, strong body odor.

Behavior: Agitated, pacing constantly, hypervigilant—frequently checking over shoulder. Initially hostile, becomes cooperative when reassured.

Speech: Rapid, pressured, loud, difficult to interrupt. Talks almost continuously.

Mood/Affect: States mood is "alert—they're watching." Affect anxious, mood-incongruent smiling when discussing threats.

Thought Process: Flight of ideas, loosely connected. Jumps from government surveillance to aliens to his neighbor's dog. Some tangentiality.

Thought Content: Persecutory delusions—believes CIA is monitoring him through satellites. Referential delusions—believes TV news contains coded messages for him. No suicidal or homicidal ideation but states he's "protecting himself."

Perception: Reports hearing voices warning him about surveillance. Voices are clear, distinct, commenting on his actions. No visual hallucinations.

Cognition: Oriented to person and place, disoriented to time (off by several days). Attention poor, easily distracted. Memory appears intact when he can focus.

Insight/Judgment: No insight—denies mental illness, attributes experiences to real surveillance. Judgment impaired—wearing foil to block signals, considering fleeing the state.

This MSE suggests acute psychosis, likely schizophrenia or substance-induced psychotic disorder. The combination of delusions, hallucinations, disorganized behavior, and lack of insight requires immediate intervention. James needs psychiatric hospitalization for stabilization and diagnosis.

Risk Assessment

Risk assessment can save lives. You identify clients at risk for suicide, homicide, or serious self-harm and take appropriate action. This assessment happens not just initially, but throughout treatment. Risk fluctuates.

Suicide Risk Assessment

Suicide is the tenth leading cause of death in the United States. Every year, over 47,000 people die by suicide. Many who die saw a healthcare provider within weeks of their death. We have opportunities to intervene—if we ask the right questions.

Risk factors increase suicide likelihood:

- Previous suicide attempt (strongest predictor)
- Mental illness, especially mood disorders, psychosis, substance use
- Recent loss—relationship, job, health, loved one
- Access to lethal means
- Family history of suicide

- History of trauma or abuse
- Chronic pain or serious medical illness
- Social isolation
- Recent discharge from psychiatric hospitalization
- Male gender, white race, older age (though rates increasing in young people and minorities)

Protective factors reduce risk:

- Strong social connections
- Reasons for living—children, pets, religious beliefs
- Access to mental health care
- Problem-solving skills
- Hope for the future

You ask directly about suicide. Research shows that asking about suicide doesn't plant ideas—it shows you care and creates opportunity for intervention. You ask progressively specific questions:

1. "Have you had thoughts that life isn't worth living?"
2. "Have you had thoughts about hurting yourself?"
3. "Have you had thoughts about killing yourself?"
4. "Have you made a plan for how you would do it?"
5. "Have you taken steps toward acting on this plan?"
6. "Is there anything stopping you from acting on these thoughts?"

The more specific the plan, the higher the risk. Vague thoughts ("Sometimes I wish I wouldn't wake up") carry less immediate risk than detailed plans ("I plan to shoot myself with my father's gun on Friday"). Access to means matters enormously. A client with a gun at home is at higher risk than one without access to lethal means.

Intent is harder to assess. Some clients with strong intent downplay it. Others with no real intent dramatize it. You look for behaviors suggesting preparation—giving away possessions, saying goodbye, suddenly seeming at peace after prolonged depression (may indicate decision made).

Imminent risk requires immediate action—hospitalization, mobile crisis team, staying with client until safe. **Elevated but not imminent risk** requires safety planning, increased contact, removal of means, and possibly higher level of care.

Safety planning is collaborative. You and the client develop a written plan:

1. Warning signs that crisis is developing

2. Internal coping strategies (things I can do myself)
3. People and social settings that provide distraction
4. People I can ask for help
5. Professionals I can contact
6. Making the environment safe (removing means)

Homicidal Risk Assessment

Homicidal ideation is less common but requires careful assessment. You consider the same elements—ideation, plan, intent, means, access to intended victim.

Tarasoff duty to warn emerged from a California case. A client told his therapist he planned to kill a woman. The therapist didn't warn her. The client killed her. Courts ruled that therapists have a duty to protect identifiable potential victims.

This creates an ethical dilemma. Confidentiality is fundamental to therapy. But safety trumps confidentiality. Most jurisdictions require warning identifiable victims and/or notifying police when clients present serious, imminent threat to specific individuals.

You assess seriousness of threat by considering:

- Specificity—vague anger versus detailed plan
- History of violence
- Current stressors and triggers
- Access to weapons
- Substance use (disinhibits violent impulses)
- Psychotic symptoms (especially command hallucinations to harm)
- Relationship to potential victim

Not every expression of anger constitutes duty to warn. Saying "My boss makes me so angry I could kill him" during a frustration discussion is different from "I'm going to shoot my boss tomorrow with my shotgun." Context matters.

Self-Harm Assessment

Non-suicidal self-injury (NSSI)—cutting, burning, hitting oneself—serves different functions than suicide attempts. People who self-harm usually don't intend to die. They're trying to:

- Regulate overwhelming emotions
- Punish themselves
- Feel something when numb

- Communicate distress
- Ground themselves when dissociating

You assess history, frequency, methods, medical severity, and function. Someone cutting superficially once monthly carries different risk than someone cutting deeply daily. But any self-harm requires attention.

You ask about suicidal intent. Most people who self-harm aren't suicidal, but some engage in both NSSI and suicidal behavior. You assess separately.

Treatment focuses on understanding function and building alternative skills. If cutting regulates emotions, you teach emotion regulation skills. If it's about self-punishment, you address underlying guilt and shame. You don't just take away the coping strategy—you build better ones.

Case Example: Sophie's Risk Assessment

Sophie, a 19-year-old college student, comes to therapy at her roommate's insistence. She's been cutting her arms and thighs for six months.

Assessment:

You ask about suicidal thoughts. Sophie says, "Sometimes I wish I could just disappear, but I'm not going to kill myself. My little sister needs me." She has no suicide plan, strong protective factors (sister, future goals), and clear intent to live.

You assess self-harm: Sophie cuts several times weekly when overwhelmed. She uses a razor blade, making superficial cuts on forearms and thighs. She's never required medical attention but scars are visible. She hides the behavior, wears long sleeves year-round.

You explore function: Sophie feels intense emotions she can't manage. Stress builds until she feels she'll "explode." Cutting releases the pressure. Afterward, she feels calm, then guilty and ashamed. The guilt triggers more cutting.

You assess current safety: Sophie is not currently suicidal but is at risk for accidental serious injury. She's developing a cutting addiction—needing it more frequently for the same relief.

Intervention:

You validate that cutting has been helpful—it's not a character flaw, it's a coping strategy that works. But it's creating problems (scars, shame, increasing frequency). You teach emotion regulation skills—identifying emotions, tolerating distress, using alternatives like ice on skin, intense exercise, talking to friends.

You create a reduction plan (not demanding immediate cessation, which could backfire). Sophie commits to trying alternatives first, cutting only if nothing else works, and calling you before cutting. You meet twice weekly initially.

Three months later, Sophie hasn't cut in six weeks. She uses alternatives successfully. She's practicing skills that will serve her for life.

Substance Use Screening and Assessment

Substance use affects mental health profoundly. Substances can cause, worsen, or mask psychiatric symptoms. You can't accurately diagnose or treat mental illness while someone is actively using. You screen for substance use with every client.

Screening identifies potential problems quickly. The **CAGE** questionnaire has four questions:

- Have you ever felt you should **C**ut down on drinking?
- Have people **A**nnoyed you by criticizing your drinking?
- Have you ever felt bad or **G**uilty about drinking?
- Have you ever had a drink first thing in the morning as an **E**ye-opener?

Two or more yes answers suggest problem drinking. But CAGE misses some problems and focuses only on alcohol. The **AUDIT** (Alcohol Use Disorders Identification Test) is more sensitive, assessing quantity, frequency, and consequences.

For drugs, the **DAST** (Drug Abuse Screening Test) or simple questions work: "How often do you use marijuana, cocaine, prescription drugs not prescribed to you, or other drugs?" If they report any use, you assess further.

Assessment goes deeper than screening. You use clinical interview and possibly biological tests (urine drug screen, blood alcohol level). You assess multiple dimensions:

Substances used: Specific substances, routes of administration, patterns of use. Poly-substance use is common and complicates treatment. Someone drinking to ease cocaine comedown has different needs than someone using alcohol alone.

Quantity and frequency: How much, how often? Daily drinking carries different implications than weekend binge drinking. Both create problems, but different problems.

Consequences: Medical (liver disease, overdoses), legal (DUIs, arrests), occupational (job loss, poor performance), social (relationship problems, isolation), psychological (depression, anxiety). Consequences indicate severity.

Dependence indicators: Tolerance (needing more for same effect), withdrawal (physical symptoms when stopping), loss of control (using more than intended), unsuccessful attempts to quit, time spent obtaining/using/recovering, giving up activities, continued use despite problems.

Motivation to change: Where is the client in the change process? Precontemplation (don't see a problem), contemplation (ambivalent), preparation (ready to change), action (actively changing), maintenance (sustaining change)? Your approach varies based on stage.

Function: Why does the client use? Self-medication for depression, anxiety, trauma? Social lubrication? Coping with boredom? Peer pressure? Understanding function guides intervention.

Risk factors: Family history of addiction, early age of first use, co-occurring mental illness, trauma history, chronic pain, easy access. These increase addiction risk and inform treatment.

Protective factors: Social support, employment, housing stability, reasons to quit, previous successful recovery periods. These support recovery and guide discharge planning.

You distinguish between **use, abuse, and dependence**. Use is consumption without significant problems. Abuse is use causing problems but without dependence. Dependence involves tolerance, withdrawal, and loss of control. The DSM-5 combined abuse and dependence into **substance use disorder** with severity levels (mild, moderate, severe) based on symptom count.

Biological testing has limitations. Urine drug screens detect recent use but don't indicate quantity, frequency, or impairment. Marijuana shows up weeks after last use. Alcohol leaves the system quickly. False positives occur. You use testing to supplement clinical assessment, not replace it.

Motivational interviewing works well for substance use assessment and early intervention. You explore ambivalence without confrontation. You help clients articulate their own reasons for change. You roll with resistance rather than challenging it directly.

Case Example: Michael's Substance Use

Michael, a 38-year-old man, enters therapy for anxiety. Initial screening reveals alcohol use. You assess further.

Use pattern: Michael drinks 6-8 beers nightly, more on weekends. He's been drinking daily for five years, increasing in past year. He occasionally drinks liquor when beer "doesn't do it anymore" (tolerance).

Consequences: Wife threatens divorce unless he stops. Boss warned him about arriving late and missing deadlines. He's gained 40 pounds. Last physical showed elevated liver enzymes. He's stopped seeing friends who don't drink.

Dependence: Clear tolerance—he used to feel drunk after three beers, now needs six. Morning shakes and sweating (withdrawal). He intends to have two beers, ends up having eight (loss of control). He's tried to quit three times, longest period was two weeks.

Function: Michael started drinking to relax after stressful workdays. It evolved into habit, then need. He now drinks to avoid withdrawal, to sleep, to feel normal. Anxiety is worse than before drinking—alcohol is causing it, not treating it.

Motivation: Michael is ambivalent. He sees problems but enjoys drinking. He's scared of losing his wife but doubts he can quit. He's in contemplation stage—aware of problem, not yet ready to change.

Intervention:

You use motivational interviewing. You don't tell Michael he's an alcoholic or demand he quit. Instead, you explore his ambivalence. "What concerns you about your drinking? What do you like about it? If you continue as you are, where will you be in five years? What would be different if you stopped?"

Michael articulates his own reasons for change: wanting to save his marriage, being there for his kids, feeling healthy again. You reinforce this change talk. You provide information about alcohol's anxiety effects—it causes the problem it seems to solve.

You discuss options: abstinence, moderation, intensive outpatient program, AA. Michael chooses to try moderation first—no more than two drinks, three times weekly. You're skeptical (his dependence suggests abstinence needed) but meet him where he is.

Two weeks later, Michael admits moderation failed. He's ready for abstinence and intensive outpatient treatment. His failed attempt wasn't wasted—it moved him from contemplation to preparation. He needed to discover for himself that moderation wouldn't work.

Practice Questions

1. In a biopsychosocial assessment, a client's genetic vulnerability to depression would be considered:

A. Biological
B. Psychological
C. Social
D. Cultural

2. Flat affect is characterized by:

A. Rapid mood swings
B. Absence of emotional expression
C. Exaggerated emotional responses
D. Emotions inappropriate to content

3. A client who jumps between unrelated ideas demonstrates:

A. Circumstantial thinking
B. Tangential thinking
C. Loose associations
D. Flight of ideas

4. The strongest predictor of future suicide attempts is:

A. Family history of suicide
B. Major depression
C. Previous suicide attempt
D. Access to firearms

5. Which question is most appropriate for initial suicide screening?

A. "You're not thinking about killing yourself, are you?"
B. "Have you had thoughts about killing yourself?"
C. "Why would you want to kill yourself?"
D. "You wouldn't do anything to hurt yourself, would you?"

6. Asking a client about suicidal thoughts:

A. Plants the idea in their mind
B. Shows you care and opens dialogue
C. Should only be done if client brings it up
D. Is primarily for documentation

7. A client reports hearing voices telling him to harm his neighbor. This raises concern for:

A. Duty to warn
B. Breach of confidentiality
C. Normal psychotic symptoms
D. No particular concern

8. Non-suicidal self-injury most commonly serves to:

A. Manipulate others
B. Seek attention
C. Regulate emotions
D. Threaten suicide

9. In the mental status exam, "mood" refers to:

A. What the client reports feeling
B. What the clinician observes
C. Emotional range
D. Appropriateness of emotions

10. Pressured speech is most associated with:

A. Depression
B. Anxiety
C. Mania
D. Schizophrenia

11. Two or more "yes" answers on the CAGE questionnaire suggest:

A. Normal drinking
B. Problem drinking
C. Definite alcoholism
D. No alcohol use

12. Tolerance in substance use means:

A. Accepting others' substance use
B. Needing more substance for same effect
C. Physical symptoms when stopping
D. Continued use despite problems

13. A client smiles while describing a traumatic assault. This suggests:

A. The assault wasn't traumatic
B. Incongruent affect
C. Appropriate coping
D. Normal response

14. Delusions are best defined as:

A. Sensory experiences without stimuli
B. Fixed false beliefs
C. Exaggerated worries
D. Intrusive thoughts

15. Disorientation to time, place, and person most suggests:

A. Depression
B. Anxiety
C. Delirium or dementia
D. Personality disorder

16. Command hallucinations are concerning because they:

A. Are always obeyed
B. May direct harmful behavior
C. Never occur in schizophrenia
D. Indicate malingering

17. In assessing suicide risk, protective factors include:

A. Access to firearms
B. Recent losses
C. Social connections
D. Previous attempts

18. A client states, "I asked my neighbor for sugar, the sugar bowl reminded me of my grandmother, she made great cookies, cookies are round like the earth." This exemplifies:

A. Loose associations
B. Circumstantial thinking
C. Thought blocking
D. Perseveration

19. Motivational interviewing for substance use focuses on:

A. Confronting denial
B. Exploring ambivalence
C. Mandating abstinence
D. Providing education only

20. Poor insight means the client:

A. Has low intelligence
B. Doesn't recognize having a problem
C. Makes poor decisions
D. Can't remember recent events

21. The biopsychosocial model recognizes that:

A. Biology is most critical
B. Psychology determines all symptoms
C. Social factors don't affect mental health
D. All three factors interact

22. Psychomotor retardation is observed as:

A. Slowed movements
B. Rapid, agitated behavior
C. Purposeless movement
D. Normal activity

23. Visual hallucinations are most commonly caused by:

A. Schizophrenia
B. Depression
C. Medical conditions or substances
D. Anxiety disorders

24. A detailed suicide plan with high lethality means indicates:

A. Low risk
B. Attention-seeking
C. High risk
D. No immediate concern

25. The Tarasoff duty to warn applies when:

A. Any violence is mentioned
B. There's serious threat to identifiable victim
C. Client is angry
D. Therapist feels uncomfortable

26. Flight of ideas is characterized by:

A. Forgetting what one was saying
B. Rapidly jumping between loosely connected thoughts
C. Slow, labored thinking
D. Repeating the same idea

27. Judgment is best assessed by:

A. IQ testing
B. Memory questions
C. Hypothetical situations
D. Orientation questions

28. In substance use assessment, "function" refers to:

A. Level of impairment
B. Why the client uses
C. How much is used
D. What substance is used

29. Labile affect means:

A. No emotional expression
B. Rapidly shifting emotions
C. Exaggerated emotions
D. Flat emotions

30. A client who suddenly seems at peace after severe depression may indicate:

A. Recovery
B. Decision to attempt suicide
C. Medication working
D. Natural mood fluctuation

31. Thought blocking is characterized by:

A. Rapid thoughts
B. Sudden stops mid-sentence
C. Organized thinking
D. Detailed explanations

32. Chronic pain is a risk factor for suicide because:

A. Pain is imaginary
B. It causes suffering and hopelessness
C. It only affects elderly
D. Medications prevent suicide

33. In the MSE, "range of affect" describes:

A. Appropriateness
B. Stability
C. Breadth of emotional expression
D. Congruence with mood

34. The DSM-5 combined substance abuse and dependence into:

A. Addiction
B. Substance use disorder
C. Chemical dependency
D. Substance misuse

35. A client gives away possessions and says goodbye to loved ones. This suggests:

A. Generosity
B. Normal behavior
C. Possible suicide preparation
D. Manic spending

36. Persecutory delusions involve beliefs that:

A. One has special powers
B. People are trying to harm you
C. TV is sending messages
D. One's body is changing

37. Cultural factors affect MSE because:

A. Mental illness is cultural
B. Eye contact norms vary by culture
C. Only Western cultures have mental illness
D. Culture doesn't matter

38. Immediate suicide risk requires:

A. Outpatient follow-up
B. Safety planning only
C. Immediate intervention
D. No action

39. In assessing self-harm, you should:

A. Ignore it unless suicidal
B. Assess separately from suicide
C. Assume it's attention-seeking
D. Hospitalize immediately

40. Withdrawal symptoms indicate:

A. Substance use disorder
B. Recreational use
C. No problem
D. Successful quitting

41. A biopsychosocial assessment of anxiety might include:

A. Only brain chemistry
B. Only traumatic thoughts
C. Only social stressors
D. All three interacting

42. Grandiose delusions involve beliefs about:

A. Persecution
B. Special powers or importance
C. Body changes
D. Reference

43. Safety planning for suicide includes:

A. Ignoring warning signs
B. Identifying coping strategies
C. Keeping means accessible
D. Avoiding support

44. The contemplation stage of change means:

A. Not seeing a problem
B. Ready to change now
C. Ambivalent about changing
D. Successfully changed

45. Tangential thinking:

A. Eventually reaches the point
B. Goes off-topic permanently
C. Involves loose associations
D. Shows thought blocking

46. A client reports "the TV is sending me personal messages." This is:

A. Grandiose delusion
B. Persecutory delusion
C. Delusion of reference
D. Somatic delusion

47. Male gender is a suicide risk factor because:

A. Men experience more depression
B. Men use more lethal means
C. Men seek help more readily
D. Men have more protective factors

48. The AUDIT screens for:

A. Depression
B. Anxiety
C. Alcohol problems
D. Drug use

49. Circumstantial thinking:

A. Never reaches the point
B. Eventually reaches the point but takes winding path
C. Shows loose associations
D. Involves rapid jumping

50. Medication side effects should be assessed because:

A. All medications are dangerous
B. They can mimic psychiatric symptoms
C. Clients always report them
D. They're unrelated to mental health

51. Recent discharge from psychiatric hospitalization is a risk factor because:

A. Hospitals cause suicide
B. Transition period involves high stress
C. Hospitalization doesn't work
D. It indicates low risk

52. Illusions differ from hallucinations in that:

A. Illusions involve misperception of real stimuli
B. Illusions are more severe
C. Illusions indicate psychosis
D. There's no difference

53. A client's inability to do simple calculations suggests problems with:

A. Mood
B. Affect
C. Cognition
D. Perception

54. Self-medication hypothesis suggests substance use:

A. Is purely recreational
B. Attempts to treat psychiatric symptoms
C. Has no function
D. Is always conscious choice

55. Asking "What would you do if you found a stamped envelope?" assesses:

A. Memory
B. Intelligence
C. Judgment
D. Orientation

56. Family history of mental illness is assessed because:

A. It proves causation
B. Genetics play a role
C. Families cause all problems
D. It's required documentation

57. A safety plan for suicide should be:

A. Developed by clinician alone
B. Collaborative with client
C. Generic for all clients
D. Focused only on hospitalization

58. Somatic delusions involve:

A. Special powers
B. Persecution
C. Body or health changes
D. Environmental messages

59. The more specific a suicide plan:

A. The lower the risk
B. The higher the risk
C. Risk is unchanged
D. It indicates no real intent

60. Polysubstance use complicates treatment because:

A. It's rare
B. Different substances interact
C. It's easier to treat
D. Assessment isn't needed

61. Restricted affect shows:

A. No emotion
B. Rapidly shifting emotions
C. Limited emotional range
D. Inappropriate emotions

62. Religious beliefs can be protective against suicide by:

A. Preventing all mental illness
B. Providing meaning and prohibitions
C. Replacing treatment
D. Eliminating risk

63. Orientation to situation means the client:

A. Knows the date
B. Knows their name
C. Understands why they're here
D. Knows the location

64. Early age of first substance use increases risk because:

A. Young people can't get addicted
B. Developing brain is vulnerable
C. It indicates maturity
D. It's protective

65. Congruent affect means:

A. Emotions don't match content
B. Emotions match content
C. No emotional expression
D. Rapid mood changes

66. Access to firearms increases suicide risk because:

A. Guns cause mental illness
B. They're a highly lethal means
C. Gun owners are depressed
D. They prevent treatment

67. Remote memory refers to:

A. Immediate recall
B. Recent events
C. Significant life events from past
D. Future planning

68. Harm reduction in substance use means:

A. Mandating abstinence
B. Reducing consequences even if use continues
C. Ignoring substance use
D. Accepting all use

69. A client who repeats the same response to different questions shows:

A. Circumstantial thinking
B. Perseveration
C. Flight of ideas
D. Loose associations

70. Social isolation is a suicide risk factor because:

A. Isolated people are weak
B. Lack of connection increases hopelessness
C. It prevents diagnosis
D. It's only concerning in elderly

71. The biopsychosocial model emerged because:

A. Medical model was sufficient
B. Single-factor explanations were inadequate
C. Biology doesn't matter
D. Social work rejects science

72. Referential delusions involve beliefs that:

A. One is being persecuted
B. Environmental cues have special meaning
C. One has special powers
D. One's body is changing

73. Recent significant loss increases suicide risk because:

A. Loss causes suicide
B. Grief and hopelessness intensify
C. Everyone who grieves is suicidal
D. Loss is protective

74. Urine drug screens have limitations including:

A. Perfect accuracy
B. Detecting all substances equally
C. False positives and varying detection windows
D. No limitations

75. Stable affect means:

A. Rapidly changing emotions
B. Emotions remain consistent
C. No emotions
D. Inappropriate emotions

Answer Key with Detailed Explanations

1. A. Biological
Genetic vulnerability to depression is a biological factor in the biopsychosocial model. This includes inherited susceptibility, family history, and neurobiological predisposition. Biological factors work in combination with psychological factors (thoughts, coping patterns) and social factors (relationships, stressors) to influence mental health outcomes.

2. B. Absence of emotional expression
Flat affect describes complete or near-complete absence of emotional expression—the person shows no facial expression, has monotone voice, and displays no emotional reactions even to emotionally charged content. This is common in schizophrenia and severe depression. It differs from restricted affect (limited range) and blunted affect (diminished but present emotional expression).

3. C. Loose associations
Loose associations occur when the client jumps between unrelated ideas with no clear connection. This differs from flight of ideas (rapid jumping but with some connection), tangential thinking (going off-topic), and circumstantial thinking (eventually reaching point but taking winding path). Loose associations suggest thought disorder, often seen in schizophrenia.

4. C. Previous suicide attempt
Previous suicide attempt is the strongest single predictor of future attempts. People who have attempted before are at significantly higher risk than those who haven't, regardless of other risk factors. This doesn't mean all previous attempters will attempt again, but it requires close monitoring and intervention. Other factors like depression and family history are also significant but less predictive than past attempts.

5. B. "Have you had thoughts about killing yourself?"
Direct, clear questions work best for suicide screening. This question is straightforward, uses clear language, and doesn't suggest the answer. Options A and D suggest the expected answer is "no," potentially leading clients to minimize. Option C asks "why" before establishing "if," which can feel judgmental. Research shows direct questioning doesn't increase suicide risk and often provides relief that someone is willing to discuss it.

6. B. Shows you care and opens dialogue
Asking about suicidal thoughts demonstrates that you take the client seriously and are comfortable discussing difficult topics. Research consistently shows that asking about suicide doesn't plant ideas or increase risk. Instead, it opens dialogue, provides relief, and creates opportunity for intervention. Many clients report feeling relieved that someone finally asked directly.

7. A. Duty to warn
Command hallucinations directing harm to a specific person may trigger duty to warn obligations. If

the client presents serious, imminent threat to an identifiable victim, you may be required to warn the intended victim and/or notify police. This creates an exception to confidentiality when safety is at stake. You need to assess seriousness—not all violent thoughts require warning, but command hallucinations with identified victim and means warrant action.

8. C. Regulate emotions
Non-suicidal self-injury most commonly serves to regulate overwhelming emotions. People describe feeling intense emotional pain that builds until cutting or burning releases it. The physical pain replaces emotional pain, which feels more controllable. While some may use it for other reasons, emotion regulation is the primary function. Understanding this function guides treatment toward building alternative emotion regulation skills.

9. A. What the client reports feeling
Mood is the client's subjective report of their emotional state—"I feel depressed," "I'm anxious," "I'm happy." Affect is what the clinician observes—the visible expression of emotion. These don't always match. A client might report feeling fine (mood) while appearing tearful and sad (affect). The discrepancy provides clinical information about insight, denial, or disconnect between internal experience and external expression.

10. C. Mania
Pressured speech—rapid, difficult to interrupt speech where the person feels driven to keep talking—is characteristic of mania. The rate is increased, the person is hard to interrupt, and there's urgency to the communication. Depressed clients typically show slowed, monotone speech. Anxious clients may speak rapidly but usually can be interrupted. Schizophrenia may show disordered content but not necessarily pressured rate.

11. B. Problem drinking
Two or more "yes" answers on CAGE suggest problem drinking warranting further assessment. It's a screening tool, not diagnostic. It identifies potential problems quickly but can miss some problems and doesn't assess severity. Positive screen leads to comprehensive assessment. CAGE has limitations—it's less sensitive to early problems and in certain populations, so clinical judgment is always needed.

12. B. Needing more substance for same effect
Tolerance means needing increasing amounts of a substance to achieve the desired effect, or experiencing diminished effect with continued use of the same amount. This is a sign of physiological adaptation to the substance and indicates developing dependence. Tolerance alone doesn't mean addiction, but it's one criterion for substance use disorder. It's distinct from withdrawal (symptoms when stopping) and behavioral aspects of addiction.

13. B. Incongruent affect
Affect is incongruent when emotional expression doesn't match the content being discussed. Smiling while describing trauma suggests disconnect between content and emotion—possibly due to dissociation, psychosis, or severe defense mechanisms. It raises clinical concerns and warrants further exploration. Congruent affect would show sadness or distress when discussing trauma.

14. B. Fixed false beliefs
Delusions are fixed false beliefs that persist despite contradictory evidence and aren't explained by cultural or religious background. They're held with conviction even when evidence clearly contradicts them. Hallucinations are sensory experiences without stimuli. Obsessions are intrusive thoughts. Delusions are a thought content problem, indicating altered reality testing seen in psychotic disorders.

15. C. Delirium or dementia
Disorientation to time, place, and person most strongly suggests delirium (acute confusion often from medical causes) or dementia (chronic cognitive decline). Orientation is typically preserved in depression, anxiety, and personality disorders unless symptoms are extremely severe. Disorientation requires medical evaluation to rule out underlying medical conditions, medication effects, or substance intoxication/withdrawal.

16. B. May direct harmful behavior
Command hallucinations—voices telling the person what to do—are concerning because they may direct harmful behavior. Commands to harm self or others require immediate risk assessment. Not all commands are obeyed, but people with psychosis may feel compelled to follow them, especially if they believe the voices have authority. Assessment includes content of commands, person's relationship to voices, and history of following commands.

17. C. Social connections
Social connections are protective factors that reduce suicide risk. Strong relationships, sense of belonging, and people to turn to for support buffer against suicidal ideation and behavior. Other protective factors include effective coping skills, reasons for living, hope for future, and access to care. Risk factors include access to firearms, recent losses, and previous attempts—the question asks for protective factors.

18. B. Circumstantial thinking
Circumstantial thinking takes a winding, detailed path but eventually reaches the point. The client includes excessive, unnecessary detail and makes tangents, but there's underlying logic and they return to the original topic. This differs from tangential thinking (goes off-topic, never returns) and loose associations (no logical connection between ideas). Circumstantial thinking can be normal in some people or indicate anxiety, mania, or cognitive issues when excessive.

19. B. Exploring ambivalence
Motivational interviewing focuses on exploring the client's ambivalence about change in a non-confrontational way. You help clients articulate their own reasons for change rather than imposing yours. You roll with resistance instead of challenging it directly. This approach is more effective than confrontation for substance use, as it reduces defensiveness and helps clients resolve their own ambivalence toward change.

20. B. Doesn't recognize having a problem
Poor insight means the client doesn't recognize they have a problem or understand how it affects their life. They may deny symptoms, attribute them to external causes, or not see the need for treatment. This is common in psychosis, mania, and some personality disorders. It's different from intelligence (cognitive ability), judgment (decision-making), or memory (information retention).

21. D. All three factors interact
The biopsychosocial model recognizes that biological, psychological, and social factors all contribute to mental health and interact in complex ways. No single factor alone explains mental illness. A person might have genetic vulnerability (biological) that's triggered by trauma (psychological) in the context of poverty and isolation (social). Effective assessment and treatment address all three levels.

22. A. Slowed movements
Psychomotor retardation describes slowed physical movements and speech, commonly seen in depression. The person moves slowly, speaks slowly, and may have delayed responses. This differs from psychomotor agitation (restless, excessive movement seen in anxiety and mania) and purposeless movement (seen in some psychotic and neurological conditions). Observing motor activity is part of the behavioral component of MSE.

23. C. Medical conditions or substances
Visual hallucinations are more commonly caused by medical conditions (delirium, neurological problems, brain injury) or substance use (intoxication, withdrawal, hallucinogens) than primary psychiatric disorders. Auditory hallucinations are most characteristic of schizophrenia. Visual hallucinations in psychiatric settings always warrant medical evaluation to rule out underlying physical causes.

24. C. High risk
A detailed suicide plan with high lethality means (gun, hanging, jumping from height) indicates high risk requiring immediate intervention. Specificity of plan and lethality of chosen method are key risk factors. Vague thoughts carry less immediate risk than detailed plans with accessible means. This doesn't mean the client will definitely attempt, but it requires safety measures—possibly hospitalization, definitely safety planning and increased monitoring.

25. B. There's serious threat to identifiable victim
Tarasoff duty to warn applies when a client presents a serious, imminent threat to a specific, identifiable person. The threat must be more than vague anger—it requires credible threat, identified victim, and means/opportunity. When these conditions are met, you may be legally required to warn the intended victim and/or notify police. Not every expression of anger triggers this duty; context and seriousness matter.

26. B. Rapidly jumping between loosely connected thoughts
Flight of ideas involves rapid movement between thoughts that have some connection but are loosely related. Ideas flow rapidly, jumping from topic to topic with minimal links. This is characteristic of mania. It differs from loose associations (no connection between ideas) and thought blocking (sudden stopping). The rapid flow and loose but present connections distinguish flight of ideas.

27. C. Hypothetical situations
Judgment is best assessed through hypothetical situations: "What would you do if you found a stamped envelope?" or "What would you do if you saw smoke in a theater?" These questions assess decision-making ability and social judgment. Responses reveal whether the person can think through situations and make reasonable decisions. IQ tests measure intelligence, not judgment. Memory and orientation questions assess cognitive functions other than decision-making.

28. B. Why the client uses
Function refers to why the client uses substances—what purpose it serves. Self-medication for anxiety? Coping with trauma? Social lubrication? Boredom? Peer pressure? Understanding function is critical for treatment planning because you need to address the underlying need the substance meets. If someone drinks to manage anxiety, treatment must address anxiety and teach alternative coping skills.

29. B. Rapidly shifting emotions
Labile affect describes rapidly shifting emotions—crying one moment, laughing the next, then angry. Emotions change quickly and sometimes without clear external trigger. This can indicate borderline personality disorder, neurological conditions, or sometimes substance use. It differs from flat affect (no emotion), restricted affect (limited range), or stable affect (consistent emotional tone).

30. B. Decision to attempt suicide
When someone who has been severely depressed suddenly seems at peace or happy, this can indicate they've made a decision to attempt suicide and feel relief at having an "answer" to their pain. This sudden improvement without intervention is a red flag requiring immediate assessment. It doesn't always mean suicide decision, but it warrants careful inquiry about suicidal thoughts and plans.

31. B. Sudden stops mid-sentence
Thought blocking occurs when the person suddenly stops speaking mid-sentence, as if their thoughts have been taken away. After a pause, they may resume speaking but can't recall what they were saying. This suggests thought disorder and is seen in schizophrenia. It differs from just losing one's train of thought—it's abrupt, complete stopping with inability to resume the original thought.

32. B. It causes suffering and hopelessness
Chronic pain is a suicide risk factor because it causes ongoing suffering, reduces quality of life, limits activities, and can create hopelessness about the future. Pain is real, not imaginary. It affects people of all ages. While pain medications can increase risk (if used for overdose), the primary risk comes from the suffering and despair that chronic pain creates.

33. C. Breadth of emotional expression
Range of affect describes the breadth of emotional expression—from broad (full range of emotions) to restricted (limited range) to flat (no expression). This is distinct from appropriateness (does affect match content), stability (does affect shift), and congruence (does affect match stated mood). Range tells you how much emotional expression the person can display.

34. B. Substance use disorder
DSM-5 combined the previous categories of substance abuse and dependence into substance use disorder, with severity specifiers (mild, moderate, severe) based on number of criteria met. This recognizes that substance problems exist on a continuum rather than as distinct categories. Severity is determined by symptom count: 2-3 symptoms = mild, 4-5 = moderate, 6+ = severe.

35. C. Possible suicide preparation
Giving away possessions and saying goodbye can indicate suicide preparation. The person is "putting affairs in order" and saying final goodbyes. Not everyone who does this is suicidal (someone moving

away might do this), but in the context of depression or suicidal ideation, it's a serious warning sign requiring immediate assessment. The sudden giving away of valued possessions is particularly concerning.

36. B. People are trying to harm you
Persecutory delusions involve beliefs that people or organizations are trying to harm you—being followed, poisoned, spied on, plotted against. These are among the most common delusions in schizophrenia and can be highly distressing. They differ from grandiose delusions (special powers), referential delusions (environmental messages), and somatic delusions (body changes).

37. B. Eye contact norms vary by culture
Cultural factors affect MSE interpretation because behaviors have different meanings across cultures. Direct eye contact is respectful in some cultures, disrespectful in others. What appears as avoidance in one culture is appropriate deference in another. Emotional expression, personal space, communication style—all vary by culture. You must interpret MSE findings within cultural context to avoid misdiagnosis.

38. C. Immediate intervention
Immediate suicide risk requires immediate intervention—psychiatric hospitalization, mobile crisis team, staying with the client until they're safe. You don't schedule an outpatient appointment for someone expressing imminent intent to die. Safety planning alone isn't sufficient for imminent risk. The client needs a safe environment and intensive monitoring until risk decreases.

39. B. Assess separately from suicide
Self-harm should be assessed separately from suicide because it usually serves different functions and requires different intervention. Most people who self-harm aren't trying to die—they're trying to cope with emotions, punish themselves, or feel something when numb. However, some people engage in both self-harm and suicidal behavior, so you assess both. Assuming all self-harm is attention-seeking or requiring hospitalization would be incorrect.

40. A. Substance use disorder
Withdrawal symptoms—physical or psychological symptoms when substance use stops or reduces—indicate physiological dependence and are one criterion for substance use disorder. Withdrawal doesn't occur with pure recreational use (though tolerance might develop). Its presence suggests the body has adapted to the substance and requires it to function normally. Withdrawal can be dangerous and may require medical management.

41. D. All three interacting
A biopsychosocial assessment of anxiety would examine biological factors (genetics, medical conditions affecting anxiety, brain chemistry), psychological factors (trauma history, thought patterns, coping skills), and social factors (stressors, relationships, work environment)—and most important, how these factors interact to create and maintain anxiety. Single-factor explanations miss the complexity of mental health problems.

42. B. Special powers or importance
Grandiose delusions involve inflated beliefs about oneself—having special powers, being extremely

important, having a special relationship with famous people or God, having made great discoveries. These are common in mania and can occur in schizophrenia. They differ from persecutory (persecution), referential (environmental messages), and somatic (body changes) delusions.

43. B. Identifying coping strategies
Safety planning includes identifying warning signs, internal coping strategies (what I can do myself), people and places that provide distraction, people to ask for help, professionals to contact, and ways to make the environment safe (removing means). It's a concrete, written plan developed collaboratively. Ignoring warning signs, keeping means accessible, and avoiding support would increase rather than reduce risk.

44. C. Ambivalent about changing
The contemplation stage (from Stages of Change model) describes ambivalence—the person sees the problem but isn't yet ready to change. They're weighing pros and cons, considering change but not committed. Precontemplation means not seeing a problem. Preparation means ready to change soon. Action means actively changing. Maintenance means sustaining changes already made.

45. B. Goes off-topic permanently
Tangential thinking goes off-topic and never returns to the original point. The person starts answering a question but veers onto a tangent and stays there. This differs from circumstantial thinking (eventually reaches point) and loose associations (no logical connection). Thought blocking is sudden stopping. Tangential thinking can indicate thought disorder or sometimes just anxiety-driven rambling.

46. C. Delusion of reference
Delusions of reference involve beliefs that environmental cues have special personal meaning—TV talking to you specifically, songs containing messages for you, strangers' conversations referring to you. The person believes neutral stimuli are specifically directed at them. This differs from grandiose (special powers), persecutory (harm), and somatic (body) delusions.

47. B. Men use more lethal means
Males have higher suicide completion rates primarily because they tend to use more lethal means (firearms, hanging) versus methods with higher survival rates (overdose, cutting). Women actually attempt suicide more often, but men complete more often due to method lethality. This gender difference in method choice, not differences in depression rates or help-seeking, accounts for the higher male suicide rate.

48. C. Alcohol problems
AUDIT (Alcohol Use Disorders Identification Test) is a screening tool specifically for alcohol problems. It assesses consumption patterns, dependence symptoms, and alcohol-related problems. It's more sensitive than CAGE and can identify problematic drinking before severe dependence develops. Different tools screen for different substances—DAST screens for drugs, various tools screen for mental health conditions.

49. B. Eventually reaches the point but takes winding path
Circumstantial thinking includes excessive detail and takes tangents but eventually returns to and

answers the original question. There's underlying logic, just inefficient. The person can't get to the point directly but gets there eventually. This differs from tangential (never reaches point), loose associations (no logic), and flight of ideas (rapid jumping). It can be normal or indicate anxiety, mania, or cognitive issues when excessive.

50. B. They can mimic psychiatric symptoms
Medication side effects can mimic psychiatric symptoms—depression from beta-blockers, anxiety from steroids, cognitive problems from anticholinergics, psychosis from certain medications. This is why medication review is part of every assessment. You can't know if symptoms are primary psychiatric illness or medication effects without reviewing all medications. Many clients don't realize common medications can affect mental status.

51. B. Transition period involves high stress
Recent psychiatric discharge is a high-risk period for suicide because of the stress of transition, potential for decompensation when intensive support ends, possible medication changes, and adjustment back to community stressors. The immediate post-discharge period requires careful monitoring and support. It's not that hospitalization doesn't work, but that transition from hospital to community is vulnerable.

52. A. Illusions involve misperception of real stimuli
Illusions are misperceptions of real stimuli—seeing a coat rack as a person, hearing wind as voices. There's an actual stimulus being misperceived. Hallucinations are perceptions without any external stimulus—hearing voices when no one is there, seeing things that don't exist. Illusions can occur in normal people (especially when tired or anxious), while hallucinations more strongly suggest pathology.

53. C. Cognition
Inability to perform simple calculations (serial 7s, simple addition/subtraction) suggests cognitive problems—difficulty with concentration, attention, or mental processing. This is part of cognitive assessment, which includes orientation, attention, concentration, memory, and fund of knowledge. Mood and affect describe emotional state. Perception involves sensory experiences.

54. B. Attempts to treat psychiatric symptoms
Self-medication hypothesis proposes that people use substances to alleviate psychiatric symptoms—drinking to reduce anxiety, using stimulants to manage depression, using marijuana to sleep. It's not always conscious or the only reason for use, but many people with co-occurring disorders report that substance use initially helped symptoms. Understanding this helps with treatment—you must address the underlying symptoms the substance was treating.

55. C. Judgment
Hypothetical questions like "What would you do if you found a stamped envelope?" assess judgment—the ability to think through situations and make reasonable decisions. Expected response is "mail it" or "take it to the post office." Bizarre responses (eat it, sell it) or indecision suggest impaired judgment. This differs from memory (information retention), intelligence (cognitive ability), and orientation (awareness of self and environment).

56. B. Genetics play a role
Family history is assessed because many mental illnesses have genetic components. Having a first-degree relative with depression, bipolar disorder, or schizophrenia increases risk. This doesn't mean it's deterministic—genetics create vulnerability, not certainty. Environmental factors also matter enormously. But family history helps assess risk and sometimes guides treatment choices (medications that worked for relatives might work for client).

57. B. Collaborative with client
Effective safety plans are developed collaboratively with the client, not imposed by the clinician. The client must believe in the plan and commit to following it. Generic plans copied from templates don't work—the plan must be specific to the individual's warning signs, coping strategies, and supports. Collaboration increases buy-in and effectiveness. The clinician provides structure and suggestions, but the client's input is essential.

58. C. Body or health changes
Somatic delusions involve false beliefs about body or health—organs rotting, being infested with parasites, body parts not working, having a serious disease despite negative tests. These differ from health anxiety (where the person fears they might be sick) in that delusions are fixed beliefs unshaken by evidence. They're seen in psychotic depression, schizophrenia, and sometimes dementia.

59. B. The higher the risk
The more specific and detailed the suicide plan, the higher the risk. Vague thoughts ("I wish I were dead") carry less immediate risk than specific plans ("I plan to hang myself in my garage on Friday using the rope I bought yesterday"). Specificity indicates more serious intent and planning. Combined with access to means and lack of protective factors, detailed plans require immediate intervention.

60. B. Different substances interact
Polysubstance use complicates treatment because different substances have different effects, withdrawal symptoms, and treatment needs. They also interact—alcohol and benzodiazepines both depress respiration, stimulants and alcohol interact dangerously. Someone using multiple substances needs coordinated treatment addressing all substances, not just focusing on one. Assessment must identify all substances used and their patterns.

61. C. Limited emotional range
Restricted or constricted affect shows limited emotional range—the person expresses some emotion but less variety than expected. They might show sadness but not joy, or mild emotions but nothing intense. This is less severe than flat affect (no emotion) but more limited than normal range. It can indicate depression, schizophrenia, or neurological conditions.

62. B. Providing meaning and prohibitions
Religious beliefs can be protective by providing sense of meaning and purpose, community support, and moral prohibitions against suicide. Many religions explicitly prohibit suicide, creating a barrier for religious individuals. Spirituality can provide hope and reasons for living. However, religion doesn't prevent mental illness or eliminate risk—it's one protective factor among many, and religious individuals can and do experience suicidal ideation.

63. C. Understands why they're here
Orientation to situation means the client understands the current situation—why they're meeting with you, what's happening. Someone might know the date (time), their name (person), and location (place) but be confused about why they're in the hospital or meeting with a therapist. This can indicate confusion, psychosis, denial, or cognitive impairment distinct from other orientation spheres.

64. B. Developing brain is vulnerable
Early age of first substance use (particularly before age 15) increases addiction risk because the developing adolescent brain is more vulnerable to substance effects and more likely to develop dependence. Earlier use predicts more severe substance problems and more difficulty achieving recovery. The adolescent brain's reward system is more sensitive to substances while impulse control systems are still developing.

65. B. Emotions match content
Congruent affect means emotional expression matches the content being discussed—appearing sad when discussing losses, happy when discussing joyful events. This is normal and expected. Incongruent affect (emotions don't match content) suggests problems with reality testing, dissociation, or severe defense mechanisms. Congruence is one aspect of affect assessment along with range, stability, and intensity.

66. B. They're a highly lethal means
Firearms are the most lethal suicide method with very low survival rates. Access to firearms dramatically increases suicide death risk, not because guns cause suicidal thoughts but because they make attempts more likely to be fatal. Many suicide attempts are impulsive—easy access to highly lethal means during a crisis moment significantly increases risk of death. Removing access is a critical safety intervention.

67. C. Significant life events from past
Remote memory refers to recall of significant events from the distant past—childhood experiences, where you went to school, major life events. This differs from immediate memory (repeat three words right away), recent memory (recall those words 5 minutes later), and prospective memory (future planning). Remote memory tends to be preserved longer in dementia than recent memory, which deteriorates earlier.

68. B. Reducing consequences even if use continues
Harm reduction accepts that not everyone will achieve abstinence and focuses on reducing negative consequences of substance use. This might include needle exchange programs, drinking only at home not while driving, or switching to less dangerous substances. It's not ignoring use or accepting all use uncritically—it's pragmatically reducing harm while working toward reduced use or abstinence. It meets people where they are.

69. B. Perseveration
Perseveration is repeating the same response to different questions, or continuing a response long after it's appropriate. The person seems stuck on an idea or response and repeats it regardless of new questions. This can indicate organic brain conditions, schizophrenia, or severe cognitive impairment. It differs from circumstantial thinking (winding but logical) and other thought process problems.

70. B. Lack of connection increases hopelessness
Social isolation increases suicide risk because lack of meaningful connections increases hopelessness, removes protective relationships, eliminates sources of support and reasons for living. Humans need connection—isolation creates despair. This affects people of all ages, not just elderly. Isolation isn't about weakness—it's a genuine risk factor that treatment must address by helping clients build connections.

71. B. Single-factor explanations were inadequate
The biopsychosocial model emerged because single-factor explanations (purely biological, purely psychological, purely social) couldn't adequately explain mental illness. The interaction of multiple factors better accounts for the complexity of human problems. Medical model focused too narrowly on biology. Social work's biopsychosocial approach recognizes that biology matters, but so do psychology and social context—all three interact.

72. B. Environmental cues have special meaning
Referential delusions (or delusions of reference) involve believing that environmental cues—TV, radio, strangers' conversations, songs—contain special messages directed at you. The person thinks neutral events refer specifically to them. "The news anchor is talking to me," "That song is about my life." This differs from persecution (harm), grandiosity (special powers), and somatic (body) delusions.

73. B. Grief and hopelessness intensify
Recent significant loss (relationship, job, loved one, health) increases suicide risk because grief intensifies emotional pain and loss can create hopelessness about the future. Loss doesn't directly cause suicide—most bereaved people don't become suicidal. But loss is a significant stressor that, combined with other risk factors, increases vulnerability. The first year after major loss is particularly high risk.

74. C. False positives and varying detection windows
Urine drug screens have limitations including false positives (showing substance use when there isn't any, due to cross-reactivity with other substances), false negatives, and varying detection windows (marijuana stays detectable for weeks, cocaine for days). They detect recent use but don't indicate quantity, frequency, impairment level, or prove substance use disorder. Clinical assessment remains essential—testing supplements but doesn't replace it.

75. B. Emotions remain consistent
Stable affect means emotions remain relatively consistent during the interview—not shifting rapidly or changing without apparent trigger. This is generally normal, though context matters. Discussing emotional topics might naturally produce some changes. Stability differs from lability (rapid shifting), flatness (no emotion), or range (breadth of emotions). Stable affect usually indicates good emotional control and is expected in normal functioning.

The Work Ahead

Assessment is where everything begins. Get this right, and treatment follows logically. Miss something critical, and you might spend months addressing the wrong problem. The depressed client with untreated thyroid disease. The anxious client withdrawing from benzodiazepines. The psychotic client experiencing medication side effects.

You're building a foundation. Every question you ask, every observation you make, every connection you draw between biological, psychological, and social factors—this creates understanding that guides everything that follows.

Risk assessment can feel heavy. You hold information about someone's potential death. But you also hold the possibility of prevention. You can intervene. You can create safety. You can be the person who asks the question that opens a door to help.

Assessment isn't just paperwork or diagnosis. It's relationship. It's understanding. It's the beginning of healing. When done well, clients feel heard for the first time. They see their experiences make sense. They realize they're not crazy—they're having human responses to difficult circumstances.

The technical skills matter. You need to know DSM criteria, risk factors, and assessment tools. But the art of assessment—creating safety, asking the right questions at the right time, hearing what's not said—this comes with practice and attention.

Every client teaches you something. The woman whose thyroid explained her depression. The man whose hallucinations stemmed from sleep deprivation. The adolescent whose "behavior problems" were actually PTSD. Stay curious. Keep learning. Let clients show you what you need to understand.

What You Need to Take Forward

- Biopsychosocial assessment examines how biological, psychological, and social factors interact to create and maintain mental health problems
- Mental Status Examination provides systematic assessment of current functioning across appearance, behavior, speech, mood, affect, thought process, thought content, perception, cognition, insight, and judgment
- Risk assessment for suicide, homicide, and self-harm requires direct questioning, evaluation of multiple factors, and immediate intervention when risk is imminent
- Suicide risk factors include previous attempts, mental illness, recent losses, access to means, and social isolation—protective factors include connections, reasons for living, and hope
- Asking directly about suicide doesn't increase risk and often provides relief that someone is willing to discuss difficult topics
- Command hallucinations directing harm to identifiable persons may trigger duty to warn obligations despite confidentiality
- Non-suicidal self-injury typically serves emotion regulation functions and requires separate assessment from suicide risk
- Substance use assessment examines substances used, quantity, frequency, consequences, dependence indicators, motivation to change, and function

- Cultural factors significantly affect interpretation of mental status findings—behaviors have different meanings across cultures
- Screening tools like CAGE, AUDIT, and DAST identify potential problems but require follow-up with comprehensive clinical assessment
- Medication effects can mimic psychiatric symptoms, making medication review essential for accurate assessment
- Safety planning is collaborative, specific to the individual, and includes warning signs, coping strategies, support contacts, and means restriction

Chapter 6: DSM-5-TR Diagnosis

Diagnosis is a map, not a judgment. It names the territory your client is navigating. Good diagnosis helps—it guides treatment selection, predicts course, and helps clients understand their experiences. Poor diagnosis harms—it can lead to wrong treatment, create stigma, and miss what's actually happening.

The DSM-5-TR (Diagnostic and Statistical Manual of Mental Disorders, Fifth Edition, Text Revision) is your primary diagnostic tool. It's imperfect. It pathologizes normal human responses to abnormal circumstances. It creates categories where dimensional understanding would serve better. It reflects Western cultural biases. But it's what we have, and used thoughtfully, it helps more than it hurts.

Diagnosis requires detective work. You gather information, notice patterns, rule out alternatives, and land on the explanation that best fits the evidence. But you hold it lightly. Diagnosis can change as you learn more. The "depression" that's actually bipolar disorder. The "schizophrenia" that's actually trauma responses. Stay flexible.

Diagnostic Criteria and Differential Diagnosis

Diagnostic criteria specify what symptoms must be present, how long they must last, and what level of impairment they must cause. Meeting criteria means the person's experience matches the defined pattern closely enough for the diagnosis to apply.

Some criteria are polythetic—you need a certain number from a list, but not all. Major depression requires five of nine symptoms. This means two people with the same diagnosis might have quite different presentations. One person sleeps too much, another can't sleep. Both have depression.

Duration matters. Grief looks like depression but usually improves over weeks to months. Depression persists. Brief psychotic disorder lasts less than a month. Schizophreniform disorder lasts one to six months. Schizophrenia requires six months. The timeline helps differentiate.

Impairment matters. Many people have symptoms that don't reach diagnostic threshold. Worry becomes generalized anxiety disorder when it's excessive, uncontrollable, and causes significant distress or impairment. Sadness becomes major depression when it's severe and interferes with functioning. Diagnosis requires more than just symptoms—it requires impact.

Exclusion criteria eliminate diagnoses that don't fit. You can't diagnose major depression if symptoms are better explained by bipolar disorder. You can't diagnose panic disorder if panic attacks only occur during social situations (that's social anxiety disorder). Each diagnosis has conditions that rule it out.

Differential diagnosis is the process of distinguishing between disorders with similar presentations. Someone presents with sadness, low energy, and concentration problems. Could be:

- Major depression
- Persistent depressive disorder (dysthymia)
- Bipolar depression
- Adjustment disorder with depressed mood
- Substance-induced mood disorder
- Mood disorder due to medical condition
- Normal grief

You evaluate each possibility against the evidence. How long have symptoms lasted? What's the severity? Is there history of mania? Has the person experienced recent loss? Are they using substances? Do they have medical conditions affecting mood?

Comorbidity is common. Most people with one disorder have others. Depression and anxiety frequently co-occur. Substance use disorders commonly accompany other mental illnesses. PTSD often presents with depression. You diagnose all conditions that meet criteria, understanding they interact and affect treatment.

Medical rule-out is essential. Many medical conditions cause psychiatric symptoms. Thyroid problems cause depression and anxiety. Brain tumors can cause personality changes. Medications have psychiatric side effects. You always consider and rule out medical causes before diagnosing primary psychiatric illness.

Case Example: Differential Diagnosis

Robert, a 35-year-old man, presents with depressed mood, insomnia, poor concentration, and fatigue lasting three months. Several diagnoses are possible:

Major Depressive Disorder requires five symptoms for two weeks causing impairment. Robert has four clear symptoms (depressed mood, insomnia, concentration problems, fatigue). You ask about others: changes in appetite, feelings of worthlessness, suicidal thoughts, psychomotor changes, loss of interest. He reports increased appetite and feeling worthless. Six symptoms for three months—criteria met.

Persistent Depressive Disorder requires depressed mood most days for at least two years. Robert's symptoms started three months ago. Criteria not met.

Bipolar Depression is possible if there's history of mania or hypomania. You ask about elevated mood, decreased need for sleep, increased activity, risky behavior. Robert denies any such episodes. No evidence for bipolar disorder.

Adjustment Disorder with Depressed Mood requires symptoms developing within three months of an identifiable stressor and not meeting criteria for another disorder. Robert did lose his job four months ago. But his symptoms meet criteria for major depression, which takes precedence over adjustment disorder.

Substance-Induced Mood Disorder requires substance use that could explain symptoms. Robert drinks socially, no substance use disorder. Not substance-induced.

Mood Disorder Due to Medical Condition requires medical condition known to cause depression. Robert's physical exam and labs are normal. Not medical.

Normal Grief is possible if he experienced recent loss. The job loss could trigger grief. But grief typically doesn't include worthlessness and concentration problems to this degree. His symptoms are more severe and pervasive than normal grief.

Diagnosis: Major Depressive Disorder, single episode, moderate severity. The job loss was a precipitant, but symptoms meet criteria for clinical depression requiring treatment.

Mood Disorders

Mood disorders involve disturbances in emotional state that persist and interfere with functioning. They're among the most common mental illnesses and highly treatable when properly diagnosed.

Major Depressive Disorder (MDD) requires at least five of nine symptoms for at least two weeks:

1. Depressed mood most of the day, nearly every day
2. Markedly diminished interest or pleasure in all or almost all activities
3. Significant weight loss or gain, or appetite changes
4. Insomnia or hypersomnia
5. Psychomotor agitation or retardation observable by others
6. Fatigue or loss of energy
7. Feelings of worthlessness or excessive guilt
8. Diminished ability to think or concentrate
9. Recurrent thoughts of death or suicidal ideation

At least one symptom must be depressed mood or loss of interest/pleasure. Symptoms must cause significant distress or impairment and not be attributable to substances or medical conditions.

Depression varies in severity (mild, moderate, severe) and can occur with psychotic features (hallucinations or delusions). Some people have **melancholic features**—loss of pleasure in all activities, depression worse in morning, early morning awakening, significant weight loss, excessive guilt. Others have **atypical features**—mood reactivity (brightens in response to positive events), increased appetite, hypersomnia, leaden paralysis (heavy feeling in limbs), rejection sensitivity.

Persistent Depressive Disorder (Dysthymia) involves depressed mood for at least two years (one year in children/adolescents) plus at least two of: poor appetite or overeating, insomnia or hypersomnia, low energy, low self-esteem, poor concentration, feelings of hopelessness.

Dysthymia is chronic, low-grade depression. People often say "I've always been this way" or "This is just my personality." They may not recognize it as treatable illness. It's less severe than major depression but more persistent, significantly affecting quality of life.

Bipolar I Disorder requires at least one manic episode. **Mania** means abnormally elevated, expansive, or irritable mood and increased activity or energy for at least one week (or any duration if hospitalization required) plus at least three of (four if mood is only irritable):

1. Inflated self-esteem or grandiosity
2. Decreased need for sleep
3. More talkative than usual or pressure to keep talking
4. Flight of ideas or racing thoughts
5. Distractibility
6. Increase in goal-directed activity or psychomotor agitation
7. Excessive involvement in risky activities

Mania causes marked impairment or requires hospitalization. It's not just feeling good—it's destructive. People make terrible decisions, destroy relationships, spend money they don't have, engage in dangerous behavior. Many have psychotic features during mania.

Bipolar II Disorder requires at least one hypomanic episode and at least one major depressive episode. **Hypomania** has the same symptoms as mania but lasts at least four days (not a week), doesn't cause marked impairment, and doesn't include psychotic features.

Hypomania can feel good—productive, energetic, creative. People often don't seek treatment during hypomania. They seek help during the depression that follows. This is why careful history-taking is essential. Missing hypomanic episodes leads to misdiagnosis as unipolar depression and wrong treatment (antidepressants alone can trigger mania in bipolar disorder).

Cyclothymic Disorder involves numerous periods of hypomanic symptoms and depressive symptoms (not meeting full criteria for episodes) for at least two years. It's chronic mood instability that causes significant distress but doesn't reach threshold for bipolar I or II.

Case Example: Sarah's Bipolar II Disorder

Sarah, a 28-year-old woman, presents for depression. She describes crushing sadness, sleeping 12 hours daily, difficulty concentrating, and suicidal thoughts for the past two months. Previous therapists diagnosed major depression, but medications haven't helped.

You take careful history. Sarah describes her typical mood as moderately low. But several times yearly, something shifts. She feels "amazing"—energetic, creative, needing only 4-5 hours of sleep but feeling fully rested. She starts multiple projects, talks rapidly, has great ideas. These periods last about a week, then she crashes into depression.

During elevated periods, Sarah functions well—actually, better than usual. She's productive at work, social, active. She doesn't recognize these as problematic. "That's when I'm my best self," she says. But the crashes that follow devastate her.

You recognize the pattern: hypomanic episodes followed by major depressive episodes. This is Bipolar II Disorder, not major depression. The implications are significant:

Treatment changes: Sarah needs mood stabilizer, not just antidepressant. Antidepressants alone can worsen cycling. You adjust medications, and within weeks, the cycling stabilizes.

Understanding changes: Sarah learns to recognize hypomania warning signs. What felt like "finally being myself" was actually the beginning of a cycle. She learns to manage early signs to prevent full episodes.

Prognosis changes: Bipolar disorder is lifelong but manageable. Understanding her pattern helps Sarah make sense of years of confusing mood changes. She's not weak or broken—she has a treatable medical condition.

Accurate diagnosis changed everything for Sarah. This is why differential diagnosis matters.

Anxiety Disorders and OCD

Anxiety disorders involve excessive fear or anxiety that interferes with functioning. Fear is the emotional response to real or perceived imminent threat. Anxiety is anticipation of future threat. Both can be adaptive in appropriate contexts but become disorders when excessive, persistent, and impairing.

Generalized Anxiety Disorder (GAD) requires excessive anxiety and worry about multiple events or activities, occurring more days than not for at least six months. The worry is difficult to control and associated with at least three of: restlessness, being easily fatigued, difficulty concentrating, irritability, muscle tension, sleep disturbance.

GAD is chronic worry about everything—health, finances, work, relationships, world events. The person knows the worry is excessive but can't stop it. "What if" dominates their thinking. Physical symptoms accompany mental worry—tension, fatigue, sleep problems.

Panic Disorder involves recurrent unexpected panic attacks plus at least one month of persistent concern about additional attacks, worry about attack implications, or significant behavioral change related to attacks.

Panic attacks are abrupt surges of intense fear or discomfort reaching peak within minutes, with at least four of: palpitations, sweating, trembling, shortness of breath, feeling of choking, chest pain, nausea, dizziness, chills or heat sensations, paresthesias, derealization or depersonalization, fear of losing control, fear of dying.

Panic attacks can occur in various disorders, but panic disorder specifically involves unexpected attacks (not in response to obvious trigger) and significant worry about future attacks. People often develop agoraphobia—avoiding situations where escape might be difficult or help unavailable if a panic attack occurs.

Social Anxiety Disorder (Social Phobia) involves marked fear or anxiety about social situations where the person might be scrutinized. They fear acting in ways that will be negatively evaluated. Social situations almost always provoke fear, are avoided or endured with intense distress, and the fear is out of proportion to actual threat. Symptoms must persist for at least six months.

This isn't shyness. Social anxiety is intense fear of judgment, embarrassment, or humiliation that significantly limits life. People avoid jobs requiring public speaking, turn down promotions, skip social events. The fear of negative evaluation is overwhelming and disabling.

Specific Phobia involves marked fear or anxiety about a specific object or situation (flying, heights, animals, blood, enclosed spaces). The phobic object almost always provokes immediate fear, is actively avoided, and the fear is out of proportion to actual danger. Duration is at least six months.

Specific phobias are common and often don't require treatment unless they significantly interfere with life. Someone afraid of snakes living in a city might never encounter this problem. Someone afraid of flying who must travel for work needs treatment.

Agoraphobia involves marked fear or anxiety about at least two of: public transportation, open spaces, enclosed spaces, standing in line or being in a crowd, being outside the home alone. The person fears these situations because escape might be difficult or help might not be available if panic-like symptoms develop. The situations are actively avoided, require companion, or are endured with intense distress.

Agoraphobia often develops from panic disorder but can occur independently. At its worst, people become housebound, unable to leave home without severe anxiety.

Obsessive-Compulsive Disorder (OCD) involves obsessions, compulsions, or both. **Obsessions** are recurrent, persistent thoughts, urges, or images experienced as intrusive and unwanted, causing marked anxiety. The person attempts to ignore or suppress them or neutralize them with some other thought or action.

Compulsions are repetitive behaviors or mental acts the person feels driven to perform in response to an obsession or according to rigid rules. They're aimed at preventing or reducing anxiety or preventing a dreaded event, but they're not connected in a realistic way to what they're designed to neutralize or prevent, or they're clearly excessive.

Common obsessions include contamination concerns, need for symmetry, aggressive or horrific thoughts, sexual thoughts, religious concerns. Common compulsions include washing, checking, counting, ordering, seeking reassurance, mental rituals.

OCD is not about being neat or organized. It's about intrusive thoughts that create intense anxiety and repetitive behaviors performed to reduce that anxiety. The person often recognizes the thoughts and behaviors as excessive or unreasonable but can't stop them. OCD consumes hours daily and significantly impairs functioning.

Case Example: Marcus's OCD

Marcus, a 32-year-old accountant, presents with anxiety and "weird thoughts" he's ashamed to discuss. With gentle questioning, he reveals that for the past year, he's had intrusive thoughts about harming his baby daughter. Images of dropping her, thoughts of stabbing her, fears he'll lose control and hurt her.

Marcus is horrified by these thoughts. He knows he loves his daughter and would never hurt her. But the thoughts come constantly, especially when he's near her. He's developed compulsive checking—watching her breathe when she sleeps, checking that knives are locked away, reviewing his actions to confirm he didn't harm her.

The checking provides brief relief, then the thoughts return stronger. Marcus now avoids being alone with his daughter. He's sleeping poorly, unable to concentrate at work. He's terrified he's a terrible person or going crazy.

You explain OCD. The intrusive thoughts are obsessions—unwanted, ego-dystonic (against his values), and not reflective of actual desires. The checking and avoidance are compulsions—attempts to reduce anxiety that actually maintain the cycle. The fact that he's horrified by the thoughts proves they're OCD, not desires. People who want to harm children aren't disturbed by thoughts of harming them.

Marcus feels enormous relief understanding this. He's not evil or crazy—he has a treatable disorder. Treatment involves exposure and response prevention (ERP)—gradually facing the thoughts without performing compulsions. You also provide psychoeducation for his wife, who's been confused and frightened by his behavior.

Within months, Marcus's symptoms significantly improve. He can be alone with his daughter without overwhelming anxiety. The thoughts still come occasionally, but they no longer control his life. Understanding the diagnosis was the first step toward recovery.

Trauma and Stressor-Related Disorders

These disorders develop following exposure to traumatic or stressful events. The trauma itself doesn't cause the disorder—most people exposed to trauma don't develop these conditions. But the disorders can't develop without the exposure.

Post-Traumatic Stress Disorder (PTSD) requires exposure to actual or threatened death, serious injury, or sexual violence through: direct experience, witnessing it happen to others, learning it happened to close family or friend (actual or threatened death must have been violent or accidental), or repeated or extreme exposure to aversive details (doesn't apply to media exposure unless work-related).

Following exposure, the person must have symptoms from four clusters:

Intrusion symptoms (at least one): recurrent, involuntary intrusive distressing memories; recurrent distressing dreams; dissociative reactions (flashbacks); intense psychological distress at cues; marked physiological reactions to cues.

Avoidance symptoms (at least one): avoidance of distressing memories, thoughts, or feelings; avoidance of external reminders (people, places, conversations, activities, objects, situations).

Negative alterations in cognitions and mood (at least two): inability to remember important aspects of trauma; persistent negative beliefs about self, others, or world; persistent distorted cognitions about cause or consequences leading to blame of self or others; persistent negative emotional state; markedly diminished interest in activities; feeling detached or estranged from others; persistent inability to experience positive emotions.

Alterations in arousal and reactivity (at least two): irritable behavior and angry outbursts; reckless or self-destructive behavior; hypervigilance; exaggerated startle response; problems with concentration; sleep disturbance.

Symptoms must persist for more than one month and cause significant distress or impairment. PTSD can occur with dissociative symptoms (depersonalization or derealization) and can be specified as delayed expression if full criteria aren't met until at least six months after trauma.

Acute Stress Disorder has similar symptoms to PTSD but occurs three days to one month after trauma exposure. If symptoms persist beyond one month, diagnosis changes to PTSD.

Adjustment Disorders involve emotional or behavioral symptoms developing within three months of an identifiable stressor. Symptoms must be out of proportion to the stressor (considering cultural context) or cause significant impairment. Symptoms don't meet criteria for another mental disorder and aren't normal bereavement.

Adjustment disorders can be specified: with depressed mood, with anxiety, with mixed anxiety and depressed mood, with disturbance of conduct, with mixed disturbance of emotions and conduct. They typically resolve within six months of stressor ending, though symptoms can persist if the stressor is ongoing.

Adjustment disorder is a residual category—if symptoms meet criteria for another disorder (major depression, PTSD), you diagnose that disorder instead. But adjustment disorder recognizes that significant stressors can cause symptoms requiring treatment even when they don't meet criteria for other disorders.

Reactive Attachment Disorder and **Disinhibited Social Engagement Disorder** are childhood disorders resulting from inadequate care. They reflect the profound impact of early neglect on a child's ability to form attachments.

Case Example: Jennifer's PTSD

Jennifer, a 26-year-old nurse, presents six months after a serious car accident. She survived with minor injuries, but her passenger died. Since the accident, Jennifer's life has unraveled.

Intrusion: Jennifer has vivid, intrusive memories of the crash. She dreams about it nightly, waking in panic. Anything resembling the accident—car horns, the song that was playing, the smell of gasoline—triggers intense distress. Her heart races, she sweats, she feels she's back in the moment of impact.

Avoidance: Jennifer sold her car and refuses to drive. She avoids the street where the accident occurred, which means a 30-minute detour to work. She can't talk about the accident without breaking down, so she avoids the topic. She stopped seeing friends who knew her passenger because they remind her.

Negative cognitions and mood: Jennifer believes the accident was her fault (it wasn't—a drunk driver ran a red light). She thinks "I should have died instead." She can't remember parts of the accident, which frightens her. She feels numb most of the time, disconnected from people. Activities she loved now seem pointless. She can't imagine a future.

Arousal and reactivity: Jennifer is constantly on edge. She startles at sudden noises. She scans for danger constantly while walking. She's irritable and snaps at coworkers. She can't concentrate on tasks. Sleep is nearly impossible—she's exhausted but afraid to sleep because of nightmares.

The symptoms have persisted six months, significantly impair her functioning (she's on medical leave from work), and clearly stem from the accident. Diagnosis: PTSD with dissociative symptoms (she experiences derealization during flashbacks).

Treatment involves trauma-focused therapy—prolonged exposure and cognitive processing therapy. You help Jennifer process the trauma, challenge guilt and blame, and gradually face avoided situations. You use EMDR (Eye Movement Desensitization and Reprocessing) to help reprocess traumatic memories.

Progress is gradual. After three months, nightmares decrease. After six months, Jennifer returns to work part-time. After a year, she's driving again. The trauma doesn't disappear, but it no longer controls her life. She integrates the experience and moves forward.

Personality Disorders

Personality disorders involve enduring patterns of inner experience and behavior that deviate markedly from cultural expectations, are pervasive and inflexible, begin in adolescence or early adulthood, are stable over time, and lead to distress or impairment.

These aren't just difficult personalities—they're patterns causing significant dysfunction. The person's way of perceiving and relating to self and others is fundamentally problematic across many contexts and over long periods.

The DSM-5-TR organizes personality disorders into three clusters:

Cluster A (Odd/Eccentric): Paranoid, Schizoid, Schizotypal Personality Disorders

Paranoid Personality Disorder involves pervasive distrust and suspiciousness of others, interpreting motives as malevolent. The person suspects others are exploiting, harming, or deceiving them; doubts loyalty of friends; is reluctant to confide in others; reads hidden meanings into benign remarks; persistently bears grudges; perceives attacks on character and quickly counterattacks; has recurrent suspicions regarding fidelity of spouse or partner.

Schizoid Personality Disorder involves pervasive pattern of detachment from social relationships and restricted emotional expression. The person doesn't desire or enjoy close relationships; almost always chooses solitary activities; has little interest in sexual experiences; takes pleasure in few activities; lacks close friends; appears indifferent to praise or criticism; shows emotional coldness or flat affectivity.

Schizotypal Personality Disorder involves pervasive pattern of social and interpersonal deficits marked by acute discomfort with close relationships, cognitive or perceptual distortions, and eccentricities of behavior. Symptoms include ideas of reference; odd beliefs or magical thinking; unusual perceptual experiences; odd thinking and speech; suspiciousness or paranoid ideation; inappropriate or constricted affect; odd or eccentric behavior or appearance; lack of close friends; excessive social anxiety.

Cluster B (Dramatic/Emotional/Erratic): Antisocial, Borderline, Histrionic, Narcissistic Personality Disorders

Antisocial Personality Disorder requires pervasive pattern of disregard for and violation of the rights of others occurring since age 15, plus evidence of Conduct Disorder before age 15. The person fails to conform to social norms (repeatedly performs acts that are grounds for arrest); shows deceitfulness (lying, using aliases, conning others); demonstrates impulsivity or failure to plan ahead; shows irritability and aggressiveness (fights or assaults); demonstrates reckless disregard for safety of self or others; shows consistent irresponsibility (failure to sustain work or honor financial obligations); lacks remorse (indifferent to or rationalizes having hurt others).

Borderline Personality Disorder (BPD) involves pervasive pattern of instability in relationships, self-image, and affects, plus marked impulsivity. Symptoms include: frantic efforts to avoid real or imagined abandonment; pattern of unstable and intense interpersonal relationships (alternating idealization and devaluation); identity disturbance (unstable self-image); impulsivity in at least two areas that are self-damaging (spending, sex, substance use, reckless driving, binge eating); recurrent suicidal behavior, gestures, threats, or self-harm; affective instability (marked reactivity of mood); chronic feelings of emptiness; inappropriate, intense anger; transient, stress-related paranoid ideation or severe dissociative symptoms.

Histrionic Personality Disorder involves pervasive pattern of excessive emotionality and attention-seeking. The person is uncomfortable when not center of attention; shows inappropriately sexually seductive or provocative behavior; displays rapidly shifting and shallow emotions; uses physical appearance to draw attention; has impressionistic speech style lacking detail; shows self-dramatization and exaggerated emotional expression; is suggestible; considers relationships more intimate than they actually are.

Narcissistic Personality Disorder involves pervasive pattern of grandiosity, need for admiration, and lack of empathy. The person has grandiose sense of self-importance; is preoccupied with fantasies of unlimited success, power, brilliance, beauty, or ideal love; believes they're special and can only be understood by other special people; requires excessive admiration; has sense of entitlement; is interpersonally exploitative; lacks empathy; is often envious of others or believes others are envious of them; shows arrogant, haughty behaviors or attitudes.

Cluster C (Anxious/Fearful): Avoidant, Dependent, Obsessive-Compulsive Personality Disorders

Avoidant Personality Disorder involves pervasive pattern of social inhibition, feelings of inadequacy, and hypersensitivity to negative evaluation. The person avoids occupational activities involving significant interpersonal contact due to fear of criticism or rejection; is unwilling to get involved with people unless certain of being liked; shows restraint within intimate relationships due to fear of ridicule; is preoccupied with being criticized or rejected in social situations; is inhibited in new interpersonal situations due to feelings of inadequacy; views self as socially inept or inferior; is unusually reluctant to take personal risks or engage in new activities due to fear of embarrassment.

Dependent Personality Disorder involves pervasive and excessive need to be taken care of, leading to submissive and clinging behavior and fears of separation. The person has difficulty making everyday decisions without excessive reassurance; needs others to assume responsibility for most major areas of life; has difficulty expressing disagreement due to fear of loss of support; has difficulty initiating projects due to lack of self-confidence; goes to excessive lengths to obtain nurturance and support from others; feels uncomfortable or helpless when alone; urgently seeks another relationship when one ends; is unrealistically preoccupied with fears of being left to take care of self.

Obsessive-Compulsive Personality Disorder (OCPD) involves pervasive pattern of preoccupation with orderliness, perfectionism, and control. The person is preoccupied with details, rules, lists, order, organization, or schedules to extent that major point of activity is lost; shows perfectionism that interferes with task completion; is excessively devoted to work and productivity to exclusion of leisure and friendships; is overconscientious and inflexible about morality, ethics, or values; is unable to discard worn-out or worthless objects; is reluctant to delegate tasks unless others submit to exact way; adopts miserly spending style; shows rigidity and stubbornness.

Note that OCPD differs from OCD. OCD involves unwanted intrusive thoughts and compulsive behaviors causing distress. OCPD involves ego-syntonic (consistent with self-image) perfectionism and control that the person values, even if it causes problems.

Case Example: Lisa's Borderline Personality Disorder

Lisa, a 24-year-old woman, has been in therapy with seven different therapists over five years. Each relationship ended badly—Lisa felt abandoned, therapists felt manipulated. Her current therapist refers her to you for dialectical behavior therapy (DBT).

Lisa's history reveals the BPD pattern clearly:

Fear of abandonment: Lisa's relationships are intense and unstable. She falls in love quickly, idealizing partners. Any perceived slight triggers panic about abandonment. She's made frantic efforts to prevent breakups—threatening suicide, creating crises. When relationships end, she feels devastated and empty.

Identity disturbance: Lisa doesn't know who she is. Her interests, values, career goals, even sexual orientation shift based on who she's dating. She adopts others' preferences as her own. When alone, she feels empty and lost.

Impulsivity: Lisa engages in binge eating, reckless spending (thousands in debt), risky sexual behavior, and occasional substance use. These behaviors spike during stress.

Self-harm and suicidal behavior: Lisa cuts when overwhelmed. She's made three suicide attempts, all triggered by relationship losses. She denies current suicidal intent but acknowledges chronic suicidal thoughts.

Affective instability: Lisa's mood shifts rapidly—from okay to despondent in hours, from content to rageful over minor events. Moods are intense and reactive.

Chronic emptiness: Lisa describes feeling "hollow" most of the time. Nothing fills the void. She's constantly seeking something to make her feel whole.

Anger: Lisa experiences intense, inappropriate anger. She rages at partners over small mistakes. Afterward, she feels guilty and fears she's driven them away, which triggers more panic.

Dissociation: Under severe stress, Lisa experiences depersonalization—feeling detached from herself, watching herself from outside her body. This terrifies her.

Lisa meets criteria for BPD. The diagnosis explains her difficulties but doesn't excuse harmful behavior. Treatment involves DBT—teaching emotion regulation, distress tolerance, interpersonal effectiveness, and mindfulness skills.

You explain BPD to Lisa. She's not manipulative or attention-seeking—she's desperate for connection but terrified of abandonment. Her nervous system is dysregulated, making emotions intense and overwhelming. Self-harm and impulsivity are attempts to cope, not character flaws.

Progress is slow. Lisa tests boundaries repeatedly—calls at midnight, threatens to quit therapy, idealizes then devalues you. You maintain consistent, clear boundaries while validating her emotions. Gradually, Lisa develops skills. She learns to tolerate distress without self-harm, to regulate emotions, to build stable relationships.

Two years later, Lisa is in a stable relationship, working consistently, and hasn't self-harmed in six months. She still has BPD—it's a chronic condition—but she manages it. She has a life worth living.

Psychotic Disorders

Psychotic disorders involve loss of contact with reality, manifested through hallucinations, delusions, disorganized thinking, or disorganized behavior. These are serious mental illnesses requiring comprehensive treatment.

Schizophrenia requires at least two of the following, with at least one being 1, 2, or 3:

1. Delusions
2. Hallucinations
3. Disorganized speech
4. Grossly disorganized or catatonic behavior

5. Negative symptoms (diminished emotional expression or avolition)

Symptoms must be present for a significant portion of time during a one-month period (or less if successfully treated) and continuous signs of disturbance must persist for at least six months. The six-month period must include at least one month of active symptoms (or less if treated) and may include prodromal or residual periods with only negative symptoms or attenuated forms of positive symptoms.

Functioning must be markedly below the level achieved before onset, or if onset in childhood/adolescence, failure to achieve expected level of functioning. The disturbance can't be attributable to substances or medical conditions or better explained by another mental disorder.

Positive symptoms (excesses or distortions of normal functions): delusions, hallucinations, disorganized speech, disorganized or catatonic behavior.

Negative symptoms (diminutions or loss of normal functions): flat affect, alogia (poverty of speech), avolition (lack of motivation), anhedonia (inability to experience pleasure), asociality (lack of interest in social interactions).

Schizoaffective Disorder requires an uninterrupted period of illness during which there's a major mood episode (major depressive or manic) concurrent with criteria for schizophrenia. Delusions or hallucinations must also occur for at least two weeks in the absence of major mood episode during the lifetime duration of the illness. Mood episodes must be present for the majority of the total duration of the illness.

This diagnosis bridges schizophrenia and mood disorders. The person has both psychotic and mood symptoms, but the psychosis occurs even when mood is stable (distinguishing it from mood disorder with psychotic features).

Brief Psychotic Disorder involves one or more of delusions, hallucinations, disorganized speech, or grossly disorganized or catatonic behavior. At least one symptom must be delusions, hallucinations, or disorganized speech. Duration is at least one day but less than one month, with eventual full return to premorbid functioning.

This might occur after extreme stress (specified "with marked stressor(s)") or during postpartum period. The brief duration distinguishes it from schizophreniform disorder (1-6 months) and schizophrenia (6+ months).

Schizophreniform Disorder meets criteria for schizophrenia except duration is at least one month but less than six months. If symptoms persist beyond six months, diagnosis changes to schizophrenia.

Delusional Disorder involves one or more delusions for at least one month. Apart from the impact of the delusions, functioning isn't markedly impaired and behavior isn't obviously bizarre. If hallucinations are present, they're not prominent and are related to the delusional theme. The disturbance isn't attributable to substances, medical conditions, or better explained by other mental disorders.

Delusions can be erotomanic (someone is in love with them), grandiose (exceptional talent or discovery), jealous (partner is unfaithful), persecutory (being conspired against), somatic (physical defect or medical condition), mixed, or unspecified.

Case Example: Michael's Schizophrenia

Michael, a 22-year-old man, is brought to the emergency room by police after neighbors reported him standing in his yard at 3 AM, shouting at the sky.

History: Michael was an average student who became increasingly isolated during his senior year of high school. He dropped out of community college after one semester, saying professors were "sending signals." Over the past six months, his behavior has deteriorated. He stopped showering, stays in his room, and talks to himself.

Current presentation: Michael appears disheveled, with poor hygiene. He's suspicious and guarded. His speech is tangential and hard to follow. He explains that the CIA is monitoring him through satellites because he discovered a formula for free energy. He hears agents' voices discussing his whereabouts and actions. He must stay vigilant because they're planning to abduct him.

Positive symptoms:

- Delusions: Persecutory (CIA monitoring) and grandiose (important discovery)
- Hallucinations: Auditory (hearing agents' voices)
- Disorganized speech: Tangential, loosely connected thoughts
- Disorganized behavior: Poor self-care, bizarre behavior (shouting at sky)

Negative symptoms:

- Flat affect: Shows little emotional expression
- Avolition: No motivation for activities, dropped out of school
- Asociality: Withdrawn, isolated in room

Timeline: Prodromal symptoms (isolation, odd beliefs) began over a year ago. Active psychotic symptoms have been present for six months. Criteria for schizophrenia are met.

Treatment: Michael is hospitalized for stabilization. Antipsychotic medication reduces hallucinations and delusions. Family psychoeducation helps parents understand the illness. After discharge, Michael enters outpatient treatment combining medication, individual therapy, and social skills training.

Schizophrenia is chronic, but treatment helps many people manage symptoms and live fulfilling lives. Michael's early intervention improves his prognosis. With consistent treatment, he can return to school, develop relationships, and work toward his goals.

Substance-Related Disorders

Substance-related disorders include substance use disorders (problematic patterns of use) and substance-induced disorders (intoxication, withdrawal, and substance/medication-induced mental disorders).

Substance Use Disorder requires a problematic pattern of substance use leading to clinically significant impairment or distress, with at least two of the following in a 12-month period:

1. Substance taken in larger amounts or over longer period than intended
2. Persistent desire or unsuccessful efforts to cut down or control use
3. Great deal of time spent obtaining, using, or recovering from substance
4. Craving or strong desire to use
5. Recurrent use resulting in failure to fulfill major obligations at work, school, or home
6. Continued use despite persistent social or interpersonal problems caused or exacerbated by substance
7. Important activities given up or reduced because of use
8. Recurrent use in physically hazardous situations
9. Continued use despite knowledge of persistent physical or psychological problem caused or exacerbated by substance
10. Tolerance (need for increased amounts or diminished effect with same amount)
11. Withdrawal (characteristic withdrawal syndrome or substance taken to relieve or avoid withdrawal)

Severity is specified: Mild (2-3 symptoms), Moderate (4-5 symptoms), Severe (6+ symptoms).

Substance Intoxication requires development of a reversible substance-specific syndrome due to recent ingestion, clinically significant problematic behavioral or psychological changes, and symptoms not attributable to medical conditions or other mental disorders.

Substance Withdrawal requires development of a substance-specific syndrome due to cessation or reduction of heavy and prolonged use, causing clinically significant distress or impairment, with symptoms not attributable to medical conditions or other mental disorders.

Different substances have different intoxication and withdrawal patterns. Alcohol withdrawal can be life-threatening. Opioid withdrawal is intensely uncomfortable but rarely dangerous. Stimulant withdrawal involves depression and fatigue. Sedative withdrawal resembles alcohol withdrawal.

Substance/Medication-Induced Mental Disorders occur when a substance causes symptoms of another mental disorder. Examples: substance-induced psychotic disorder, substance-induced depressive disorder, substance-induced anxiety disorder.

The key is temporal relationship—symptoms develop during or soon after substance exposure or withdrawal, and the substance is capable of producing the symptoms. If symptoms persist for substantial time after intoxication or withdrawal ends, they may represent an independent mental disorder rather than substance-induced.

Case Example: David's Alcohol Use Disorder

David, a 42-year-old construction worker, enters outpatient treatment at his wife's ultimatum: get help or she leaves.

Criteria assessment:

1. **Larger amounts/longer**: David intends to have "a couple beers" but drinks until he passes out. Every time.
2. **Unsuccessful control**: He's tried to quit countless times. Longest period was three weeks. He's tried cutting back—never works.
3. **Time spent**: David spends evenings drinking, weekends recovering from hangovers. Alcohol dominates his time.
4. **Craving**: He thinks about drinking constantly. By noon, he's counting hours until he can drink.
5. **Failure to fulfill obligations**: He's missed work due to hangovers. His performance has deteriorated. At home, he's emotionally absent.
6. **Interpersonal problems**: His wife threatens divorce. His kids avoid him when he's drinking. Friends who don't drink have drifted away.
7. **Activities given up**: David used to coach his son's Little League team. He quit because practices interfere with drinking. He stopped hiking, fishing—anything conflicting with alcohol.
8. **Hazardous use**: He's driven drunk multiple times. Last week, he operated machinery while hungover.
9. **Continued despite problems**: His doctor warned that liver enzymes are elevated. David knows alcohol is destroying his health and relationships. He drinks anyway.
10. **Tolerance**: He used to get drunk on four beers. Now he needs eight to twelve. Same with liquor—double what it used to take.
11. **Withdrawal**: If David doesn't drink by evening, he gets shaky, sweaty, anxious. Morning drinking stops the shakes. This is withdrawal.

David meets all eleven criteria. **Diagnosis**: Alcohol Use Disorder, Severe.

Treatment involves medical detoxification (alcohol withdrawal can be dangerous), individual therapy using motivational interviewing and cognitive-behavioral approaches, family therapy to repair relationships and build support, and medication (naltrexone to reduce cravings, acamprosate to support abstinence).

David also attends AA meetings, finding support from others who understand his struggle. Recovery is difficult—he relapses twice in the first year. But he keeps trying. Two years later, he's maintained sobriety for 14 months, rebuilt his marriage, and reconnected with his children.

Substance use disorders are chronic, relapsing conditions. Treatment works, but it often requires multiple attempts and ongoing support. David's willingness to keep trying, combined with comprehensive treatment and family support, gives him the best chance for sustained recovery.

Practice Questions

1. Major Depressive Disorder requires symptoms for at least:

A. Two weeks
B. One month
C. Six months
D. One year

2. Bipolar I Disorder requires:

A. At least one major depressive episode
B. At least one manic episode
C. At least one hypomanic episode
D. Both manic and depressive episodes

3. Hypomania differs from mania primarily in:

A. Types of symptoms
B. Duration and severity
C. Treatment approach
D. Age of onset

4. Generalized Anxiety Disorder requires excessive worry for at least:

A. Two weeks
B. One month
C. Three months
D. Six months

5. Panic attacks are characterized by:

A. Gradual onset over hours
B. Peak intensity within minutes
C. Duration of several hours
D. Only physical symptoms

6. Social Anxiety Disorder involves fear of:

A. Being alone
B. Crowded spaces

C. Scrutiny by others
D. Loss of control

7. OCD obsessions are best described as:

A. Exaggerated worries
B. Intrusive, unwanted thoughts
C. Voluntary thoughts
D. Realistic concerns

8. PTSD requires trauma exposure plus symptoms from:

A. Two symptom clusters
B. Three symptom clusters
C. Four symptom clusters
D. Five symptom clusters

9. Acute Stress Disorder symptoms occur:

A. Immediately after trauma
B. 3 days to 1 month after trauma
C. 1-6 months after trauma
D. 6+ months after trauma

10. Adjustment Disorder symptoms must develop within:

A. Two weeks of stressor
B. One month of stressor
C. Three months of stressor
D. Six months of stressor

11. Borderline Personality Disorder is characterized by:

A. Distrust and suspiciousness
B. Instability in relationships, self-image, and affects
C. Social detachment
D. Grandiosity and need for admiration

12. Antisocial Personality Disorder requires evidence of Conduct Disorder before age:

A. 12
B. 15
C. 18
D. 21

13. Avoidant Personality Disorder involves:

A. Need to be taken care of
B. Disregard for others' rights

C. Social inhibition and feelings of inadequacy
D. Preoccupation with orderliness

14. Schizophrenia requires continuous signs of disturbance for at least:

A. One month
B. Three months
C. Six months
D. One year

15. Negative symptoms of schizophrenia include:

A. Delusions and hallucinations
B. Flat affect and avolition
C. Agitation and aggression
D. Rapid speech and racing thoughts

16. Schizoaffective Disorder involves:

A. Only psychotic symptoms
B. Only mood symptoms
C. Psychotic symptoms plus major mood episode
D. Brief psychotic symptoms

17. Brief Psychotic Disorder lasts:

A. Less than one day
B. At least one day but less than one month
C. 1-6 months
D. More than six months

18. Substance Use Disorder severity is based on:

A. Type of substance
B. Amount consumed
C. Number of criteria met
D. Duration of use

19. Mild Substance Use Disorder involves:

A. 2-3 symptoms
B. 4-5 symptoms
C. 6-7 symptoms
D. 8+ symptoms

20. Persistent Depressive Disorder (Dysthymia) requires depressed mood for at least:

A. Two weeks
B. One month

C. One year
D. Two years

21. A client with depression who brightens in response to positive events likely has:

A. Melancholic features
B. Atypical features
C. Psychotic features
D. Seasonal pattern

22. Bipolar II Disorder involves:

A. Manic episodes only
B. Hypomanic and major depressive episodes
C. Mixed episodes
D. Rapid cycling

23. Agoraphobia involves fear of at least:

A. One situation
B. Two situations
C. Three situations
D. Four situations

24. The key feature distinguishing OCD from OCPD is:

A. Severity of symptoms
B. OCD involves unwanted intrusive thoughts
C. OCPD is more treatable
D. Age of onset

25. PTSD avoidance symptoms include:

A. Flashbacks
B. Nightmares
C. Avoiding reminders of trauma
D. Hypervigilance

26. Narcissistic Personality Disorder involves:

A. Unstable relationships
B. Grandiosity and lack of empathy
C. Social anxiety
D. Detachment from relationships

27. Dependent Personality Disorder is characterized by:

A. Need for control
B. Excessive need to be taken care of

C. Distrust of others
D. Emotional detachment

28. Delusional Disorder involves delusions for at least:

A. One week
B. Two weeks
C. One month
D. Six months

29. Substance-induced mental disorders require:

A. Preexisting mental illness
B. Temporal relationship with substance use
C. Genetic predisposition
D. Childhood trauma

30. Schizophreniform Disorder lasts:

A. Less than one month
B. 1-6 months
C. 6-12 months
D. More than one year

31. Major Depression with psychotic features differs from Schizoaffective Disorder in that:

A. Psychosis only occurs during mood episodes
B. Depression is more severe
C. Hallucinations are visual
D. Treatment is different

32. Cyclothymic Disorder involves mood symptoms for at least:

A. Six months
B. One year
C. Two years
D. Five years

33. Specific Phobia requires symptoms lasting at least:

A. One month
B. Three months
C. Six months
D. One year

34. Paranoid Personality Disorder involves:

A. Brief episodes of paranoia
B. Pervasive distrust and suspiciousness

C. Paranoid delusions
D. Social anxiety

35. Schizoid Personality Disorder is characterized by:

A. Odd beliefs and magical thinking
B. Detachment from social relationships
C. Splitting and identity disturbance
D. Suspiciousness

36. Histrionic Personality Disorder involves:

A. Attention-seeking and excessive emotionality
B. Lack of empathy
C. Social inhibition
D. Need for control

37. Obsessive-Compulsive Personality Disorder involves:

A. Unwanted intrusive thoughts
B. Preoccupation with orderliness and control
C. Fear of contamination
D. Checking compulsions

38. The difference between adjustment disorder and normal stress response is:

A. Type of stressor
B. Symptoms are out of proportion or cause significant impairment
C. Duration only
D. Need for medication

39. Alcohol withdrawal can be life-threatening due to:

A. Depression
B. Seizures and delirium tremens
C. Insomnia
D. Anxiety

40. Tolerance in substance use means:

A. Accepting others' use
B. Needing more for same effect
C. Withdrawal symptoms
D. Loss of control

41. A manic episode requires symptoms for at least:

A. Three days
B. Four days

C. One week
D. Two weeks

42. Atypical depression features include:

A. Weight loss
B. Mood reactivity and increased appetite
C. Early morning awakening
D. Excessive guilt

43. Panic Disorder diagnosis requires:

A. Single panic attack
B. Recurrent unexpected panic attacks plus worry about attacks
C. Panic attacks in specific situations
D. Only physical symptoms

44. Command hallucinations are most concerning in:

A. Depression
B. Anxiety
C. Psychotic disorders
D. Personality disorders

45. The hallmark of Borderline Personality Disorder is:

A. Lack of empathy
B. Instability
C. Grandiosity
D. Detachment

46. Schizotypal Personality Disorder involves:

A. Psychotic episodes
B. Cognitive or perceptual distortions and eccentricities
C. Antisocial behavior
D. Mood instability

47. A client with persistent delusions but otherwise normal functioning likely has:

A. Schizophrenia
B. Brief Psychotic Disorder
C. Delusional Disorder
D. Schizoaffective Disorder

48. Substance withdrawal symptoms:

A. Are identical for all substances
B. Vary by substance

C. Are always dangerous
D. Don't require treatment

49. Differential diagnosis between Major Depression and Bipolar Disorder requires:

A. Severity assessment
B. History of manic or hypomanic episodes
C. Family history only
D. Response to medication

50. PTSD hyperarousal symptoms include:

A. Avoidance
B. Flashbacks
C. Exaggerated startle response
D. Negative beliefs

51. Antisocial Personality Disorder requires the individual to be at least:

A. 15 years old
B. 18 years old
C. 21 years old
D. 25 years old

52. A hypomanic episode lasts at least:

A. Two days
B. Four days
C. One week
D. Two weeks

53. The primary difference between worry in GAD and obsessions in OCD is:

A. Severity
B. GAD worries are about real-life concerns; OCD obsessions are intrusive and unwanted
C. Duration
D. Treatment response

54. Reactive Attachment Disorder results from:

A. Genetic factors
B. Inadequate care in childhood
C. Trauma exposure
D. Substance use

55. A client meets criteria for Major Depression but symptoms developed after job loss three months ago and are somewhat out of proportion to the stressor. The best diagnosis is:

A. Adjustment Disorder
B. Major Depressive Disorder

C. Persistent Depressive Disorder
D. Normal grief

56. Negative symptoms in schizophrenia are called "negative" because:

A. They're bad symptoms
B. They represent loss or diminishment of normal functions
C. Patients have negative attitudes
D. They don't respond to medication

57. A person who experiences full manic and major depressive symptoms simultaneously has:

A. Bipolar I with mixed features
B. Bipolar II
C. Cyclothymic Disorder
D. Schizoaffective Disorder

58. Substance use becomes a disorder when:

A. Any use occurs
B. Pattern causes significant impairment or distress
C. Daily use occurs
D. Tolerance develops

59. The key feature of Avoidant Personality Disorder is:

A. Fear of abandonment
B. Hypersensitivity to negative evaluation
C. Need for admiration
D. Lack of empathy

60. Delusions in Delusional Disorder are:

A. Always bizarre
B. Non-bizarre and possible but unlikely
C. Brief and transient
D. Always persecutory

61. A client with depression, anxiety, insomnia, and panic attacks following spouse's death two weeks ago likely has:

A. Major Depressive Disorder
B. Panic Disorder
C. Adjustment Disorder
D. Normal grief reaction

62. The presence of negative symptoms helps distinguish schizophrenia from:

A. Brief Psychotic Disorder
B. Delusional Disorder

C. Substance-induced psychosis
D. All of the above

63. Comorbidity refers to:

A. Medical complications
B. Presence of multiple disorders
C. Severe symptoms
D. Chronic conditions

64. Avolition in schizophrenia means:

A. Hearing voices
B. Lack of motivation
C. Disorganized thinking
D. Emotional flatness

65. A diagnosis of substance-induced depressive disorder requires that symptoms:

A. Preexist substance use
B. Develop during or shortly after substance exposure
C. Occur only during withdrawal
D. Last at least six months

66. The main difference between Bipolar I and Bipolar II is:

A. Severity of depression
B. Bipolar I has mania; Bipolar II has hypomania
C. Treatment approach
D. Bipolar II is more severe

67. Ego-syntonic symptoms are:

A. Experienced as alien to self
B. Consistent with self-image
C. More severe
D. Unresponsive to treatment

68. OCD compulsions are performed to:

A. Seek attention
B. Reduce anxiety from obsessions
C. Gain pleasure
D. Manipulate others

69. PTSD requires exposure to trauma involving:

A. Any stressful event
B. Actual or threatened death, serious injury, or sexual violence

C. Only combat
D. Childhood abuse only

70. Cluster B personality disorders are characterized by:

A. Anxious, fearful traits
B. Odd, eccentric traits
C. Dramatic, emotional, erratic traits
D. Psychotic features

71. A person who takes substances to relieve withdrawal symptoms meets criteria for:

A. Tolerance
B. Withdrawal
C. Both tolerance and withdrawal
D. Neither

72. Schizoaffective Disorder requires psychotic symptoms:

A. Only during mood episodes
B. For at least two weeks in absence of mood episode
C. Never without mood symptoms
D. For less than one month

73. The best way to differentiate between similar diagnoses is:

A. Trial and error
B. Careful assessment of symptom patterns, duration, and functional impact
C. Family preference
D. Insurance requirements

74. A client with moderate depression who has never had mania or hypomania is diagnosed with:

A. Bipolar I Disorder
B. Bipolar II Disorder
C. Major Depressive Disorder
D. Cyclothymic Disorder

75. Personality disorders are characterized by patterns that are:

A. Brief and situation-specific
B. Pervasive, inflexible, and stable over time
C. Easily changed with treatment
D. Always severe

76. Flight of ideas is most characteristic of:

A. Depression
B. Mania

C. Schizophrenia
D. Anxiety

77. The primary goal of differential diagnosis is to:

A. Use the most severe diagnosis
B. Identify the diagnosis that best explains symptoms
C. Diagnose as many conditions as possible
D. Avoid stigmatizing labels

78. Splitting (viewing people as all good or all bad) is characteristic of:

A. Narcissistic Personality Disorder
B. Borderline Personality Disorder
C. Antisocial Personality Disorder
D. Schizoid Personality Disorder

79. Substance-induced disorders can mimic:

A. Only mood disorders
B. Only psychotic disorders
C. Almost any psychiatric disorder
D. No other disorders

80. A person who checks locks 50 times before leaving home and recognizes this is excessive has:

A. OCPD
B. OCD
C. Paranoid Personality Disorder
D. GAD

81. The prodromal phase of schizophrenia:

A. Doesn't exist
B. Involves subtle symptoms before full psychosis
C. Always includes hallucinations
D. Lasts only days

82. Medical rule-out is important because:

A. Medical conditions never cause psychiatric symptoms
B. Many medical conditions can cause psychiatric symptoms
C. It's required by insurance
D. It's not actually important

83. A client with social anxiety, panic attacks, and depression has:

A. Three separate disorders
B. Only one disorder

C. Comorbid conditions requiring integrated treatment
D. No diagnosable condition

84. Disorganized speech in schizophrenia may include:

A. Pressured speech
B. Loose associations
C. Slow speech
D. Selective mutism

85. The difference between specific phobia and agoraphobia is:

A. Severity
B. Specific phobia involves one object/situation; agoraphobia involves multiple situations
C. Treatment approach
D. Age of onset

86. Grandiose delusions involve beliefs about:

A. Being persecuted
B. Having special powers or importance
C. Body changes
D. Infidelity

87. A person with no close relationships who prefers solitary activities and shows emotional coldness likely has:

A. Avoidant Personality Disorder
B. Schizoid Personality Disorder
C. Schizotypal Personality Disorder
D. Antisocial Personality Disorder

88. Substance use disorder diagnosis requires symptoms causing:

A. Any discomfort
B. Significant impairment or distress
C. Physical illness
D. Legal problems

89. A client who experienced trauma 8 months ago and still has nightmares, avoidance, and hypervigilance has:

A. Acute Stress Disorder
B. PTSD
C. Adjustment Disorder
D. Normal trauma response

90. The primary feature of Dependent Personality Disorder is:

A. Need for control
B. Pervasive need to be taken care of
C. Distrust
D. Social anxiety

91. Catatonic behavior in schizophrenia may include:

A. Only increased movement
B. Decreased movement or unusual postures
C. Normal movement
D. Rapid speech

92. Someone who has depressed mood plus two other symptoms for two years has:

A. Major Depressive Disorder
B. Persistent Depressive Disorder
C. Adjustment Disorder
D. Bipolar Disorder

93. Insight in psychotic disorders refers to:

A. Intelligence
B. Awareness of having a mental illness
C. Memory
D. Judgment

94. A person with intrusive thoughts about harming their baby but horrified by these thoughts has:

A. Desire to harm the baby
B. OCD (obsessions ego-dystonic)
C. Psychosis
D. Postpartum depression

95. The key to diagnosing Bipolar vs. Unipolar Depression is:

A. Severity of depression
B. History of elevated mood episodes
C. Family history only
D. Treatment response

96. Substance withdrawal syndrome:

A. Is the same for all substances
B. Is substance-specific
C. Never requires medical management
D. Indicates lack of willpower

97. A person who feels uncomfortable when not the center of attention likely has:

A. Narcissistic Personality Disorder
B. Histrionic Personality Disorder
C. Borderline Personality Disorder
D. Dependent Personality Disorder

98. PTSD intrusion symptoms include:

A. Avoidance
B. Flashbacks and nightmares
C. Hypervigilance
D. Negative beliefs

99. The most common comorbidity with Major Depressive Disorder is:

A. Schizophrenia
B. Anxiety disorders
C. Personality disorders
D. Substance use disorders

100. Diagnosing personality disorders requires:

A. Single assessment
B. Observation of pervasive, long-standing patterns
C. Family report only
D. Brief symptoms

Answer Key with Detailed Explanations

1. A. Two weeks
Major Depressive Disorder requires five of nine symptoms present for at least two weeks, representing a change from previous functioning. This duration criterion distinguishes clinical depression from transient sadness. Symptoms must be present most of the day, nearly every day during the two-week period.

2. B. At least one manic episode
Bipolar I Disorder requires at least one manic episode. Depressive episodes commonly occur but aren't required for the diagnosis. The presence of even a single manic episode defines Bipolar I, distinguishing it from Bipolar II (which requires hypomania plus depression) and Major Depressive Disorder (which involves only depressive episodes).

3. B. Duration and severity
Hypomania and mania have the same types of symptoms, but hypomania lasts at least four days (mania requires seven days or hospitalization), is less severe, doesn't cause marked impairment, and doesn't include psychotic features. Hypomania may actually feel good and increase functioning temporarily, while mania causes significant problems and often requires hospitalization.

4. D. Six months
Generalized Anxiety Disorder requires excessive anxiety and worry occurring more days than not for

at least six months, about multiple events or activities. This duration distinguishes GAD from normal worry or adjustment-related anxiety. The worry must be difficult to control and cause significant distress or impairment.

5. B. Peak intensity within minutes
Panic attacks are characterized by abrupt surge of intense fear or discomfort that reaches peak within minutes. They include both physical symptoms (heart racing, sweating, shaking) and psychological symptoms (fear of dying, losing control). The rapid onset distinguishes panic from gradual-building anxiety.

6. C. Scrutiny by others
Social Anxiety Disorder involves marked fear of social situations where the person might be scrutinized by others. The person fears acting in ways that will be negatively evaluated—showing anxiety symptoms, saying something embarrassing, being judged. This differs from agoraphobia (fear of situations where escape is difficult) and specific phobias (fear of specific objects or situations).

7. B. Intrusive, unwanted thoughts
OCD obsessions are intrusive, unwanted thoughts, urges, or images that cause marked anxiety. They're ego-dystonic (experienced as alien to the self) and the person attempts to ignore, suppress, or neutralize them. This distinguishes them from worries (which are about real-life concerns) and psychotic thoughts (which aren't recognized as coming from one's own mind).

8. C. Four symptom clusters
PTSD requires symptoms from four clusters: intrusion (at least one symptom), avoidance (at least one), negative alterations in cognitions and mood (at least two), and alterations in arousal and reactivity (at least two). All four clusters must be present for PTSD diagnosis. Symptoms must persist for more than one month.

9. B. 3 days to 1 month after trauma
Acute Stress Disorder symptoms occur three days to one month after trauma exposure. If symptoms persist beyond one month, the diagnosis changes to PTSD. The minimum three-day criterion distinguishes Acute Stress Disorder from immediate trauma responses that resolve quickly. This temporal window is the main distinction between Acute Stress Disorder and PTSD.

10. C. Three months of stressor
Adjustment Disorder symptoms must develop within three months of the onset of an identifiable stressor. This temporal relationship between stressor and symptoms is essential for the diagnosis. If symptoms develop more than three months after the stressor, another diagnosis should be considered.

11. B. Instability in relationships, self-image, and affects
Borderline Personality Disorder's hallmark is pervasive instability—in relationships (idealizing then devaluing), self-image (identity disturbance), and affects (mood swings). This instability, combined with marked impulsivity and fear of abandonment, defines BPD. The other options describe different personality disorders.

12. B. 15
Antisocial Personality Disorder requires evidence of Conduct Disorder (pattern of violating others'

rights and social norms) with onset before age 15. The individual must currently be at least age 18 for the diagnosis. This criterion ensures that antisocial patterns began in childhood/adolescence and persisted into adulthood, not just emerging in adulthood.

13. C. Social inhibition and feelings of inadequacy
Avoidant Personality Disorder involves pervasive social inhibition, feelings of inadequacy, and hypersensitivity to negative evaluation. The person wants relationships but fears criticism and rejection so intensely that they avoid social contact. This differs from Schizoid (no desire for relationships) and Dependent (fears being left to care for self) Personality Disorders.

14. C. Six months
Schizophrenia requires continuous signs of disturbance for at least six months. This must include at least one month of active-phase symptoms (or less if treated successfully) plus prodromal or residual symptoms. This duration criterion distinguishes schizophrenia from Brief Psychotic Disorder (less than one month) and Schizophreniform Disorder (1-6 months).

15. B. Flat affect and avolition
Negative symptoms represent diminishment or absence of normal functions. They include flat affect (lack of emotional expression), avolition (lack of motivation), alogia (poverty of speech), anhedonia (inability to experience pleasure), and asociality (lack of interest in social interactions). Delusions and hallucinations are positive symptoms (excesses of normal function).

16. C. Psychotic symptoms plus major mood episode
Schizoaffective Disorder involves an uninterrupted period of illness during which there's a major mood episode (depressive or manic) concurrent with schizophrenia criteria. Critically, delusions or hallucinations must occur for at least two weeks in absence of major mood episode. This distinguishes it from mood disorder with psychotic features (psychosis only during mood episodes) and schizophrenia (mood symptoms aren't prominent).

17. B. At least one day but less than one month
Brief Psychotic Disorder lasts at least one day but less than one month, with eventual full return to premorbid functioning. If symptoms persist 1-6 months, the diagnosis becomes Schizophreniform Disorder. If symptoms persist beyond six months, it becomes Schizophrenia. The brief duration is the defining characteristic.

18. C. Number of criteria met
Substance Use Disorder severity is determined by the number of criteria met from a list of 11: mild (2-3 criteria), moderate (4-5 criteria), severe (6+ criteria). Severity isn't based on type of substance, amount consumed, or duration alone—it's the pattern of problematic use across multiple domains that determines severity.

19. A. 2-3 symptoms
Mild Substance Use Disorder involves meeting 2-3 of the 11 criteria. This might include taking larger amounts than intended and spending considerable time using, but without severe life disruption. Moderate is 4-5 criteria, severe is 6 or more. This dimensional approach recognizes substance problems exist on a continuum.

20. D. Two years
Persistent Depressive Disorder (Dysthymia) requires depressed mood for most of the day, more days than not, for at least two years in adults (one year in children/adolescents), plus at least two additional symptoms. This chronic, low-grade depression is less severe than Major Depression but more persistent, significantly affecting quality of life over years.

21. B. Atypical features
Atypical depression features include mood reactivity (brightening in response to positive events), along with increased appetite/weight gain, hypersomnia, leaden paralysis, or rejection sensitivity. This differs from melancholic depression (no mood reactivity, worse mood in morning, early awakening, significant weight loss). Understanding features guides treatment selection.

22. B. Hypomanic and major depressive episodes
Bipolar II Disorder requires at least one hypomanic episode and at least one major depressive episode. There must never have been a manic episode (which would make it Bipolar I). People with Bipolar II often seek treatment during depressive episodes and may not report hypomanic periods, which feel good. Careful history-taking is essential.

23. B. Two situations
Agoraphobia involves marked fear or anxiety about at least two of five situations: public transportation, open spaces, enclosed spaces, standing in line/being in crowds, or being outside home alone. The person fears these because escape might be difficult or help unavailable if panic-like symptoms develop. The multiple situations criterion distinguishes agoraphobia from specific phobia.

24. B. OCD involves unwanted intrusive thoughts
OCD involves ego-dystonic (unwanted, distressing) intrusive thoughts (obsessions) and compulsive behaviors to reduce anxiety. OCPD involves ego-syntonic (consistent with self-image) perfectionism, orderliness, and control that the person values. OCD causes distress; OCPD causes problems for others more than self. They're completely different disorders despite similar names.

25. C. Avoiding reminders of trauma
PTSD avoidance symptoms include efforts to avoid distressing memories, thoughts, or feelings about the trauma, and avoidance of external reminders (people, places, conversations, activities, objects, situations). Flashbacks and nightmares are intrusion symptoms. Hypervigilance is an arousal/reactivity symptom. Understanding symptom clusters guides assessment and treatment.

26. B. Grandiosity and lack of empathy
Narcissistic Personality Disorder involves pervasive grandiosity, need for admiration, and lack of empathy. The person has inflated sense of self-importance, fantasies of unlimited success, believes they're special, requires excessive admiration, has sense of entitlement, exploits others, lacks empathy, and shows arrogant behaviors. This differs from other Cluster B disorders.

27. B. Excessive need to be taken care of
Dependent Personality Disorder involves pervasive, excessive need to be taken care of, leading to submissive, clinging behavior and fears of separation. The person has difficulty making decisions,

needs others to assume responsibility for major life areas, has difficulty expressing disagreement (fears loss of support), and urgently seeks new relationships when one ends.

28. C. One month
Delusional Disorder requires one or more delusions for at least one month. Apart from the impact of delusions, functioning isn't markedly impaired and behavior isn't obviously bizarre. If hallucinations are present, they're not prominent. This duration distinguishes Delusional Disorder from Brief Psychotic Disorder (less than one month).

29. B. Temporal relationship with substance use
Substance-induced mental disorders require temporal relationship between substance use and symptom development—symptoms develop during or shortly after substance exposure or withdrawal. The substance must be capable of producing the symptoms. If symptoms persist substantially beyond intoxication/withdrawal, they may represent independent mental disorder rather than substance-induced.

30. B. 1-6 months
Schizophreniform Disorder meets criteria for schizophrenia except duration is at least one month but less than six months. It's essentially a provisional diagnosis—if symptoms persist beyond six months, diagnosis changes to schizophrenia. If symptoms resolve before six months with full return to functioning, it remains schizophreniform.

31. A. Psychosis only occurs during mood episodes
In Major Depression with psychotic features, psychotic symptoms occur only during the depressive episode. In Schizoaffective Disorder, psychotic symptoms occur for at least two weeks in the absence of major mood episode. This is the key distinction—timing of psychosis relative to mood symptoms determines which diagnosis applies.

32. C. Two years
Cyclothymic Disorder requires numerous periods of hypomanic symptoms and depressive symptoms (not meeting full criteria for episodes) for at least two years in adults (one year in children/adolescents). It's chronic mood instability without reaching full episode thresholds. The person hasn't been without symptoms for more than two months at a time during the two-year period.

33. C. Six months
Specific Phobia requires marked fear or anxiety about a specific object or situation that persists for at least six months. This duration criterion ensures the fear isn't transient. The phobic object almost always provokes immediate fear, is actively avoided or endured with intense distress, and the fear is out of proportion to actual danger.

34. B. Pervasive distrust and suspiciousness
Paranoid Personality Disorder involves pervasive, long-standing pattern of distrust and suspiciousness where others' motives are interpreted as malevolent. This is personality-based suspiciousness, not paranoid delusions (which would be psychotic). The person suspects others are exploiting or deceiving them, doubts loyalty, reads hidden meanings into benign remarks, and bears grudges.

35. B. Detachment from social relationships
Schizoid Personality Disorder involves pervasive detachment from social relationships and restricted emotional expression. The person doesn't desire or enjoy close relationships, almost always chooses solitary activities, has little interest in sex, takes pleasure in few activities, lacks close friends, appears indifferent to praise/criticism, and shows emotional coldness. This differs from Schizotypal (which includes cognitive/perceptual distortions).

36. A. Attention-seeking and excessive emotionality
Histrionic Personality Disorder involves pervasive excessive emotionality and attention-seeking. The person is uncomfortable when not center of attention, shows inappropriately seductive behavior, displays rapidly shifting shallow emotions, uses physical appearance to draw attention, has impressionistic speech, shows self-dramatization, is suggestible, and considers relationships more intimate than they are.

37. B. Preoccupation with orderliness and control
Obsessive-Compulsive Personality Disorder involves pervasive preoccupation with orderliness, perfectionism, and control, at the expense of flexibility and efficiency. The person is preoccupied with details/rules/lists, shows perfectionism interfering with completion, is excessively devoted to work, is overconscientious about morality, can't discard worthless objects, is reluctant to delegate, adopts miserly spending, and shows rigidity. This is ego-syntonic, unlike OCD.

38. B. Symptoms are out of proportion or cause significant impairment
Adjustment Disorder differs from normal stress response in that symptoms are either out of proportion to the stressor (considering cultural context) or cause significant impairment in functioning. Normal stress responses are proportionate and don't cause marked impairment. If symptoms meet criteria for another disorder (like Major Depression), that diagnosis takes precedence.

39. B. Seizures and delirium tremens
Alcohol withdrawal can be life-threatening due to risk of seizures and delirium tremens (severe confusion, hallucinations, autonomic instability). Withdrawal from alcohol and benzodiazepines can be medically dangerous, unlike most other substance withdrawals. This is why medical detoxification is often necessary for severe alcohol dependence. Untreated severe alcohol withdrawal has significant mortality risk.

40. B. Needing more for same effect
Tolerance means needing markedly increased amounts of substance to achieve desired effect, or experiencing markedly diminished effect with continued use of the same amount. This represents physiological adaptation to the substance and is one criterion for Substance Use Disorder. Tolerance alone doesn't mean addiction but indicates physical dependence is developing.

41. C. One week
A manic episode requires abnormally elevated, expansive, or irritable mood and increased activity or energy for at least one week (or any duration if hospitalization is required). This distinguishes mania from hypomania (which requires only four days but is less severe). The one-week duration ensures symptoms aren't just brief mood fluctuations.

42. B. Mood reactivity and increased appetite
Atypical depression features include mood reactivity (mood brightens in response to actual or potential positive events), along with at least two of: significant weight gain or increased appetite, hypersomnia, leaden paralysis (heavy feeling in limbs), or long-standing pattern of rejection sensitivity. This differs significantly from melancholic features, which include lack of mood reactivity and decreased appetite.

43. B. Recurrent unexpected panic attacks plus worry about attacks
Panic Disorder requires recurrent unexpected panic attacks plus at least one month of concern about additional attacks, worry about implications of attacks (having heart attack, going crazy), or significant behavioral change related to attacks. Single panic attacks can occur in many contexts and don't constitute Panic Disorder. The persistent concern distinguishes the disorder.

44. C. Psychotic disorders
Command hallucinations—voices telling the person what to do, especially to harm self or others—are most concerning in psychotic disorders. The person may feel compelled to obey the voices. Assessment includes content of commands, person's relationship to voices (does person feel must obey?), and history of following commands. Commands to harm require immediate risk assessment.

45. B. Instability
The hallmark of Borderline Personality Disorder is pervasive instability—in relationships (intense, unstable, alternating idealization and devaluation), self-image (identity disturbance, unstable sense of self), and affects (marked mood reactivity, emotional lability). This instability, combined with impulsivity and frantic efforts to avoid abandonment, defines BPD and distinguishes it from other personality disorders.

46. B. Cognitive or perceptual distortions and eccentricities
Schizotypal Personality Disorder involves pervasive social and interpersonal deficits with acute discomfort in close relationships, plus cognitive or perceptual distortions and behavioral eccentricities. This includes ideas of reference, odd beliefs, unusual perceptual experiences, odd thinking/speech, suspiciousness, inappropriate affect, odd behavior/appearance, lack of close friends, and social anxiety. It's more severe than Schizoid but doesn't include psychotic episodes.

47. C. Delusional Disorder
Delusional Disorder involves persistent delusions (at least one month) with otherwise relatively normal functioning. Apart from impact of delusions, the person functions normally and behavior isn't obviously bizarre. This distinguishes it from schizophrenia (which includes negative symptoms and more functional impairment) and Brief Psychotic Disorder (duration less than one month).

48. B. Vary by substance
Withdrawal symptoms are substance-specific. Alcohol/sedative withdrawal includes tremors, sweating, anxiety, possible seizures. Opioid withdrawal includes muscle aches, nausea, anxiety. Stimulant withdrawal involves depression and fatigue. Some withdrawals (alcohol, benzodiazepines) can be medically dangerous. Others (opioids) are intensely uncomfortable but rarely life-threatening. Treatment approaches vary by substance.

49. B. History of manic or hypomanic episodes
Differentiating Major Depression from Bipolar Depression requires careful assessment of history for manic or hypomanic episodes. Depression episodes may look identical, but history of elevated mood episodes changes the diagnosis to Bipolar and significantly affects treatment (mood stabilizers needed, antidepressants alone can trigger mania). Many people with Bipolar II don't report hypomania because it feels good.

50. C. Exaggerated startle response
PTSD hyperarousal/reactivity symptoms include irritable behavior and angry outbursts, reckless or self-destructive behavior, hypervigilance, exaggerated startle response, problems with concentration, and sleep disturbance. Avoidance is a separate symptom cluster. Flashbacks are intrusion symptoms. Negative beliefs are part of the cognition/mood cluster. Understanding symptom organization guides assessment.

51. B. 18 years old
Antisocial Personality Disorder requires the individual to be at least age 18, though they must have evidence of Conduct Disorder before age 15. This ensures antisocial patterns began in childhood/adolescence and persisted into adulthood. Before age 18, Conduct Disorder is diagnosed instead, recognizing that not all youth with conduct problems develop Antisocial Personality Disorder.

52. B. Four days
A hypomanic episode requires at least four consecutive days of abnormally elevated, expansive, or irritable mood and increased activity. This is shorter than manic episodes (one week or hospitalization). Combined with lesser severity and lack of marked impairment, the four-day minimum distinguishes hypomania from brief mood fluctuations while differentiating it from full mania.

53. B. GAD worries are about real-life concerns; OCD obsessions are intrusive and unwanted
GAD worry focuses on real-life concerns (finances, health, work, family) that are excessive but based in reality. OCD obsessions are intrusive, unwanted thoughts that are often unrealistic or bizarre (contamination fears out of proportion to actual risk, aggressive thoughts contrary to values). OCD is ego-dystonic (thoughts feel alien); GAD worry is ego-syntonic (consistent with concerns).

54. B. Inadequate care in childhood
Reactive Attachment Disorder and Disinhibited Social Engagement Disorder result from insufficient care—typically severe neglect, frequent changes in caregivers, or institutional rearing with high child-to-caregiver ratios. These disorders reflect the profound impact of early attachment disruption. They don't result from trauma alone or substance use—they specifically require inadequate caregiving during critical developmental periods.

55. B. Major Depressive Disorder
When symptoms meet criteria for Major Depression, that diagnosis takes precedence over Adjustment Disorder, even if there's an identifiable stressor. Adjustment Disorder is diagnosed only when symptoms don't meet criteria for another disorder. The fact that symptoms followed a stressor doesn't prevent Major Depression diagnosis—many depressive episodes are triggered by stressors.

56. B. They represent loss or diminishment of normal functions
Negative symptoms are called "negative" because they represent absence or diminishment of functions normally present—loss of emotional expression (flat affect), motivation (avolition), speech (alogia), pleasure capacity (anhedonia), and social interest (asociality). This contrasts with positive symptoms (delusions, hallucinations), which are excesses or distortions of normal functions. The terminology isn't about good/bad.

57. A. Bipolar I with mixed features
When full criteria for both manic and major depressive episodes occur simultaneously or in rapid alternation, this is specified as "with mixed features." The person might have depressed mood alongside increased energy and racing thoughts, or euphoric mood alongside suicidal thoughts. Mixed features are associated with higher risk and often require different treatment approaches.

58. B. Pattern causes significant impairment or distress
Substance use becomes a disorder when the pattern of use causes clinically significant impairment or distress. This includes failure to fulfill obligations, social/interpersonal problems, dangerous use, continued use despite problems, plus physiological signs like tolerance and withdrawal. Use alone doesn't equal disorder—the pattern must cause meaningful problems in functioning.

59. B. Hypersensitivity to negative evaluation
Avoidant Personality Disorder's key feature is hypersensitivity to negative evaluation, leading to social inhibition and feelings of inadequacy. The person wants relationships but fears criticism, rejection, and humiliation so intensely that they avoid social contact. They view themselves as socially inept and inferior. This differs from social anxiety (situational fear) in being pervasive and affecting sense of self.

60. B. Non-bizarre and possible but unlikely
Delusions in Delusional Disorder are non-bizarre—situations that could conceivably occur but are false (being followed, being deceived by spouse, having disease). This contrasts with bizarre delusions in schizophrenia (organs being stolen, thoughts inserted by aliens). Delusional Disorder delusions persist at least one month and can be persecutory, jealous, erotomanic, somatic, or grandiose.

61. D. Normal grief reaction
Following spouse's death two weeks ago, depression, anxiety, and even panic symptoms can be part of normal grief. While these symptoms overlap with mental disorders, they're expected in early bereavement. Normal grief includes emotional pain, yearning, preoccupation with deceased, but typically improves over weeks to months. If symptoms persist unchanged for many months or include specific features (worthlessness, suicidal ideation), disorder diagnosis becomes appropriate.

62. D. All of the above
Negative symptoms (flat affect, avolition, alogia, anhedonia, asociality) help distinguish schizophrenia from other psychotic presentations. Brief Psychotic Disorder and substance-induced psychosis typically don't include prominent negative symptoms. Delusional Disorder involves delusions without negative symptoms or marked functional impairment. Prominent negative symptoms suggest schizophrenia specifically.

63. B. Presence of multiple disorders

Comorbidity refers to presence of two or more disorders in the same person at the same time. Comorbidity is common in mental health—depression and anxiety frequently co-occur, substance use disorders often accompany other mental illnesses. Understanding comorbidity is essential because disorders interact, affect each other's course, and require integrated treatment.

64. B. Lack of motivation

Avolition in schizophrenia means lack of motivation to initiate and sustain purposeful activities. The person may sit for hours doing nothing, show poor hygiene, lack energy for work or social activities. This isn't laziness—it's a negative symptom reflecting brain dysfunction. Avolition significantly impairs functioning and is distinct from depression (which includes other mood symptoms).

65. B. Develop during or shortly after substance exposure

Substance-induced disorders require symptoms developing during or shortly after substance exposure (intoxication) or withdrawal. The temporal relationship is key—symptoms begin with substance use or withdrawal. If symptoms persist substantially beyond the expected duration of intoxication/withdrawal, they may represent independent mental disorder rather than substance-induced. The substance must be capable of producing the symptoms.

66. B. Bipolar I has mania; Bipolar II has hypomania

The fundamental difference is that Bipolar I involves at least one manic episode (severe, causing marked impairment or requiring hospitalization), while Bipolar II involves hypomanic episodes (less severe, four days minimum, no marked impairment) plus major depressive episodes. Both have depression, but the type of elevated mood episode distinguishes them. Bipolar I is not necessarily more severe overall—Bipolar II often involves more time spent depressed.

67. B. Consistent with self-image

Ego-syntonic symptoms are consistent with the person's self-image and values. The person doesn't experience them as problematic or foreign. OCPD is ego-syntonic—the person values their perfectionism and control. This contrasts with ego-dystonic symptoms (like OCD obsessions), which feel alien and distressing. Ego-syntonicity affects treatment because people don't seek to change symptoms they value.

68. B. Reduce anxiety from obsessions

OCD compulsions are performed to reduce anxiety or distress caused by obsessions, or to prevent a feared event according to rigid rules. The person feels driven to perform compulsions and experiences temporary anxiety relief afterward. Compulsions aren't for pleasure or attention—they're attempts to manage overwhelming anxiety. Understanding this function guides treatment (exposure and response prevention).

69. B. Actual or threatened death, serious injury, or sexual violence

PTSD requires exposure to trauma involving actual or threatened death, serious injury, or sexual violence through direct experience, witnessing, learning it happened to close others (if violent/accidental), or repeated exposure to aversive details (first responders, not media exposure). Not all stressful events qualify as PTSD trauma. The specific types of exposure and trauma determine if PTSD criteria can be met.

70. C. Dramatic, emotional, erratic traits
Cluster B personality disorders (Antisocial, Borderline, Histrionic, Narcissistic) are characterized by dramatic, emotional, or erratic traits. Cluster A (Paranoid, Schizoid, Schizotypal) involves odd/eccentric traits. Cluster C (Avoidant, Dependent, Obsessive-Compulsive) involves anxious/fearful traits. These clusters help organize understanding of personality disorder patterns.

71. B. Withdrawal
Taking substances to relieve or avoid withdrawal symptoms is one of the withdrawal criteria for Substance Use Disorder. This indicates physiological dependence—the body has adapted to the substance and experiences distress when it's absent. People may use in the morning to stop shakes, drink to prevent anxiety, or use opioids to avoid withdrawal sickness. This cycle maintains addiction.

72. B. For at least two weeks in absence of mood episode
Schizoaffective Disorder's defining feature is that delusions or hallucinations occur for at least two weeks in the absence of a major mood episode during the lifetime duration of illness. This distinguishes it from mood disorder with psychotic features (psychosis only during mood episodes) and from schizophrenia (mood symptoms aren't prominent). Psychotic symptoms must occur both with and without mood episodes.

73. B. Careful assessment of symptom patterns, duration, and functional impact
Effective differential diagnosis requires systematic assessment of specific symptom patterns, duration of symptoms, degree and type of functional impairment, temporal relationships, and ruling out medical causes and substance effects. Diagnosis isn't trial and error—it's careful detective work matching clinical presentation to diagnostic criteria while considering alternative explanations.

74. C. Major Depressive Disorder
A client with moderate depression and no history of mania or hypomania has Major Depressive Disorder (assuming symptoms meet criteria). Bipolar I requires manic episode. Bipolar II requires hypomanic episode plus depression. Cyclothymic involves numerous periods of hypomanic and depressive symptoms not meeting full episode criteria. Absence of elevated mood history rules out bipolar diagnoses.

75. B. Pervasive, inflexible, and stable over time
Personality disorders are enduring patterns that are pervasive (across many contexts), inflexible (doesn't adapt to situations), and stable over time (typically traceable to adolescence or early adulthood). They're not situational or brief. This chronicity and pervasiveness distinguish personality disorders from other mental disorders and from normal personality variations.

76. B. Mania
Flight of ideas—rapid flow of thoughts jumping between loosely connected topics—is characteristic of manic episodes. Thoughts race faster than the person can speak. Topics shift rapidly with tangential connections. This differs from loose associations in schizophrenia (no logical connection) and pressured speech (rapid rate). Flight of ideas reflects the accelerated thinking of mania.

77. B. Identify the diagnosis that best explains symptoms
The primary goal of differential diagnosis is identifying the diagnosis that best accounts for the

client's symptoms and presentation. This involves considering multiple possibilities, evaluating each against the evidence, and selecting the explanation that best fits. It's not about finding the most severe diagnosis or diagnosing everything possible—it's about accurate explanation.

78. B. Borderline Personality Disorder
Splitting—viewing people (including self) as all good or all bad with rapid shifts between these extremes—is characteristic of Borderline Personality Disorder. A person is idealized as perfect, then one disappointment triggers viewing them as completely bad. This black-and-white thinking reflects identity disturbance and contributes to relationship instability. It's a defense mechanism against the anxiety of seeing people as complex.

79. C. Almost any psychiatric disorder
Substance-induced disorders can mimic almost any psychiatric condition—psychotic disorders, mood disorders, anxiety disorders, cognitive disorders. Alcohol can cause depressive disorder. Stimulants can cause psychotic disorder. Sedatives can cause anxiety disorder during withdrawal. This is why substance use assessment and medical rule-out are essential before diagnosing primary psychiatric disorders.

80. B. OCD
Checking locks 50 times while recognizing this is excessive indicates OCD. The behavior is compulsive (driven by obsessive anxiety about safety), ego-dystonic (the person recognizes it's excessive and wants to stop), and time-consuming. OCPD would involve valuing orderliness and checking, not seeing it as excessive. The recognition that behavior is unreasonable is typical of OCD with good insight.

81. B. Involves subtle symptoms before full psychosis
The prodromal phase of schizophrenia involves subtle changes before full psychotic symptoms emerge—social withdrawal, odd beliefs, perceptual disturbances, declining functioning, unusual thoughts. This phase can last months to years. Recognizing prodromal symptoms allows early intervention, which improves outcomes. Not everyone with prodromal symptoms develops schizophrenia, but it's a high-risk period.

82. B. Many medical conditions can cause psychiatric symptoms
Medical rule-out is critical because numerous medical conditions can cause or mimic psychiatric symptoms—thyroid disorders cause mood and anxiety symptoms, brain tumors can cause personality changes, infections can cause psychosis, medications have psychiatric side effects. Treating psychiatric symptoms without ruling out medical causes can miss serious medical problems and provide ineffective treatment.

83. C. Comorbid conditions requiring integrated treatment
A client with social anxiety, panic attacks, and depression has comorbid (co-occurring) conditions. Each disorder meets diagnostic criteria and each requires attention in treatment. Comorbidity is common and requires integrated treatment addressing all conditions, understanding how they interact and affect each other. Treating only one disorder often leaves the person still significantly impaired.

84. B. Loose associations
Disorganized speech in schizophrenia may include loose associations (jumping between unrelated ideas), tangentiality (going off-topic), circumstantiality (overly detailed, eventually reaching point), neologisms (made-up words), or incoherence (incomprehensible speech). The speech reflects disorganized thinking—thoughts don't connect logically. This is distinct from pressured speech (rapid rate) or slow speech (psychomotor change).

85. B. Specific phobia involves one object/situation; agoraphobia involves multiple situations
Specific phobia involves marked fear of one specific object or situation (flying, heights, animals, blood, enclosed spaces). Agoraphobia involves fear of at least two of five situation types (public transit, open spaces, enclosed spaces, lines/crowds, being outside home alone). The multiple situations and fear of inability to escape during panic-like symptoms distinguish agoraphobia.

86. B. Having special powers or importance
Grandiose delusions involve inflated beliefs about one's own importance, power, knowledge, or identity—believing one has special powers, has made great discoveries, has special relationship with God or famous people, is actually someone famous. These occur in mania and can occur in schizophrenia. They differ from persecutory (being harmed), referential (messages directed at self), and somatic (body changes) delusions.

87. B. Schizoid Personality Disorder
A person with no close relationships, preference for solitary activities, and emotional coldness most likely has Schizoid Personality Disorder. The key feature is detachment from social relationships and restricted emotional range. They don't desire or enjoy closeness, choose solitary activities, take pleasure in few things, lack friends, and appear indifferent. This differs from Avoidant (wants relationships but fears rejection) and Schizotypal (includes cognitive/perceptual distortions).

88. B. Significant impairment or distress
Substance use disorder requires that the pattern of use causes clinically significant impairment or distress. At least two of 11 criteria must be met within 12 months. The impairment might be social, occupational, health-related, or manifest through continued use despite problems. Use alone without impairment or distress doesn't meet disorder criteria—the substance use must cause meaningful problems.

89. B. PTSD
Trauma occurred 8 months ago with persistent symptoms—this is PTSD, not Acute Stress Disorder (which occurs 3 days to 1 month post-trauma). PTSD requires symptoms for more than one month. Eight months of nightmares, avoidance, and hypervigilance following trauma clearly meets PTSD criteria. This isn't normal trauma response—symptoms should have improved significantly by this point.

90. B. Pervasive need to be taken care of
Dependent Personality Disorder's primary feature is pervasive, excessive need to be taken care of, leading to submissive behavior and fears of separation. The person has difficulty making decisions, needs others to assume responsibility, has trouble expressing disagreement (fears rejection), feels

helpless alone, and urgently seeks new relationships when one ends. They fear being left to care for themselves.

91. B. Decreased movement or unusual postures
Catatonic behavior in schizophrenia can include decreased motor activity (stupor), excessive motor activity, extreme negativism or mutism, peculiarities of movement (unusual postures, grimacing, stereotypies), or echolalia/echopraxia (repeating others' words or movements). Catatonia represents severe psychomotor disturbance and can occur in schizophrenia, mood disorders, and medical conditions.

92. B. Persistent Depressive Disorder
Depressed mood for two years plus at least two additional symptoms (from a specific list) without meeting full Major Depression criteria indicates Persistent Depressive Disorder (Dysthymia). This is chronic, low-grade depression—less severe than Major Depression but more persistent. The person may say "I've always been depressed" or "This is just how I am." It significantly affects quality of life and is treatable.

93. B. Awareness of having a mental illness
Insight in psychotic disorders refers to awareness that one has a mental illness and that symptoms are pathological, not real. Poor insight means the person doesn't recognize they're ill—they believe delusions are true, hallucinations are real. Good insight means recognizing "I'm hearing voices because I have schizophrenia, not because there are actually voices." Insight affects treatment adherence and prognosis.

94. B. OCD (obsessions ego-dystonic)
Intrusive thoughts about harming a loved one that horrify the person indicate OCD, not desire to harm. The thoughts are ego-dystonic—alien to the person's values and distressing. Parents with these obsessions love their children and would never harm them. The horror at the thoughts proves they're unwanted intrusions, not desires. This is a common OCD presentation requiring specific treatment (exposure and response prevention).

95. B. History of elevated mood episodes
The key to differentiating Bipolar from Unipolar Depression is careful assessment for history of manic or hypomanic episodes. Depression episodes may appear identical, but history of elevated mood changes the diagnosis and treatment dramatically. Many people with Bipolar II don't report hypomania spontaneously because it feels good. Asking specifically about periods of elevated mood, decreased sleep need, increased activity is essential.

96. B. Is substance-specific
Withdrawal syndromes are substance-specific—alcohol withdrawal involves tremors, sweating, anxiety, possible seizures and delirium. Opioid withdrawal involves muscle aches, nausea, diarrhea, anxiety. Stimulant withdrawal involves depression, fatigue, increased appetite. Understanding substance-specific withdrawal guides treatment. Some withdrawals require medical management; others are uncomfortable but not dangerous.

97. B. Histrionic Personality Disorder
Feeling uncomfortable when not the center of attention is characteristic of Histrionic Personality Disorder. The person shows excessive emotionality and attention-seeking—using physical appearance to draw attention, displaying rapidly shifting shallow emotions, being inappropriately seductive, showing self-dramatization, and considering relationships more intimate than they are. The constant need for attention distinguishes this disorder.

98. B. Flashbacks and nightmares
PTSD intrusion symptoms include recurrent involuntary intrusive distressing memories, distressing dreams about trauma, dissociative reactions (flashbacks), intense psychological distress at trauma cues, and marked physiological reactions to cues. These represent trauma memories intruding into consciousness against the person's will. Avoidance is a separate cluster. Hypervigilance is arousal/reactivity. Negative beliefs are cognition/mood changes.

99. B. Anxiety disorders
The most common comorbidity with Major Depressive Disorder is anxiety disorders. The two frequently co-occur—many people with depression also have generalized anxiety, panic disorder, or social anxiety. Substance use disorders also commonly co-occur with depression. Understanding common comorbidities helps with comprehensive assessment and integrated treatment planning.

100. B. Observation of pervasive, long-standing patterns
Diagnosing personality disorders requires observing pervasive, long-standing patterns of inner experience and behavior across many contexts. Single assessments are often insufficient—collateral information, longitudinal observation, and assessment across multiple domains (relationships, work, emotional regulation, reality testing) are necessary. Patterns must be stable over time and traceable to adolescence or early adulthood.

What Matters Most

Diagnosis is a tool, not an identity. The person sitting across from you is more than their diagnosis. But accurate diagnosis helps—it guides treatment, predicts course, and helps people understand their experiences.

You'll make diagnostic mistakes. You'll miss bipolar disorder hidden behind depression. You'll diagnose substance-induced psychosis that turns out to be schizophrenia. You'll see personality disorder where there's actually complex PTSD. This is part of learning. Stay humble. Revise diagnoses as you learn more.

Use diagnosis to help, not to label or limit. The person with schizophrenia who's told they'll never work or have relationships may give up trying. The person with borderline personality disorder who's dismissed as "manipulative" may stop seeking help. Your words and attitudes shape how people see themselves and their possibilities.

Diagnosis opens doors to understanding and treatment. Use it wisely.

What You Must Carry With You

- Major Depressive Disorder requires five of nine symptoms for two weeks including depressed mood or loss of interest causing significant impairment
- Bipolar I requires at least one manic episode while Bipolar II requires hypomania plus major depression—careful history-taking distinguishes them
- Generalized Anxiety Disorder involves excessive worry about multiple concerns for six months that's difficult to control
- OCD involves ego-dystonic intrusive thoughts (obsessions) and repetitive behaviors (compulsions) performed to reduce anxiety
- PTSD requires trauma exposure plus symptoms from four clusters (intrusion, avoidance, negative cognitions/mood, arousal/reactivity) lasting over one month
- Borderline Personality Disorder's hallmark is pervasive instability in relationships, self-image, and affects with marked impulsivity
- Schizophrenia requires psychotic symptoms for at least one month within six months of continuous disturbance including negative symptoms
- Substance Use Disorder diagnosis requires problematic pattern with at least two of eleven criteria causing significant impairment
- Differential diagnosis requires systematic assessment of symptom patterns, duration, functional impact, temporal relationships, and medical rule-out
- Comorbidity is common—most people with one disorder have others that interact and require integrated treatment
- Medical conditions and substance effects can mimic almost any psychiatric disorder making thorough assessment essential
- Personality disorders involve pervasive, inflexible, long-standing patterns across contexts that are stable since adolescence or early adulthood
- Diagnosis is a clinical tool to guide treatment and understanding, not a label that defines or limits the person
- Hold diagnoses tentatively and revise as you learn more—diagnostic humility prevents errors and improves care

Chapter 7: Treatment Planning

A diagnosis tells you what's wrong. A treatment plan tells you what to do about it. You've assessed thoroughly, ruled out medical causes, arrived at accurate diagnosis. Now the real work begins—translating understanding into action that creates change.

Treatment planning isn't filling out forms to satisfy insurance requirements. It's collaborative problem-solving with your client. You bring expertise about interventions. They bring expertise about their life, values, and goals. Together, you create a roadmap from current suffering toward desired future.

Good treatment plans are specific, realistic, and measurable. Bad plans are vague ("Client will feel better"), unachievable ("Client will never feel anxious again"), or imposed without client input ("Client will attend AA five times weekly" when client works nights).

Treatment planning is both science and art. Science provides evidence about what works. Art involves adapting those interventions to this specific person, in this specific context, with these specific goals and constraints.

Collaborative Goal Setting

Treatment planning starts with goals, and goals start with the client. What do they want to change? What would make their life better? What does success look like?

Client-centered goals reflect what matters to the client, not what you think should matter. A client with depression might care more about returning to work than about eliminating every symptom. A client with anxiety might prioritize being able to attend their child's school events over feeling completely calm. Your job is helping them achieve their goals, not imposing yours.

SMART goals are Specific, Measurable, Achievable, Relevant, and Time-bound. Compare these goal statements:

Vague: "Client will feel less depressed."

SMART: "Client will reduce depression symptoms from severe to moderate range as measured by PHQ-9 scores, decreasing from current score of 22 to below 15 within three months."

Vague: "Client will improve relationships."

SMART: "Client will have at least two positive interactions with spouse weekly without conflict, as tracked in mood log, within six weeks."

The SMART version tells you exactly what you're working toward and how you'll know if you're making progress.

Short-term and long-term goals provide structure. Long-term goals describe the desired end state—major changes requiring months. Short-term goals are stepping stones—smaller changes achievable within weeks that build toward long-term goals.

For a client with social anxiety:

Long-term goal: "Client will attend social gatherings without overwhelming anxiety and participate in conversations comfortably within six months."

Short-term goals:

- "Client will identify three negative automatic thoughts related to social situations within two weeks."
- "Client will practice one conversation with a stranger in a low-stakes situation (cashier, neighbor) weekly for four weeks."
- "Client will attend one small social gathering for at least 30 minutes within eight weeks."

Each short-term goal builds capacity and confidence for the next step.

Behavioral goals describe observable actions. "Client will feel better" isn't behavioral. "Client will get out of bed by 9 AM on five of seven days" is behavioral. You can observe it, measure it, and track progress.

Symptom reduction goals target specific symptoms. Depression treatment might include: "Client will report sleeping 7-8 hours nightly at least five nights per week" or "Client will engage in at least three previously enjoyable activities weekly."

Functional goals focus on life roles and activities. These often matter most to clients: returning to work, caring for children, maintaining relationships, pursuing education, engaging in hobbies. "Client will return to work part-time within two months" or "Client will attend daughter's soccer games without panic attacks within six weeks."

Barriers to goal achievement must be identified and addressed. A client wants to attend therapy weekly but has no transportation. A client wants to exercise daily but works 12-hour shifts. A client wants to reduce drinking but all their friends drink heavily. You help identify barriers and problem-solve around them.

Case Example: Collaborative Goal Setting with Tom

Tom, a 45-year-old man with Major Depressive Disorder, enters therapy. You complete assessment and now begin treatment planning.

Your initial attempt: "Our goal is to reduce your depression. You'll practice cognitive restructuring and behavioral activation."

Tom looks confused and disengaged. This plan came from you, not him. It uses jargon he doesn't understand. It doesn't connect to what matters in his life.

Collaborative approach: "Tom, you've told me about the depression—the low mood, fatigue, difficulty concentrating. If we work together successfully, what would be different in your life six months from now? What would tell you that things are better?"

Tom thinks. "I'd be back at work. I've been on disability for three months, and I'm going crazy at home. I'd have energy to do things with my kids—right now, I just lie on the couch. And I'd feel like myself again, not this fog I'm living in."

Now you have real goals that matter to Tom:

Long-term goals (six months):

1. Return to work full-time with ability to concentrate and complete tasks effectively
2. Engage in meaningful activities with children at least twice weekly
3. Experience improved mood and energy most days

Short-term goals (four to eight weeks):

1. Establish regular sleep schedule (in bed by 11 PM, up by 7 AM) at least five nights weekly
2. Engage in one previously enjoyable activity (woodworking, which Tom mentioned) for 30 minutes twice weekly
3. Take 15-minute walk three times weekly
4. Identify and challenge three negative thoughts daily using thought log
5. Attend all scheduled therapy sessions

Objectives (specific, measurable steps):

- Week 1-2: Create sleep routine, begin thought log
- Week 3-4: Add walks, resume woodworking for short periods
- Week 5-6: Increase activity duration, plan one activity with children
- Week 7-8: Do one activity with children, evaluate readiness for return to work planning

You explain how each short-term goal connects to his long-term goals. Regular sleep and activity combat fatigue, improving energy for kids and work. Thought logs address the "fog" by challenging depressive thinking. Gradual activity increase rebuilds capacity for work.

Tom understands and agrees. These are his goals, using his words, addressing what matters to him. He's invested because the plan makes sense and connects to his values.

Two months later, Tom is sleeping regularly, taking daily walks, doing woodworking weekly, and had two good afternoons with his kids. His PHQ-9 score dropped from 22 to 14. He's ready to discuss return-to-work planning. The collaborative goals guided effective treatment because they meant something to Tom.

Evidence-Based Treatment Selection

Evidence-based practice integrates best research evidence, clinical expertise, and client values/circumstances. You don't just pick treatments you like or learned first. You select interventions shown effective for the specific problem.

Cognitive-Behavioral Therapy (CBT) has strong evidence for depression, anxiety disorders, OCD, PTSD, eating disorders, insomnia, and substance use. CBT focuses on changing problematic thought patterns and behaviors. It's time-limited (typically 12-20 sessions), structured, and skills-focused.

For depression, CBT addresses negative automatic thoughts, cognitive distortions, and behavioral patterns that maintain depression. A client thinks "I'm worthless" (negative thought). You help them examine evidence, identify cognitive distortions (overgeneralization, all-or-nothing thinking), and develop balanced alternative thoughts. You also use behavioral activation—increasing activities that provide pleasure and mastery to counter depressive withdrawal.

For anxiety, CBT uses exposure—gradually facing feared situations while learning anxiety decreases naturally. A client with social anxiety might practice brief conversations, then longer conversations, then small group interactions, building comfort at each level before advancing.

Dialectical Behavior Therapy (DBT) was developed for Borderline Personality Disorder but helps with emotion dysregulation across diagnoses. DBT teaches four skill modules: mindfulness, distress tolerance, emotion regulation, and interpersonal effectiveness.

DBT involves individual therapy plus weekly skills group. Individual sessions address motivation, apply skills to specific situations, and reduce therapy-interfering behaviors. Skills group teaches and practices the four modules systematically.

Prolonged Exposure (PE) has strong evidence for PTSD. PE involves imaginal exposure (repeatedly recounting trauma memory in therapy) and in vivo exposure (gradually approaching trauma-related situations avoided). Clients initially fear that focusing on trauma will overwhelm them, but exposure allows reprocessing of traumatic memories and reduces avoidance maintaining PTSD.

Cognitive Processing Therapy (CPT) also treats PTSD effectively. CPT focuses on how trauma affected beliefs about self, others, and the world. Clients examine "stuck points"—problematic beliefs like "It was my fault" or "The world is completely dangerous"—and develop more balanced beliefs.

Eye Movement Desensitization and Reprocessing (EMDR) treats trauma through bilateral stimulation (eye movements, taps, or sounds) while processing traumatic memories. EMDR helps reprocess memories so they're less distressing and no longer intrusive.

Motivational Interviewing (MI) addresses ambivalence about change, particularly effective for substance use. Rather than confronting denial, MI explores ambivalence, elicits the person's own reasons for change, and strengthens commitment to change. You roll with resistance, express empathy, develop discrepancy between current behavior and values, and support self-efficacy.

Interpersonal Therapy (IPT) treats depression by addressing interpersonal problems. IPT focuses on four areas: grief, role disputes, role transitions, or interpersonal deficits. Treatment helps resolve these interpersonal issues, which alleviates depression.

Acceptance and Commitment Therapy (ACT) uses acceptance, mindfulness, and commitment strategies to increase psychological flexibility. Rather than fighting uncomfortable thoughts and feelings, clients learn to accept them while committing to valued actions. ACT is effective for depression, anxiety, chronic pain, and other conditions.

Medication treats many mental health conditions effectively. Antidepressants (SSRIs, SNRIs) treat depression and anxiety. Mood stabilizers treat bipolar disorder. Antipsychotics treat schizophrenia and acute mania. Anxiolytics provide short-term anxiety relief. As a social worker, you don't prescribe but you collaborate with prescribers and help clients understand medications.

Integrative approaches combine treatments. Depression might be treated with CBT plus medication. PTSD might receive CPT plus medication for sleep and anxiety. Borderline Personality Disorder might involve DBT plus medication for mood symptoms. You select and combine treatments based on evidence, client preference, and practical considerations.

Client factors affect treatment selection. A client with transportation barriers might do better with telehealth CBT than weekly in-person sessions. A client who's highly intellectual might benefit from CPT's cognitive focus. A client who struggles with abstract thinking might need more behavioral, concrete approaches. A client from a culture where discussing emotions is stigmatized might initially engage better with problem-focused interventions.

Case Example: Evidence-Based Treatment Selection

Three clients present with different problems requiring different treatment approaches:

Client 1: Jessica—Panic Disorder

Jessica, 28, has panic disorder with agoraphobia. She has panic attacks multiple times weekly and avoids driving, shopping, and anywhere she might feel trapped. She's missed work due to panic and stopped socializing.

Evidence-based options: CBT for panic disorder has strongest evidence. This includes psychoeducation about panic, breathing retraining, cognitive restructuring of catastrophic thoughts about panic, and interoceptive exposure (deliberately inducing feared physical sensations to learn they're not dangerous) plus situational exposure (gradually approaching avoided situations).

Treatment plan: 12-16 sessions of CBT. You teach Jessica that panic attacks are uncomfortable but not dangerous. You help her understand the panic cycle—sensations trigger catastrophic thoughts ("I'm having a heart attack"), which increase fear, which increases sensations. You practice breathing techniques. You use cognitive restructuring to challenge thoughts like "If I panic in the store, I'll lose control and everyone will think I'm crazy."

You implement gradual exposure—first, Jessica drives short distances. Then longer distances. Then to the grocery store parking lot. Then into the store briefly. Then for longer shopping trips. At each step, her anxiety initially rises then falls, teaching her that she can handle the situation and anxiety decreases naturally.

After three months, Jessica's panic attacks decreased from 8-10 per week to 1-2 per month. She drives regularly and shops without panic. She understands panic attacks and has tools to manage them. The evidence-based approach worked.

Client 2: Michael—PTSD from Combat

Michael, 34, is a veteran with PTSD from combat exposure. He has intrusive memories, nightmares, hypervigilance, avoids reminders of deployment, and believes "The world is completely dangerous" and "I should have saved my buddy."

Evidence-based options: PE, CPT, and EMDR all have strong evidence for PTSD. You discuss options with Michael. PE involves repeatedly recounting trauma, which Michael finds too daunting initially. EMDR's bilateral stimulation approach interests him less. CPT's focus on examining beliefs appeals to him.

Treatment plan: 12 sessions of CPT. Michael writes about the trauma's impact on beliefs about safety, trust, power/control, esteem, and intimacy. He identifies stuck points: "It was my fault my buddy died" and "I can never let my guard down or something terrible will happen."

You help Michael examine evidence for and against these beliefs. Was he actually responsible for his buddy's death, or did circumstances beyond his control lead to it? Is the world as dangerous here as it was in combat? Through Socratic questioning and written exercises, Michael develops more balanced beliefs: "I did everything I could in an impossible situation" and "While bad things can happen, I don't need to be hypervigilant every moment."

His PTSD symptoms decrease significantly. He sleeps better, feels less on edge, and stops avoiding reminders. The evidence-based trauma-focused treatment addressed the core problem.

Client 3: Carlos—Borderline Personality Disorder

Carlos, 25, has BPD with emotional instability, self-harm, unstable relationships, and chronic suicidal thoughts. He's been in therapy multiple times but never made lasting progress.

Evidence-based options: DBT has the strongest evidence for BPD. Standard CBT alone isn't adequate for the emotion dysregulation and self-harm. Medication can help mood symptoms but doesn't address core problems.

Treatment plan: Comprehensive DBT including individual therapy weekly and skills group weekly for at least six months. You teach Carlos mindfulness (observing emotions without being overwhelmed), distress tolerance (surviving crises without self-harm), emotion regulation (understanding and modifying intense emotions), and interpersonal effectiveness (asking for what he needs, saying no, maintaining relationships).

When Carlos has urges to self-harm, you conduct chain analysis—examining the sequence from trigger through thoughts, emotions, and actions to consequence. You identify intervention points. Carlos learns to use skills instead of self-harm—holding ice, intense exercise, calling support people.

Progress is slower than with anxiety or depression. Carlos relapses several times. But gradually, self-harm decreases. Relationships stabilize. Emotional storms still happen but pass more quickly. The evidence-based DBT approach addresses his specific needs better than generic therapy.

Treatment Plan Development

Treatment plans document the roadmap from assessment to goals. They include diagnosis, goals, interventions, timeline, and progress measurement. Good plans are living documents that evolve as treatment progresses.

Components of a treatment plan:

1. **Problem statements** describe specific issues requiring attention. These come from your assessment and client's concerns. "Client experiences panic attacks 8-10 times weekly with avoidance of driving and shopping, interfering with work and social functioning."

2. **Long-term goals** describe desired outcomes. "Client will reduce panic attack frequency to less than one per month and resume normal driving and shopping activities within six months."

3. **Short-term goals** are stepping stones toward long-term goals. "Client will understand panic cycle and practice breathing techniques within two weeks." "Client will complete one graduated exposure activity weekly for eight weeks."

4. **Interventions** specify what you'll do. "Provide psychoeducation about panic disorder and panic cycle." "Teach diaphragmatic breathing and practice in session." "Develop exposure hierarchy collaboratively and implement graduated exposure."

5. **Responsible party** identifies who does what. Usually you and the client share responsibility. "Therapist will provide psychoeducation. Client will practice breathing techniques daily."

6. **Target dates** provide timeline. Short-term goals typically have 4-8 week timeframes. Long-term goals might be 3-6 months or longer.

7. **Progress measurement** specifies how you'll know if goals are met. "Client will report panic attack frequency weekly. Success = reduction from 8-10 to fewer than 4 within eight weeks."

Treatment plan format varies by setting, but all plans include these core elements. Some use problem-oriented format (separate sections for each problem). Others use goal-oriented format (organized by goals). Most include space for progress notes documenting movement toward goals.

Treatment plan example for depression:

Diagnosis: Major Depressive Disorder, moderate

Problem 1: Client experiences depressed mood daily with loss of interest in previously enjoyed activities, poor sleep, low energy, difficulty concentrating, affecting work performance and relationships.

Long-term goal: Client will reduce depression symptoms from moderate to mild range, resume meaningful activities, and maintain consistent work performance within three months.

Short-term goals:

1. Client will establish regular sleep schedule (in bed by 11 PM, up by 7 AM) five nights weekly within two weeks
2. Client will identify and challenge negative automatic thoughts using thought log daily within two weeks
3. Client will engage in three previously enjoyed activities weekly within four weeks
4. Client will attend all scheduled work commitments and meetings within four weeks

Interventions:

- CBT focusing on cognitive restructuring and behavioral activation
- Psychoeducation about depression and sleep hygiene
- Teach thought record technique and practice in session
- Develop activity schedule collaboratively
- Monitor mood and activity weekly using PHQ-9 and activity log

Responsible party:

- Therapist: Provide CBT, teach skills, monitor progress
- Client: Complete thought logs daily, implement sleep routine, engage in scheduled activities, attend sessions weekly

Target dates:

- Short-term goals: 2-4 weeks
- Long-term goal: 3 months
- Review and revise plan: 6 weeks

Progress measurement: PHQ-9 completed every two weeks (success = score below 10). Activity log tracking engagement in activities (success = 3+ activities weekly). Self-report of sleep (success = 5+ nights meeting schedule). Work attendance tracking (success = no missed days).

This plan is specific, measurable, and actionable. You and the client both know what you're working toward and how you'll know if you're making progress.

Revision and adaptation happen throughout treatment. You review progress regularly and adjust the plan. If a goal is achieved early, you develop new goals. If progress stalls, you examine barriers and modify interventions. If a new problem emerges, you address it in the plan.

Treatment plans aren't static documents filed away after the first session. They guide ongoing work and evolve with the client's changing needs.

Progress Monitoring and Outcome Measures

How do you know if treatment is working? You measure. Regular progress monitoring improves outcomes because it helps you identify when treatment isn't working and adjust course before the client drops out or fails.

Standardized measures provide objective tracking:

PHQ-9 (Patient Health Questionnaire-9) measures depression severity. Nine items corresponding to DSM criteria, scored 0-3. Total scores: 0-4 minimal, 5-9 mild, 10-14 moderate, 15-19 moderately severe, 20-27 severe. Administer every 2-4 weeks to track depression change.

GAD-7 (Generalized Anxiety Disorder-7) measures anxiety severity. Seven items scored 0-3. Total scores: 0-4 minimal, 5-9 mild, 10-14 moderate, 15-21 severe. Quick screening and monitoring tool for anxiety.

PCL-5 (PTSD Checklist for DSM-5) measures PTSD symptoms. Twenty items corresponding to DSM-5 criteria, scored 0-4. Tracks intrusion, avoidance, negative alterations, and arousal symptoms. Used to assess PTSD severity and monitor treatment progress.

OQ-45 (Outcome Questionnaire-45) measures overall distress, interpersonal relationships, and social role functioning. Broader measure of mental health and quality of life. Tracks general therapeutic progress.

Self-report tracking uses logs and journals:

Mood logs track daily mood ratings (0-10 scale), activities, thoughts, and events. Reveals patterns connecting thoughts, activities, and mood. Used in CBT for depression and anxiety.

Thought records capture situations, automatic thoughts, emotions, and alternative thoughts. Documents cognitive work and shows progress in identifying and challenging negative thinking.

Activity schedules track daily activities and associated pleasure/mastery ratings. Shows relationship between activity level and mood. Guides behavioral activation.

Panic logs record panic attack frequency, intensity, duration, triggers, and coping used. Tracks panic disorder progress as attacks decrease in frequency and intensity.

Functional measures track real-world outcomes:

Work attendance documents days worked versus missed. Depression treatment should improve ability to work consistently.

Social engagement tracks social activities per week. Social anxiety or depression treatment should increase social participation.

Sleep quality monitors hours slept, number of awakenings, morning fatigue. Insomnia or depression treatment should improve sleep.

Substance use tracks days abstinent, amount used, triggers, cravings. Substance use disorder treatment monitors reduction in use or maintenance of abstinence.

Goal attainment scaling measures progress toward individualized goals. For each goal, you define levels: -2 (worse than baseline), -1 (baseline), 0 (expected outcome), +1 (better than expected), +2 (much better than expected). You rate where the client is at each measurement point.

Session-by-session monitoring tracks progress after every session. Brief measures (PHQ-9, GAD-7) take minutes but provide continuous feedback. Research shows therapists who use session-by-session monitoring have better outcomes—they catch deterioration early and adjust treatment.

Clinical significance differs from statistical significance. A client might show statistically significant improvement (PHQ-9 drops from 22 to 18) but still be moderately depressed. You want clinically significant change—moving from clinical range to normal functioning range.

Reliable Change Index calculates whether change exceeds measurement error. Small score changes might just reflect normal variation. Reliable change means the person has genuinely improved beyond random fluctuation.

When progress stalls:

If a client isn't improving after reasonable time with adequate dose of evidence-based treatment, you assess what's happening:

- **Is the diagnosis correct?** Treating unipolar depression when it's actually bipolar will fail. Reassess.
- **Is the client actually doing the treatment?** If they're not completing homework, attending irregularly, or not engaging, treatment won't work. Address barriers and motivation.
- **Are there maintaining factors you missed?** Unaddressed substance use, domestic violence, medical problems, or severe stressors can prevent progress.
- **Is this the right treatment approach?** Maybe the evidence-based treatment for the diagnosis doesn't fit this client. Consider alternatives.
- **Does treatment need to be more intensive?** Maybe weekly outpatient isn't enough. Consider intensive outpatient or higher level of care.
- **Are you implementing the treatment competently?** Honest self-assessment—are you trained adequately in this approach? Consider consultation or supervision.

Case Example: Progress Monitoring with Emma

Emma, 32, enters treatment for Major Depression with initial PHQ-9 score of 21 (severe). You implement CBT with behavioral activation.

Week 2: PHQ-9 = 19. Slight improvement but still severe. Emma completed some thought logs but struggled with behavioral activation. She says she's "too tired" to do activities. You problem-solve barriers—she's trying to do too much at once. You scale back to just one 15-minute activity daily.

Week 4: PHQ-9 = 18. Minimal change after four sessions. This isn't expected progress. You reassess. Emma reveals she's drinking 4-5 glasses of wine nightly to help sleep. This wasn't disclosed initially. Alcohol is maintaining depression and interfering with treatment.

You address substance use, explaining how alcohol worsens depression. Emma agrees to cut back. You connect her with substance use resources. You add sleep hygiene work because the drinking was self-medication for insomnia.

Week 6: PHQ-9 = 15 (moderately severe). Progress! Reducing alcohol helped. Emma's sleeping better without wine, has more energy for activities. Thought logs show less negative thinking. You continue current approach.

Week 8: PHQ-9 = 12 (moderate). Good progress. Emma is engaging in activities regularly, sleep is improved, mood is better. You begin preparing for termination and relapse prevention.

Week 12: PHQ-9 = 7 (mild). Clinically significant improvement. Emma meets goals. You terminate with relapse prevention plan and offer booster sessions if needed.

Without progress monitoring, you might have continued CBT for weeks while Emma struggled, missing the substance use issue. Regular measurement helped you identify the problem and adjust treatment, leading to good outcomes.

Case Formulation

Case formulation integrates assessment information into a coherent explanation of how this person developed these problems and what maintains them. It guides treatment by explaining mechanisms to target.

CBT case formulation identifies:

- **Precipitating factors**: What triggered current problems? Job loss, relationship ending, trauma, medical diagnosis?
- **Predisposing factors**: What vulnerabilities existed before? Genetic risk, childhood adversity, previous episodes, personality factors?
- **Perpetuating factors**: What maintains problems now? Avoidance, negative thinking patterns, substance use, relationship patterns, lack of coping skills?
- **Protective factors**: What resources exist? Social support, employment, strengths, previous successful coping, reasons for living?

Core beliefs are fundamental assumptions developed early in life that shape how we see ourselves, others, and the world. Positive core beliefs support resilience: "I'm competent," "People are trustworthy," "The world is safe." Negative core beliefs create vulnerability: "I'm inadequate," "People will abandon me," "The world is dangerous."

Intermediate beliefs include rules ("I must be perfect or I'm worthless") and assumptions ("If I show weakness, people will reject me"). These flow from core beliefs and guide behavior.

Automatic thoughts are situation-specific thoughts that pop into consciousness. They're shaped by core and intermediate beliefs. Someone with core belief "I'm inadequate" has automatic thoughts like "I'll fail this presentation" or "Everyone thinks I'm stupid."

Behavioral patterns maintain problems. Depression leads to withdrawal, which reduces opportunities for positive experiences, which worsens depression. Anxiety leads to avoidance, which prevents learning that feared situations are safe, which maintains anxiety.

Case formulation example for social anxiety:

Precipitating factors: Client was humiliated giving a presentation in college (dropped notes, went blank, classmates laughed). Since then, social anxiety has worsened.

Predisposing factors: Shy temperament as child, critical parents who emphasized how others judge us, history of being bullied in middle school for being quiet.

Perpetuating factors:

- **Cognitive**: Core belief "I'm socially incompetent." Automatic thoughts like "Everyone will think I'm boring/stupid," "I'll embarrass myself," "They're judging me negatively."
- **Behavioral**: Avoids social situations, which prevents learning that social interactions can go well and that anxiety decreases with exposure. Safety behaviors (staying quiet, rehearsing everything beforehand) maintain anxiety.
- **Physiological**: High baseline anxiety, interprets normal anxiety sensations (blushing, shaking) as evidence of incompetence.

Protective factors: Intelligent, successful career in field requiring minimal social interaction, supportive spouse, motivated for change, previous therapy experience.

Formulation: Client developed core belief "I'm socially incompetent" through childhood experiences (shy temperament, critical parents, bullying). College presentation trauma confirmed this belief. Now, automatic thoughts predict social failure. Client avoids social situations (prevents disconfirmation of beliefs) and uses safety behaviors (prevents natural engagement). Avoidance maintains anxiety by preventing new learning. Treatment will address beliefs through cognitive restructuring and avoidance through graduated exposure.

This formulation explains how social anxiety developed and what maintains it, guiding treatment targets. You'll challenge the core belief, modify automatic thoughts, and use exposure to break the avoidance cycle.

Formulation guides intervention selection. If formulation emphasizes cognitive factors (negative thinking patterns), cognitive restructuring is central. If it emphasizes behavioral factors (avoidance), exposure is primary. If it involves emotion dysregulation, skills training is needed. If it involves interpersonal patterns, interpersonal work is important.

Sharing formulation with clients helps them understand their problems. Many clients feel confused about why they're suffering. Formulation makes sense of their experience. "You're not weak or broken. Here's how this developed and why it persists. And here's how we'll address it."

Case Example: Formulation-Driven Treatment

Marcus, 40, presents with depression and anger outbursts that threaten his marriage. He's "always been this way"—irritable, quick to anger, but also periodically depressed and withdrawn.

Your formulation:

Precipitating: Recent job stress (new supervisor who micromanages) triggered increased irritability and depression.

Predisposing:

- Grew up with alcoholic, rageful father who was unpredictably violent
- Learned early that expressing needs led to punishment or neglect
- Developed belief "I must be tough and self-reliant; needing others is weakness"
- Learned to suppress vulnerable emotions (sadness, fear, loneliness) but expressed through anger

Perpetuating:

- **Cognitive**: Core beliefs "I must be in control or I'm weak," "People will let me down." Automatic thoughts "She's trying to control me," "He doesn't respect me."
- **Emotional**: Can't identify or express vulnerable emotions. Sadness and fear are experienced as anger. Depression manifests as irritability.
- **Behavioral**: Anger pushes people away, creating the abandonment he fears. Withdrawal when depressed prevents connection and support. Never asks for help or shows vulnerability.
- **Interpersonal**: Pattern of conflict in relationships. People walk on eggshells around him. Wife is exhausted and considering leaving.

Protective factors: Intelligent, successful career, loves his family, motivated to save marriage, capable of insight.

Formulation: Marcus learned in childhood that vulnerability is dangerous and expressing needs leads to rejection. He developed hyper-independence and emotion suppression. Vulnerable emotions (sadness, fear, loneliness) are experienced and expressed as anger—the one emotion that felt safe.

Depression presents as irritability. Anger and withdrawal maintain problems by preventing genuine connection, which he desperately needs but can't ask for.

Treatment plan:

1. Help Marcus identify emotions beneath anger. When he feels angry, what else might he be feeling? Sad? Afraid? Hurt?
2. Teach emotional vocabulary and expression. Marcus literally doesn't have words for vulnerable emotions.
3. Challenge beliefs about vulnerability and needs. "Needing others is human, not weakness."
4. Develop alternative communication. Express needs directly instead of through anger or withdrawal.
5. Couple sessions to help wife understand and rebuild connection.

This formulation-driven treatment addresses core issues rather than just managing symptoms. After six months, Marcus's depression has improved, anger outbursts decreased dramatically, and his marriage is strengthening. He's learning that vulnerability creates connection, not rejection—the opposite of what he learned as a child.

Practice Questions

1. SMART goals are:

A. General aspirations
B. Specific, Measurable, Achievable, Relevant, Time-bound
C. Selected by the therapist
D. Symptom-focused only

2. Collaborative goal setting means:

A. Therapist decides goals
B. Client decides everything
C. Goals are developed jointly based on client values and clinical expertise
D. Goals come from insurance requirements

3. Evidence-based practice integrates:

A. Research evidence only
B. Clinical expertise only
C. Research evidence, clinical expertise, and client values
D. Whatever the therapist prefers

4. CBT has strongest evidence for:

A. Personality disorders only
B. Depression and anxiety disorders
C. Schizophrenia
D. Dementia

5. DBT was originally developed for:

A. Depression
B. Anxiety
C. Borderline Personality Disorder
D. Psychosis

6. Prolonged Exposure therapy treats:

A. Depression
B. PTSD
C. OCD
D. Panic Disorder

7. Motivational Interviewing is particularly effective for:

A. Psychosis
B. Ambivalence about change
C. Cognitive impairment
D. Mania

8. A behavioral goal is:

A. "Client will feel better"
B. "Client will understand depression"
C. "Client will attend work five days weekly"
D. "Client will have better relationships"

9. Short-term goals typically have timeframes of:

A. 1-2 days
B. 4-8 weeks
C. 6-12 months
D. Several years

10. Progress monitoring improves outcomes because:

A. It satisfies insurance requirements
B. It identifies when treatment isn't working so adjustments can be made
C. It creates paperwork
D. It's required by law

11. The PHQ-9 measures:

A. Anxiety
B. Depression
C. Psychosis
D. Personality

12. A PHQ-9 score of 15-19 indicates:

A. Minimal depression
B. Mild depression
C. Moderate depression
D. Moderately severe depression

13. Case formulation explains:

A. Only current symptoms
B. How problems developed and what maintains them
C. Insurance billing codes
D. Legal issues

14. Core beliefs are:

A. Situation-specific thoughts
B. Fundamental assumptions about self, others, and world
C. Always positive
D. Easy to change

15. In CBT formulation, perpetuating factors are:

A. Historical causes
B. What maintains problems currently
C. Future predictions
D. Unimportant

16. Exposure therapy for anxiety works by:

A. Avoiding feared situations
B. Gradually facing fears while learning anxiety decreases
C. Eliminating all anxiety
D. Using medication only

17. Behavioral activation treats depression by:

A. Analyzing childhood
B. Increasing engagement in meaningful activities
C. Avoiding difficult situations
D. Only using medication

18. The GAD-7 measures:

A. Depression
B. Anxiety
C. PTSD
D. Mania

19. Treatment plans should be:

A. Developed once and never changed
B. Written by insurance companies
C. Living documents that evolve with progress
D. Kept secret from clients

20. Clinically significant change means:

A. Any improvement
B. Statistical significance
C. Moving from clinical range to normal functioning
D. Client feels slightly better

21. If progress stalls, you should:

A. Continue same approach indefinitely
B. Blame the client
C. Assess barriers and modify treatment
D. Give up

22. Cognitive restructuring involves:

A. Brain surgery
B. Examining and modifying negative thought patterns
C. Avoiding thoughts
D. Medication only

23. A long-term goal for social anxiety might be:

A. "Client will feel calm always"
B. "Client will attend social events comfortably within six months"
C. "Client will become extroverted"
D. "Client will never feel anxious"

24. Graduated exposure means:

A. Facing biggest fear first
B. Avoiding all fears
C. Gradually approaching feared situations starting with easiest
D. Using medication instead

25. The PCL-5 measures:

A. Depression
B. Anxiety
C. PTSD symptoms
D. Substance use

26. Dialectical Behavior Therapy teaches:

A. Only medication management
B. Mindfulness, distress tolerance, emotion regulation, interpersonal effectiveness
C. Psychoanalysis
D. No specific skills

27. Automatic thoughts are:

A. Always accurate
B. Situation-specific thoughts influenced by core beliefs
C. Impossible to change
D. The same as emotions

28. Behavioral goals describe:

A. Internal feelings only
B. Vague aspirations
C. Observable, measurable actions
D. Diagnosis

29. Evidence-based treatment for panic disorder includes:

A. Avoiding all situations
B. CBT with exposure
C. Medication only
D. No treatment works

30. Problem statements in treatment plans:

A. Blame the client
B. Are vague and general
C. Describe specific issues requiring attention
D. Are written by insurance

31. Motivational Interviewing involves:

A. Confronting denial aggressively
B. Exploring ambivalence and eliciting client's own reasons for change
C. Telling clients what to do
D. Ignoring substance use

32. Thought records track:

A. Only positive thoughts
B. Situations, automatic thoughts, emotions, and alternative thoughts
C. Nothing useful
D. Only behaviors

33. A good treatment plan includes:

A. Vague goals with no timeline
B. Goals imposed by therapist
C. Specific goals, interventions, timeline, and progress measurement
D. No client input

34. EMDR treats trauma through:

A. Avoiding trauma memories
B. Bilateral stimulation while processing traumatic memories
C. Medication only
D. Hypnosis

35. When selecting treatment, you should consider:

A. Only what insurance covers
B. Only what you learned first
C. Evidence, client factors, and practical considerations
D. Random choice

36. Functional goals focus on:

A. Symptoms only
B. Life roles and activities
C. Diagnosis
D. Insurance requirements

37. Session-by-session monitoring:

A. Wastes time
B. Helps catch deterioration early
C. Isn't necessary
D. Only for research

38. Core beliefs develop:

A. In adulthood only
B. Early in life through experiences
C. Randomly
D. Only from trauma

39. Cognitive Processing Therapy for PTSD focuses on:

A. Avoiding trauma memories
B. How trauma affected beliefs and examining stuck points
C. Medication only
D. Hypnosis

40. If a client isn't improving, you should assess:

A. Only client motivation
B. Nothing, just continue
C. Diagnosis accuracy, treatment engagement, maintaining factors, treatment fit
D. Only medication

41. Activity scheduling helps depression by:

A. Keeping client busy without purpose
B. Increasing activities that provide pleasure and mastery
C. Avoiding difficult situations
D. Replacing therapy

42. Interpersonal Therapy treats depression by addressing:

A. Only thoughts
B. Interpersonal problems
C. Only biology
D. Nothing specific

43. Target dates in treatment plans:

A. Are unnecessary
B. Provide timeline for goal achievement
C. Should be decades away
D. Don't matter

44. Safety behaviors in anxiety:

A. Help anxiety decrease
B. Are necessary for safety
C. Prevent natural anxiety reduction and maintain anxiety
D. Should be encouraged

45. A treatment plan for depression should include:

A. Only medication
B. Goals for symptom reduction and functional improvement
C. No specific interventions
D. Vague aspirations

46. Intermediate beliefs include:

A. Only emotions
B. Rules and assumptions flowing from core beliefs
C. Behaviors only
D. Diagnosis

47. Progress toward goals should be measured:

A. Never
B. Only at termination
C. Regularly throughout treatment
D. Only if insurance requires

48. Acceptance and Commitment Therapy focuses on:

A. Eliminating all uncomfortable thoughts
B. Acceptance and commitment to valued actions
C. Avoiding emotions
D. Medication only

49. Exposure therapy should:

A. Be done all at once (flooding)
B. Avoid any anxiety
C. Be graduated and allow anxiety to decrease naturally
D. Never be used

50. Treatment planning is most effective when:

A. Therapist decides everything
B. Client has no input
C. It's collaborative and based on client values
D. It follows a rigid protocol

51. Chain analysis in DBT:

A. Examines sequence from trigger through actions to consequence
B. Is unnecessary
C. Blames the client
D. Only looks at current moment

52. When treatment isn't working, consider:

A. It's always the client's fault
B. Only one possible explanation
C. Multiple factors including diagnosis, engagement, maintaining factors, treatment fit
D. Nothing, just continue

53. A good short-term goal is:

A. "Client will be happy"
B. "Client will practice breathing techniques daily for two weeks"
C. "Client will never feel anxious"
D. "Client will understand everything"

54. Cognitive distortions are:

A. Always accurate
B. Patterns of biased thinking
C. Signs of psychosis
D. Untreatable

55. Treatment intensity should:

A. Always be weekly outpatient
B. Be matched to problem severity and client needs
C. Never change
D. Be minimal regardless of need

56. The goal of exposure therapy is:

A. Eliminating all anxiety forever
B. Learning anxiety decreases and situations are manageable
C. Avoiding anxiety completely
D. Increasing anxiety

57. Behavioral activation is based on the idea that:

A. Activity doesn't affect mood
B. Increasing meaningful activities improves mood
C. Avoidance helps depression
D. Only medication works

58. Goal attainment scaling:

A. Only uses pass/fail
B. Measures progress toward individualized goals on a continuum
C. Isn't useful
D. Only for research

59. Treatment plans should be:

A. Hidden from clients
B. Shared and discussed with clients
C. Written in professional jargon
D. Never revised

60. Distress tolerance skills teach:

A. How to avoid all distress
B. How to survive crises without making things worse
C. That distress is bad
D. To always act on emotions

61. Predisposing factors in formulation are:

A. Current maintaining factors
B. Vulnerabilities that existed before problems developed
C. Future predictions
D. Unimportant

62. Progress monitoring helps you:

A. Create more paperwork
B. Identify what's working and what needs adjustment
C. Bill insurance
D. Avoid talking to clients

63. Emotion regulation skills help clients:

A. Eliminate all emotions
B. Understand and modify intense emotions
C. Suppress emotions
D. Only feel positive emotions

64. A functional goal for someone with social anxiety might be:

A. "Never feel anxious"
B. "Attend daughter's school events within six weeks"
C. "Become completely comfortable with everyone"
D. "Understand why I'm anxious"

65. Precipitating factors are:

A. Long-term vulnerabilities
B. What triggered current problems
C. Maintaining factors
D. Protective factors

66. Interpersonal effectiveness skills teach:

A. How to manipulate others
B. How to ask for needs, say no, maintain relationships
C. How to avoid people
D. Nothing specific

67. If a client achieves goals early, you should:

A. Continue treatment indefinitely
B. Develop new goals or prepare for termination
C. Stop immediately
D. Change diagnosis

68. Cognitive restructuring challenges:

A. All thoughts equally
B. Negative automatic thoughts and cognitive distortions
C. Only positive thoughts
D. Nothing

69. Treatment fidelity means:

A. Being faithful to your spouse
B. Implementing treatment as designed and tested
C. Never adapting treatment
D. Random approach

70. Mindfulness skills teach:

A. Avoiding present moment
B. Observing without judgment
C. Suppressing thoughts
D. Controlling everything

71. Treatment goals should reflect:

A. Only therapist priorities
B. Insurance requirements only
C. What matters to the client
D. What's easiest

72. Systematic desensitization combines:

A. Relaxation training with graduated exposure
B. Medication only
C. Avoidance strategies
D. Nothing specific

73. Protective factors in formulation:

A. Don't matter
B. Are resources and strengths supporting recovery
C. Are the same as symptoms
D. Only include medication

74. Relapse prevention planning:

A. Isn't necessary
B. Prepares client for managing future challenges
C. Means treatment failed
D. Is only for substance use

75. The most important factor in treatment planning is:

A. Insurance approval
B. Collaboration between therapist and client
C. Following rigid protocol
D. Speed of planning

Answer Key with Detailed Explanations

1. B. Specific, Measurable, Achievable, Relevant, Time-bound
SMART goals are Specific (clearly defined), Measurable (you can track progress), Achievable (realistic given resources and constraints), Relevant (meaningful to the client), and Time-bound (have a target date). This framework ensures goals are actionable and progress can be evaluated. Vague goals like "feel better" don't guide treatment effectively. SMART goals like "reduce PHQ-9 score from 22 to below 15 within three months" provide clear direction.

2. C. Goals are developed jointly based on client values and clinical expertise
Collaborative goal setting means therapist and client work together. The client brings expertise about their life, values, and priorities. The therapist brings clinical expertise about what's achievable and what interventions can help. Neither imposes goals unilaterally. This collaboration increases client investment and ensures goals are meaningful, increasing treatment success.

3. C. Research evidence, clinical expertise, and client values
Evidence-based practice integrates three elements: best available research evidence about what works, clinical expertise to adapt interventions appropriately, and client values and circumstances to ensure treatment fits the individual. Using research evidence alone ignores individual differences. Using only clinical expertise ignores scientific knowledge. Using only client preference might miss effective treatments. Integration of all three optimizes outcomes.

4. B. Depression and anxiety disorders
CBT has strongest evidence for depression, various anxiety disorders (GAD, panic, social anxiety, specific phobias), OCD, PTSD, eating disorders, insomnia, and substance use. While CBT has some applications to other conditions, the strongest evidence base is for mood and anxiety disorders. This means you can confidently recommend CBT for these problems, knowing it's likely to help.

5. C. Borderline Personality Disorder
DBT was specifically developed by Marsha Linehan for Borderline Personality Disorder, particularly for individuals with chronic suicidal behavior and self-harm. It addresses emotion dysregulation, which is core to BPD. While DBT is now used for other conditions involving emotion dysregulation, it was originally designed for and has strongest evidence for BPD.

6. B. PTSD
Prolonged Exposure (PE) is an evidence-based treatment specifically for PTSD. It involves imaginal exposure (repeatedly recounting trauma in therapy) and in vivo exposure (gradually approaching trauma-related situations that are safe but avoided). PE helps process traumatic memories and reduce avoidance. While exposure is used for anxiety disorders too, PE specifically refers to the PTSD protocol.

7. B. Ambivalence about change
Motivational Interviewing was developed to address ambivalence—the mixed feelings people have about changing behavior. It's particularly effective for substance use because people often want to quit but also want to continue using. MI explores this ambivalence non-judgmentally, helping clients articulate their own reasons for change rather than having change imposed. This increases intrinsic motivation and reduces resistance.

8. C. "Client will attend work five days weekly"
Behavioral goals describe observable, measurable actions. You can observe and count work attendance. You can't directly observe "feeling better," "understanding," or "better relationships" without specific behavioral indicators. Behavioral goals allow objective progress measurement and clear evaluation of goal achievement.

9. B. 4-8 weeks
Short-term goals typically span 4-8 weeks—long enough to make meaningful progress but short enough to maintain focus and adjust course if needed. Long-term goals span months. Very short timeframes (days) don't allow enough time for change. Very long timeframes (years) are too distant to guide immediate action.

10. B. It identifies when treatment isn't working so adjustments can be made
Regular progress monitoring improves outcomes because it provides feedback about whether treatment is working. If a client isn't improving, you know early and can adjust approach before they drop out or fail. Without monitoring, you might continue ineffective treatment for months. While monitoring helps with documentation, the primary benefit is clinical—it improves care.

11. B. Depression
The PHQ-9 (Patient Health Questionnaire-9) measures depression severity using nine items corresponding to DSM diagnostic criteria. Scores range 0-27 with cutoffs for minimal, mild, moderate, moderately severe, and severe depression. It's quick to administer (2-3 minutes) and provides standardized measurement for tracking depression throughout treatment.

12. D. Moderately severe depression
PHQ-9 severity levels: 0-4 minimal, 5-9 mild, 10-14 moderate, 15-19 moderately severe, 20-27 severe. A score of 15-19 indicates moderately severe depression—significant symptoms requiring treatment, more severe than moderate but less severe than the highest category. Understanding these cutoffs helps evaluate symptom severity and track meaningful change.

13. B. How problems developed and what maintains them
Case formulation integrates assessment information to explain how problems developed (predisposing

and precipitating factors) and what maintains them currently (perpetuating factors). It's not just symptom description—it's explanation of mechanisms. This explanation guides treatment by identifying what to target. A good formulation makes clinical sense and guides intervention selection.

14. B. Fundamental assumptions about self, others, and world
Core beliefs are fundamental assumptions developed early in life through experiences. They shape how we interpret situations and guide emotions and behavior. Examples: "I'm competent/incompetent," "People are trustworthy/untrustworthy," "The world is safe/dangerous." Core beliefs aren't situation-specific—they're broad, pervasive views. They're resistant to change but can be modified with sustained therapeutic work.

15. B. What maintains problems currently
In CBT formulation, perpetuating factors are what maintains problems in the present—avoidance patterns, negative thinking, substance use, relationship dynamics, lack of skills. These are treatment targets because changing maintaining factors allows problems to resolve. Historical factors explain how problems developed but may not be changeable. Current maintaining factors are actionable targets.

16. B. Gradually facing fears while learning anxiety decreases
Exposure therapy works through habituation—anxiety naturally decreases with sustained exposure to feared situations. The person learns that feared outcomes don't occur and that they can tolerate anxiety. Avoidance prevents this learning. Graduated exposure starts with easier situations and progresses to harder ones. The goal isn't eliminating anxiety but learning to manage it and that situations are safe.

17. B. Increasing engagement in meaningful activities
Behavioral activation treats depression by increasing engagement in activities that provide pleasure and/or a sense of mastery. Depression causes withdrawal, which reduces positive experiences, which worsens depression. Breaking this cycle by scheduling and completing activities—even when you don't feel like it—improves mood. This isn't just staying busy—activities must be meaningful and provide pleasure or accomplishment.

18. B. Anxiety
The GAD-7 (Generalized Anxiety Disorder-7) measures anxiety severity using seven items. Scores range 0-21 with cutoffs for minimal, mild, moderate, and severe anxiety. While originally developed for generalized anxiety, it's a good general anxiety screener. It's quick to administer and provides standardized measurement for tracking anxiety.

19. C. Living documents that evolve with progress
Treatment plans should be living documents that evolve as treatment progresses. You review goals regularly and adjust based on progress. If goals are achieved, you develop new ones or prepare for termination. If progress stalls, you modify approach. Plans aren't static documents filed after the first session—they guide ongoing work and change with client needs.

20. C. Moving from clinical range to normal functioning
Clinically significant change means moving from clinical impairment to normal functioning range—

not just improvement, but meaningful recovery. Statistical significance (p-value) doesn't ensure clinical meaning—a small improvement might be statistically significant but leave the person still impaired. Clinical significance means real-world improvement that matters in the person's life.

21. C. Assess barriers and modify treatment
When progress stalls, assess why: Is diagnosis correct? Is client engaging in treatment? Are there missed maintaining factors (substance use, trauma, medical problems)? Is this the right treatment approach? Does intensity need increasing? Are you implementing competently? Once you identify barriers, modify treatment accordingly. Continuing ineffective treatment wastes time and may lead to dropout.

22. B. Examining and modifying negative thought patterns
Cognitive restructuring involves identifying negative automatic thoughts, examining evidence for and against them, identifying cognitive distortions, and developing more balanced alternative thoughts. It's not just positive thinking—it's developing realistic, evidence-based thinking. The process challenges thoughts like "Everyone thinks I'm stupid" by examining actual evidence and generating alternatives like "Some people probably like me, some don't, most aren't thinking about me at all."

23. B. "Client will attend social events comfortably within six months"
This goal is specific (attend social events), measurable (you can track attendance and self-reported comfort), achievable (with treatment), relevant (addresses client's social anxiety), and time-bound (six months). Options A, C, and D are unrealistic—complete elimination of anxiety or personality change isn't achievable or necessary. The goal is managing anxiety and functioning well, not eliminating normal human emotions.

24. C. Gradually approaching feared situations starting with easiest
Graduated exposure creates a hierarchy of feared situations from least to most anxiety-provoking. Treatment starts with easier situations, practicing until anxiety decreases, then progresses to harder situations. This builds tolerance and confidence. Starting with the hardest situation (flooding) can be overwhelming and cause dropout. Gradual progression is more tolerable and effective for most people.

25. C. PTSD symptoms
The PCL-5 (PTSD Checklist for DSM-5) measures PTSD symptoms using 20 items corresponding to DSM-5 criteria. It assesses all four symptom clusters: intrusion, avoidance, negative alterations in cognitions and mood, and alterations in arousal and reactivity. It's used to screen for PTSD and monitor treatment progress, showing which symptom clusters are most problematic.

26. B. Mindfulness, distress tolerance, emotion regulation, interpersonal effectiveness
DBT teaches four skill modules: mindfulness (observing present moment without judgment), distress tolerance (surviving crises without making things worse), emotion regulation (understanding and modifying intense emotions), and interpersonal effectiveness (asking for needs, saying no, maintaining relationships). These skills address emotion dysregulation core to BPD and other conditions.

27. B. Situation-specific thoughts influenced by core beliefs
Automatic thoughts are thoughts that pop into consciousness in specific situations. They're called "automatic" because they occur spontaneously without deliberate reasoning. They're influenced by underlying core beliefs and intermediate beliefs. In social anxiety, core belief "I'm socially incompetent" generates automatic thoughts like "Everyone thinks I'm boring." Automatic thoughts aren't always accurate—they're interpretations influenced by beliefs.

28. C. Observable, measurable actions
Behavioral goals describe what the person will do—observable, measurable actions. "Client will get out of bed by 9 AM five days weekly," "Client will attend therapy sessions weekly," "Client will practice breathing exercises daily." These can be observed and counted. Vague aspirations ("feel better") or internal states ("understand") aren't behavioral unless specified through observable indicators.

29. B. CBT with exposure
Evidence-based treatment for panic disorder is CBT including psychoeducation about panic, breathing retraining, cognitive restructuring of catastrophic thoughts, interoceptive exposure (inducing feared physical sensations), and situational exposure (approaching avoided situations). Medication can help but CBT addresses underlying mechanisms. Avoidance maintains panic—exposure breaks the cycle. Treatment works well when properly implemented.

30. C. Describe specific issues requiring attention
Problem statements in treatment plans describe specific issues identified in assessment—symptoms, functional impairments, relationship problems. Good problem statements are descriptive, not blaming: "Client experiences panic attacks 8-10 times weekly with avoidance of driving and shopping" rather than "Client is avoidant." Problem statements explain what needs to change, guiding goal development.

31. B. Exploring ambivalence and eliciting client's own reasons for change
Motivational Interviewing explores ambivalence non-judgmentally, helping clients articulate their own reasons for change rather than having reasons imposed. You express empathy, develop discrepancy between current behavior and values, roll with resistance (don't argue), and support self-efficacy. This increases intrinsic motivation. Confrontation and telling clients what to do typically increase resistance.

32. B. Situations, automatic thoughts, emotions, and alternative thoughts
Thought records capture: situation (what happened), automatic thoughts (what went through your mind), emotions (what you felt), evidence for and against thoughts, alternative thoughts (more balanced interpretations), and outcome (how you feel after developing alternatives). This documents cognitive work and shows progress in identifying and modifying thinking patterns. It makes the cognitive restructuring process concrete and trackable.

33. C. Specific goals, interventions, timeline, and progress measurement
Good treatment plans include: specific, measurable goals; interventions to achieve goals; timeline for goal achievement; responsible parties; and methods for measuring progress. Plans are collaborative—

developed with client input. They're clear enough that anyone reading them understands what you're working toward and how. They provide roadmap from current problems toward desired outcomes.

34. B. Bilateral stimulation while processing traumatic memories
EMDR (Eye Movement Desensitization and Reprocessing) involves bilateral stimulation—typically eye movements following therapist's fingers, but also taps or sounds—while the client processes traumatic memories. The bilateral stimulation is thought to facilitate reprocessing of memories so they become less distressing. EMDR has evidence for PTSD treatment and includes preparation, reprocessing, and integration phases.

35. C. Evidence, client factors, and practical considerations
Treatment selection should consider: research evidence (what's shown effective for this problem), client factors (preferences, strengths, limitations, cultural background), and practical considerations (availability, cost, time, transportation). You can't use treatment with no evidence hope it works. You can't ignore client factors and practical barriers. Effective selection integrates all considerations.

36. B. Life roles and activities
Functional goals focus on real-world roles and activities—work, relationships, parenting, self-care, hobbies, social engagement. These often matter most to clients: "Return to work full-time," "Attend children's activities," "Maintain friendships." Functional goals complement symptom goals. A person might still have some symptoms but function well, which is meaningful success.

37. B. Helps catch deterioration early
Session-by-session monitoring using brief measures (PHQ-9, GAD-7) after each session provides continuous feedback. Research shows therapists using regular monitoring have better outcomes—they identify deterioration early and adjust treatment. Without monitoring, therapists often don't realize clients aren't improving until they've struggled for weeks or dropped out. Brief measurement takes minutes but improves care.

38. B. Early in life through experiences
Core beliefs typically develop in childhood through experiences with caregivers, peers, and significant events. A child with responsive, supportive caregivers develops beliefs like "I'm competent" and "People are trustworthy." A child with neglectful, critical caregivers develops beliefs like "I'm inadequate" and "People will abandon me." While beliefs can form or change in adulthood, foundational ones typically develop early and persist.

39. B. How trauma affected beliefs and examining stuck points
Cognitive Processing Therapy for PTSD focuses on how trauma affected beliefs about safety, trust, power/control, esteem, and intimacy. Clients identify "stuck points"—problematic beliefs like "It was my fault" or "I can never trust anyone"—and examine evidence for and against them. Through Socratic questioning and written exercises, clients develop more balanced, adaptive beliefs. This reduces PTSD symptoms by changing trauma's meaning.

40. C. Diagnosis accuracy, treatment engagement, maintaining factors, treatment fit
When clients aren't improving, systematically assess: Is diagnosis correct? (Treating unipolar depression when it's bipolar won't work.) Is client engaging? (If not attending or completing

homework, treatment can't work.) Are there missed maintaining factors? (Substance use, domestic violence, medical problems can block progress.) Is this the right treatment approach? (Maybe evidence-based treatment for the diagnosis doesn't fit this client.) Then modify accordingly.

41. B. Increasing activities that provide pleasure and mastery
Activity scheduling in behavioral activation involves planning specific activities that provide pleasure (enjoyment) and/or mastery (sense of accomplishment). Depression causes withdrawal, reducing positive experiences, worsening mood. Scheduling activities—even when you don't feel like it—breaks this cycle. Activities must be meaningful, not just busywork. The client tracks activities and associated mood, showing the activity-mood connection.

42. B. Interpersonal problems
Interpersonal Therapy (IPT) treats depression by addressing interpersonal problems in four areas: grief (loss of important relationship), role disputes (conflicts in significant relationships), role transitions (life changes like retirement, becoming parent), or interpersonal deficits (social isolation, difficulties forming relationships). IPT helps resolve these problems, which alleviates depression. It's time-limited (12-16 sessions) and focused specifically on interpersonal issues.

43. B. Provide timeline for goal achievement
Target dates in treatment plans specify when goals should be achieved—short-term goals in 4-8 weeks, long-term goals in 3-6 months. Timelines create accountability, allow progress evaluation, and help pace treatment. Without timelines, treatment can drift indefinitely. Timelines aren't rigid—you adjust based on progress—but they provide structure and benchmarks for evaluating whether treatment is on track.

44. C. Prevent natural anxiety reduction and maintain anxiety
Safety behaviors are subtle avoidance strategies that prevent anxiety from decreasing naturally. Examples: gripping steering wheel tightly while driving (thinking this prevents accidents), rehearsing everything before social interaction (thinking this prevents embarrassment), carrying phone "in case of emergency." Safety behaviors maintain anxiety by preventing learning that feared outcomes don't occur and situations are safe. Effective exposure eliminates safety behaviors.

45. B. Goals for symptom reduction and functional improvement
Depression treatment plans should include both symptom goals (reduce depression severity, improve sleep, increase energy) and functional goals (return to work, engage in activities, maintain relationships). Complete symptom elimination may not be achievable or necessary—meaningful success is reduced symptoms plus improved functioning. Plans specify interventions (CBT, behavioral activation, possibly medication) and measurement methods (PHQ-9 scores, activity tracking).

46. B. Rules and assumptions flowing from core beliefs
Intermediate beliefs include rules ("I must be perfect or I'm worthless") and assumptions ("If I show weakness, people will reject me") that flow from core beliefs. Someone with core belief "I'm inadequate" develops rules about needing to compensate through perfection. Intermediate beliefs are more accessible to consciousness than core beliefs and are often targets in cognitive therapy before addressing deeper core beliefs.

47. C. Regularly throughout treatment
Progress should be measured regularly—ideally every session or every 2-4 weeks depending on measure. Regular measurement provides feedback about whether treatment is working, allows early identification of problems, guides treatment adjustments, and documents outcomes. Measuring only at termination misses opportunities to modify treatment. Progress monitoring should be routine, not just when required by external parties.

48. B. Acceptance and commitment to valued actions
Acceptance and Commitment Therapy (ACT) uses acceptance and mindfulness strategies combined with commitment and behavior change to increase psychological flexibility. Rather than fighting uncomfortable thoughts and feelings (which often increases distress), clients learn to accept them while committing to actions aligned with values. You can feel anxious and still attend the party. You can have sad thoughts and still engage in meaningful activities. Acceptance plus commitment creates psychological flexibility.

49. C. Be graduated and allow anxiety to decrease naturally
Effective exposure therapy is graduated (starting with easier situations and progressing), prolonged (staying in situation long enough for anxiety to decrease), and repeated (practicing multiple times). The person learns that anxiety decreases naturally without escape, that feared outcomes don't occur, and that they can handle situations. Rushing (flooding) can overwhelm. Brief exposure doesn't allow habituation. Safety behaviors prevent learning.

50. C. It's collaborative and based on client values
Treatment planning is most effective when collaborative—therapist and client jointly develop goals based on client values and priorities, using therapist's clinical expertise. This increases client investment, ensures goals are meaningful, and improves adherence. Therapist-imposed plans may address problems the therapist values but client doesn't, reducing motivation. Collaboration respects client autonomy while providing clinical guidance.

51. A. Examines sequence from trigger through actions to consequence
Chain analysis in DBT examines the sequence of events leading to problematic behavior (like self-harm): vulnerability factors (baseline conditions), prompting event (trigger), links in chain (thoughts, feelings, actions leading to target behavior), target behavior, and consequences. This detailed analysis identifies intervention points—places to interrupt the chain. It's not about blame but about understanding so the client can make different choices.

52. C. Multiple factors including diagnosis, engagement, maintaining factors, treatment fit
When treatment isn't working, consider multiple possibilities systematically: Wrong diagnosis? Treatment won't work if you're treating the wrong problem. Poor engagement? Treatment can't work if client isn't participating. Missed maintaining factors? Substance use, medical problems, trauma can block progress. Wrong treatment approach? Maybe evidence-based treatment for diagnosis doesn't fit this client. More intensive treatment needed? Once you identify problems, modify accordingly.

53. B. "Client will practice breathing techniques daily for two weeks"
This goal is specific (breathing techniques), measurable (daily practice trackable), achievable (two weeks is realistic), relevant (helps with anxiety management), and time-bound (two weeks). It

describes observable behavior. Options A, C, and D are vague or unrealistic. Good short-term goals are concrete, achievable stepping stones toward larger objectives.

54. B. Patterns of biased thinking
Cognitive distortions are patterns of biased, inaccurate thinking: all-or-nothing thinking (seeing things as black or white), overgeneralization (broad conclusions from single events), mental filter (focusing on negatives), discounting positives, jumping to conclusions, magnification/minimization, emotional reasoning (feeling means it's true), should statements, labeling, personalization. These patterns maintain depression and anxiety. Cognitive therapy identifies and challenges these distortions.

55. B. Be matched to problem severity and client needs
Treatment intensity should match problem severity and client needs. Mild depression might respond to brief therapy. Severe depression with suicidal ideation might require intensive outpatient or hospitalization. Active psychosis requires intensive treatment. Intensity can change—start intensive then step down, or increase if outpatient isn't sufficient. Match intensity to need rather than providing one-size-fits-all weekly therapy.

56. B. Learning anxiety decreases and situations are manageable
The goal of exposure therapy isn't eliminating anxiety—some anxiety is normal and adaptive. The goal is learning that: anxiety decreases naturally without escape (habituation), feared catastrophic outcomes don't actually occur, you can tolerate anxiety, and situations are manageable. This learning happens through experience, not through insight or reassurance. Exposure provides the experience that changes beliefs and reduces avoidance.

57. B. Increasing meaningful activities improves mood
Behavioral activation is based on the idea that increasing engagement in meaningful activities—those providing pleasure (enjoyment) or mastery (accomplishment)—improves mood. Depression causes withdrawal, which reduces positive experiences and reinforces depression. Breaking this cycle by scheduling and completing activities (even before you feel like it) improves mood through increased positive reinforcement. Activity change can drive mood change.

58. B. Measures progress toward individualized goals on a continuum (continued)
Goal Attainment Scaling measures progress on individualized goals using a scale: -2 (worse than baseline), -1 (baseline), 0 (expected outcome), +1 (better than expected), +2 (much better than expected). This allows measurement of progress on goals that don't have standardized measures. It's more nuanced than pass/fail and captures gradations of change. You define what each level looks like for each specific goal, making it highly individualized.

59. B. Shared and discussed with clients
Treatment plans should be shared with clients and developed collaboratively. Clients need to understand what you're working toward, how you'll get there, and how you'll measure progress. This transparency builds trust, increases engagement, and ensures you're addressing what matters to the client. Plans written in jargon and hidden from clients reduce collaboration and engagement. Treatment planning should be a joint process, not something done to the client.

60. B. How to survive crises without making things worse
Distress tolerance skills in DBT teach how to survive crises without engaging in behaviors that make things worse (self-harm, substance use, impulsive actions). Skills include distraction, self-soothing, improving the moment, and pros/cons. The goal isn't eliminating distress—it's getting through intense moments without destructive actions. Once the crisis passes, the person can use other skills or solve problems. Distress tolerance bridges the gap between crisis and effective action.

61. B. Vulnerabilities that existed before problems developed
Predisposing factors are vulnerabilities present before the current problem developed—genetic risk, temperament, childhood adversity, previous episodes, personality traits, learned patterns. These don't directly cause current problems but create susceptibility. Understanding predisposing factors helps explain why this person developed this problem and informs treatment (addressing underlying vulnerabilities, not just current symptoms).

62. B. Identify what's working and what needs adjustment
Progress monitoring provides feedback about whether treatment is effective. If measures show improvement, you know your approach is working. If they show no change or deterioration, you know something needs adjustment. This feedback loop—measure, evaluate, adjust—improves outcomes. Without monitoring, you continue approaches that aren't working or miss opportunities to build on success. Monitoring makes treatment responsive to the individual.

63. B. Understand and modify intense emotions
Emotion regulation skills in DBT help clients identify emotions accurately, understand what triggers them, reduce vulnerability to negative emotions (through sleep, nutrition, exercise, treating physical illness), increase positive emotions, and manage current emotions when they arise. The goal isn't eliminating emotions or only feeling positive—it's understanding emotions, reducing frequency of overwhelming emotions, and managing them effectively when they occur.

64. B. "Attend daughter's school events within six weeks"
This functional goal addresses a real-world activity that matters to the client—being present in their child's life. It's specific, measurable, achievable, relevant, and time-bound. It focuses on functioning (attending events) rather than just symptom elimination. Someone might still feel some anxiety but can function well—that's meaningful success. Unrealistic goals like "never feel anxious" or "be comfortable with everyone" aren't achievable or necessary.

65. B. What triggered current problems
Precipitating factors are events or circumstances that triggered the current episode—job loss, relationship ending, trauma, medical diagnosis, death of loved one. Not everyone who experiences these triggers develops problems (which is why predisposing factors matter), but precipitants explain timing—why now? Understanding precipitants helps with treatment (addressing grief, adjusting to change, processing trauma) and relapse prevention (preparing for future stressors).

66. B. How to ask for needs, say no, maintain relationships
Interpersonal effectiveness skills in DBT teach how to ask for what you need (while maintaining self-respect and relationship), say no to unwanted requests, and handle conflict effectively. This includes skills like DEAR MAN (Describe, Express, Assert, Reinforce, stay Mindful, Appear confident,

Negotiate) for asking for needs, and GIVE (be Gentle, act Interested, Validate, use an Easy manner) for maintaining relationships. These skills address interpersonal problems common in emotion dysregulation.

67. B. Develop new goals or prepare for termination
If a client achieves goals earlier than expected, you have options: develop new goals addressing other concerns, work on relapse prevention and skill consolidation, or prepare for termination if all significant concerns are addressed. You don't continue treatment indefinitely without purpose—that wastes resources and can create dependence. Celebrate success and determine next steps collaboratively.

68. B. Negative automatic thoughts and cognitive distortions
Cognitive restructuring specifically targets negative automatic thoughts (situation-specific negative interpretations) and cognitive distortions (patterns of biased thinking like all-or-nothing thinking, catastrophizing, overgeneralization). The process examines evidence for and against thoughts, identifies distortions, and develops more balanced alternatives. Not all thoughts are challenged—just problematic ones contributing to distress. Positive thoughts and realistic negative thoughts don't need challenging.

69. B. Implementing treatment as designed and tested
Treatment fidelity means implementing treatment as it was designed and tested in research—following the protocol, using specified techniques, maintaining intended structure and duration. High fidelity increases likelihood of achieving outcomes shown in research. Low fidelity (doing something quite different while calling it CBT or DBT) may not work as well. Some adaptation to individuals is necessary, but core elements should be maintained.

70. B. Observing without judgment
Mindfulness skills teach observing present moment experience without judgment—noticing thoughts, emotions, and sensations without trying to change, avoid, or cling to them. This includes observing (noticing), describing (putting words to experience), and participating (fully engaging). Mindfulness doesn't mean controlling or suppressing thoughts—it means being aware and accepting of present experience. This reduces suffering that comes from fighting reality.

71. C. What matters to the client
Treatment goals should reflect what matters to the client—their values, priorities, and desired outcomes. Goals imposed by therapist or insurance may not be meaningful to the client, reducing motivation and engagement. You provide expertise about what's achievable and how to get there, but the destination should be client-chosen. What would make their life better? What would success look like? Their answers guide goal development.

72. A. Relaxation training with graduated exposure
Systematic desensitization, developed by Joseph Wolpe, combines progressive muscle relaxation with graduated exposure to feared situations (initially through imagination, then in reality). The person learns to associate relaxation with previously feared stimuli. While classic systematic desensitization is less commonly used now (exposure alone is often sufficient), the principle of pairing relaxation with exposure remains useful for some clients, particularly those with very high anxiety.

73. B. Are resources and strengths supporting recovery
Protective factors are strengths, resources, and positive influences that support recovery—social support, employment, stable housing, effective coping skills, reasons for living, previous successful treatment, cultural identity, spirituality. Identifying protective factors helps you build on strengths rather than only addressing problems. Treatment that activates protective factors (strengthening relationships, connecting to community, building on existing skills) tends to be more effective and empowering.

74. B. Prepares client for managing future challenges
Relapse prevention planning prepares clients for managing future challenges and setbacks. You identify warning signs of relapse, develop strategies for managing them, create plan for what to do if symptoms return, and sometimes schedule booster sessions. Relapse prevention acknowledges that setbacks can occur but provides tools for managing them. It's not just for substance use—it applies to depression, anxiety, and other conditions with potential for recurrence.

75. B. Collaboration between therapist and client
The most critical factor in treatment planning is collaboration between therapist and client. Research consistently shows that the therapeutic relationship and client engagement predict outcomes more strongly than specific techniques. Collaborative planning—where both parties contribute expertise and work together—builds the alliance, increases client investment, ensures goals are meaningful, and improves adherence. Without collaboration, even evidence-based treatments may fail.

Bringing It Together

Treatment planning transforms assessment and diagnosis into action. You've identified the problems. You've understood how they developed and what maintains them. Now you create the roadmap from current suffering toward desired future.

The best plans are collaborative. You bring clinical expertise—knowledge of what works, understanding of change processes, awareness of obstacles. Your client brings personal expertise—knowledge of their life, clarity about values and priorities, awareness of resources and constraints. Together, you develop goals that matter and strategies that work.

Plans must be specific enough to guide action but flexible enough to adapt. Life happens. Circumstances change. New problems emerge. Unexpected barriers appear. Your plan evolves with these changes, always keeping sight of ultimate goals while adjusting the route.

Progress monitoring keeps treatment on track. You measure regularly, evaluate honestly, and adjust accordingly. When treatment works, you document success and build on it. When it doesn't, you problem-solve and modify. This feedback loop—plan, implement, measure, adjust—is treatment planning in action.

Never forget that behind every goal, every intervention, every progress measure is a person hoping for change. They're trusting you to help them build a better life. Honor that trust with careful planning, genuine collaboration, and persistent effort to help them achieve what matters most to them.

Core Principles to Guide Your Work

- SMART goals (Specific, Measurable, Achievable, Relevant, Time-bound) provide clear direction and allow objective evaluation of progress
- Collaborative goal setting between therapist and client increases engagement, ensures goals are meaningful, and improves treatment success
- Evidence-based practice integrates research evidence, clinical expertise, and client values to select treatments most likely to help
- CBT has strong evidence for depression and anxiety disorders while DBT was specifically developed for emotion dysregulation in BPD
- Exposure therapy gradually faces fears to learn that anxiety decreases naturally and situations are safe, not to eliminate all anxiety
- Behavioral activation increases meaningful activities to improve mood by breaking the withdrawal-reduced positive experiences cycle
- Treatment plans include problem statements, long and short-term goals, specific interventions, responsible parties, timelines, and progress measures
- Progress monitoring using standardized measures (PHQ-9, GAD-7, PCL-5) identifies what's working and guides treatment adjustments
- Case formulation explains how problems developed and what maintains them, guiding selection of treatment targets
- Core beliefs are fundamental assumptions developed early in life that shape automatic thoughts and emotional responses
- When progress stalls, systematically assess diagnosis accuracy, treatment engagement, maintaining factors, and treatment fit
- Functional goals focusing on life roles and activities often matter most to clients and represent meaningful recovery
- Treatment intensity should match problem severity and client needs, increasing or decreasing as appropriate
- Regular progress measurement throughout treatment improves outcomes by identifying problems early and guiding modifications
- The therapeutic relationship and collaborative planning predict outcomes as strongly as specific treatment techniques

Chapter 8: Special Populations Assessment

Assessment principles remain consistent across populations, but specific groups require adapted approaches. Children think differently than adults. Older adults face unique challenges. Couples present relational dynamics. Crisis situations demand immediate action. You adjust your assessment while maintaining core clinical skills.

Understanding developmental stages, cultural contexts, relationship patterns, and crisis dynamics allows you to assess accurately and intervene effectively. The same presenting problem—depression, for example—looks different and requires different assessment in a seven-year-old, a 45-year-old couple, and an 80-year-old with dementia.

Children and Adolescents

Assessing children and adolescents requires understanding normal development, gathering information from multiple sources, and recognizing that children's symptoms often differ from adult presentations. You can't just use adult assessment tools with younger wording—children's problems manifest differently.

Developmental considerations affect every aspect of assessment. A behavior that's concerning at age 10 might be developmentally normal at age 3. Temper tantrums are typical in toddlers, concerning in teenagers. Separation anxiety is normal at 18 months, problematic at 8 years. You must know developmental norms to distinguish problems from normal development.

Language and cognitive development affect the interview. Young children can't provide detailed histories or abstract descriptions of internal states. A seven-year-old can't explain "I've been depressed for three months with anhedonia and psychomotor retardation." They might say "I feel sad" or "Nothing is fun anymore." You adjust language, use concrete examples, and observe behavior.

Play-based assessment works when verbal skills are limited. Children communicate through play. A child who can't articulate trauma might reenact it with dolls. A child who can't describe anger might show it through aggressive play. You provide toys—dolls, puppets, art materials—and observe themes, emotions, and patterns in play.

Multiple informants are essential. Children may not recognize or report problems. Parents provide history and describe behaviors at home. Teachers report academic functioning and peer relationships. Each perspective reveals different aspects. Discrepancies between reports are common and provide clinical information—why does the child act differently at school than home?

Rating scales completed by parents and teachers standardize assessment. The **Child Behavior Checklist (CBCL)** assesses internalizing problems (anxiety, depression, somatic complaints, withdrawal) and externalizing problems (aggression, rule-breaking, attention problems). The **Conners**

Rating Scale assesses ADHD symptoms. The **Children's Depression Inventory (CDI)** and **Screen for Child Anxiety Related Disorders (SCARED)** assess specific symptoms.

Trauma assessment requires particular care. Children may not have words for traumatic experiences. They might not understand what happened. They may be afraid to tell. You create safety, use age-appropriate language, and don't push too hard. Signs of trauma include: regression (loss of previously achieved skills), reenactment in play, nightmares, hypervigilance, avoidance, clinging or fearfulness, aggression, sexualized behavior inappropriate for age.

Family dynamics profoundly affect children. You assess parent-child relationships, family structure, discipline approaches, parental mental health, family stress, and support systems. A child's problems often reflect family dysfunction. Treatment frequently involves family work, not just individual child therapy.

School functioning reveals much about development and adjustment. How are grades? Does the child complete homework? Do they have friends? Any behavioral problems? Learning difficulties? Bullying? School is a major context for children—problems there indicate significant issues.

Case Example: Assessment of Eight-Year-Old Mia

Mia, age 8, is referred by her pediatrician for behavioral problems. Her mother reports that Mia has become defiant, has frequent tantrums, refuses to do schoolwork, and fights with her younger brother constantly.

Assessment approach: You can't just interview Mia—she's eight. You gather information from multiple sources and use developmentally appropriate methods.

Parent interview: Mother describes escalating behavior over six months. Tantrums involve screaming, throwing things, occasionally hitting. Mia refuses to do homework, saying "I'm stupid" and "I can't do it." She used to play with her brother; now she's mean to him. Sleep is poor—she comes to mother's bed nightly saying she has bad dreams. Appetite is good. No recent losses or traumas that mother identifies.

You ask about family history. Mother has history of depression, currently struggling. Father travels frequently for work, gone 3-4 days weekly. Parents argue about parenting—mother feels overwhelmed and father thinks she's "too soft." Maternal grandmother died six months ago—she had been very close to Mia and provided childcare.

Child interview: Mia is initially reserved but warms up. You use simple language and concrete questions. She can identify feeling "sad" and "mad" but has limited emotional vocabulary. When asked what she wishes could be different, she says "I wish Grandma was here" and tears up. She says school is "too hard" and other kids are "mean." She describes bad dreams about "something chasing me."

Play observation: You provide art materials. Mia draws a picture of a house with stick figures. When asked to tell you about it, she points to small figure alone in a corner: "That's me. I'm in my room because I was bad." The other figures are distant. The drawing suggests isolation and negative self-perception.

Teacher report: Teacher completes Conners rating scale showing elevated scores for oppositional behavior and attention problems, but not at ADHD threshold. Teacher notes Mia seems "sad" and has withdrawn from friends. Academic performance has declined—she was a strong student, now struggles with assignments and gives up easily.

Behavioral observation: In session, Mia shows signs of depression—sad affect, low energy, self-critical statements. She's not oppositional with you, though mother describes frequent defiance at home. This discrepancy is clinically significant—behavior problems often manifest primarily at home when rooted in family dynamics or when the child feels safest expressing distress with parents.

Formulation: Mia is experiencing Major Depressive Disorder triggered by her grandmother's death (precipitating factor). Predisposing factors include genetic vulnerability (mother's depression) and possibly insecure attachment (father often absent, mother overwhelmed). Perpetuating factors include unresolved grief, family stress (parents' conflicts, father's absence), and mother's depression affecting parenting. Mia's "behavioral problems" are actually depression manifesting as irritability and defiance (common in children) plus grief.

Treatment plan:

- Individual therapy for Mia focusing on grief work and depression
- Parent guidance helping mother understand Mia's depression and improve parenting consistency
- Referral for mother to address her own depression
- Family session with father about his role and co-parenting
- Consultation with school about supporting Mia academically during this difficult period
- Possible medication evaluation if therapy alone isn't sufficient

Outcome: With treatment addressing the underlying depression and grief, Mia's "behavior problems" improve significantly. The problems weren't actually behavioral—they were depression presenting through irritability and acting out, which is common in children. Treating the depression and grief resolved the symptoms.

Adolescent assessment differs from younger children. Teens have cognitive capacity for abstract thinking and self-reflection but face unique developmental challenges.

Identity formation is central to adolescence. Teens ask: Who am I? What do I believe? What will I become? Problems during this period often relate to identity struggles—experimenting with different styles, values, friend groups.

Peer relationships gain enormous significance. Adolescents often care more about peer opinions than parent opinions—this isn't rejection of parents but normal developmental need to establish identity separate from family. Peer problems (bullying, rejection, social struggles) can trigger serious mental health problems.

Risk-taking increases due to brain development—reward systems mature faster than impulse control. Teens aren't stupid or self-destructive; their brains weight rewards differently. Assessment includes risk behaviors: substance use, sexual activity, dangerous driving, self-harm.

Parent-adolescent conflict is common and usually normal. Teens need to separate and assert autonomy. Parents struggle to let go while maintaining appropriate limits. You assess whether conflict is normative (disagreements about chores, curfew, friends) or problematic (violence, complete breakdown of relationship, severe defiance).

Confidentiality with adolescents requires balancing teen's need for privacy with parents' right to information and responsibility for safety. You explain limits of confidentiality upfront: what stays private, what you must share (imminent danger to self or others, abuse). You encourage teens to include parents in appropriate ways while respecting their need for some private space.

Substance use screening is essential with adolescents. Even if not the presenting problem, substance use affects mental health and development. Many teens experiment; you assess frequency, consequences, and whether use has become problematic.

Academic and legal problems often accompany mental health issues in adolescents. Declining grades, truancy, suspensions, or legal involvement signal significant problems requiring assessment.

Older Adults

Assessing older adults requires understanding normal aging, distinguishing aging from pathology, recognizing atypical symptom presentations, and addressing unique challenges this population faces.

Normal aging includes gradual changes that aren't pathological: some cognitive slowing (but not dementia), physical changes and chronic conditions, losses of loved ones and roles. You distinguish normal aging from mental health problems requiring treatment.

Depression in older adults often presents atypically. Rather than reporting sadness, older adults may present with:

- Somatic complaints (pain, fatigue, gastrointestinal problems)
- Cognitive complaints ("I think I have dementia")
- Irritability or anxiety rather than sadness
- Social withdrawal
- Neglect of self-care

Traditional depression screening might miss these presentations. You ask about sleep, appetite, energy, interest in activities, social engagement—not just "Are you depressed?" which older adults may deny.

Cognitive assessment distinguishes depression from dementia, which commonly co-occur. Depression can cause "pseudodementia"—cognitive problems that resolve with depression treatment. True dementia involves progressive cognitive decline that doesn't improve with mood treatment.

Mini-Mental State Examination (MMSE) briefly screens cognition: orientation, registration, attention/calculation, recall, language. Scores 24-30 suggest normal cognition, 18-23 mild impairment, 0-17 severe impairment. The **Montreal Cognitive Assessment (MoCA)** is more sensitive for detecting mild cognitive impairment.

Medication review is critical. Older adults take multiple medications; interactions and side effects can cause psychiatric symptoms. Anticholinergic medications cause confusion. Steroids trigger mood changes. Beta-blockers contribute to depression. Benzodiazepines increase fall risk and cognitive impairment. You obtain complete medication list including over-the-counter and supplements.

Medical comorbidities are common and affect mental health. Chronic pain causes depression. Heart disease affects mood and cognition. Diabetes complications include cognitive changes. Hypothyroidism mimics depression. You can't assess mental health in older adults without considering medical health.

Social support and isolation significantly affect older adults' mental health. Assess: living situation (alone or with others), social contacts (frequency of contact with family and friends), transportation access, ability to manage activities of daily living, financial resources. Isolation predicts poor outcomes; strong support predicts better ones.

Grief and loss are common. Older adults face loss of spouse, friends, health, independence, familiar roles. Multiple losses compound. Grief is normal, but prolonged complicated grief or major depression require treatment. You assess timing, intensity, and functional impact of grief.

Suicide risk is high in older adults, especially older white men. Risk factors include depression, chronic illness, chronic pain, isolation, recent losses, access to firearms. Older adults who attempt suicide are more likely to complete—they use more lethal means and are more serious about dying. You assess suicide risk carefully and directly.

Polypharmacy describes taking multiple medications. Older adults average 7-8 medications. More medications mean more side effects, more interactions, more confusion about regimens, more costs. You assess medication adherence and understanding—can the person explain what each medication is for and how to take it?

Elder abuse includes physical abuse, emotional abuse, financial exploitation, and neglect. Risk factors include cognitive impairment, physical dependence, social isolation, caregiver stress, and substance use. Signs include unexplained injuries, fearfulness around caregiver, poor hygiene, malnutrition, unpaid bills despite adequate income. You screen routinely and report suspicions as mandated.

Capacity assessment evaluates ability to make specific decisions—medical treatment, financial management, living arrangements. Capacity is decision-specific (someone might have capacity for some decisions but not others) and fluctuating (confusion might worsen at night or during illness). Legal competency determinations are made by courts, but you provide clinical input about capacity.

Case Example: Assessment of 75-Year-Old William

William, age 75, is brought to therapy by his daughter who's concerned about his memory and mood. William lives alone after his wife died one year ago. Daughter says he seems "not himself"—forgetful, no longer interested in golf, sometimes seems confused.

Clinical interview: William is cooperative but somewhat vague. He knows the date and location but struggles to recall recent events. He says he's "fine" but admits to poor sleep and decreased appetite. He misses his wife but says "that's life." He denies depression, saying "I'm not one to complain."

You ask specific questions about function:

- How's sleep? "Not good. I wake up early."
- How's appetite? "Nothing tastes good anymore."
- Do you still play golf? "No, I lost interest."
- Do you see friends? "Not really. Haven't felt like it."
- How do you spend your days? "I just sit mostly. Watch TV."
- Any physical pain? "My back hurts, my knees hurt. Getting old."

These responses suggest depression, not just aging.

Cognitive screening: You administer the MoCA. William scores 22/30—below normal cutoff of 26, suggesting mild cognitive impairment. He struggles with delayed recall and visuospatial tasks but does reasonably well on orientation and language.

Collateral information: Daughter provides crucial information. William has gotten lost driving twice—once to the grocery store he's been going to for 20 years. Bills are piling up unpaid, which is unlike him. He's not showering regularly. The house is messy, with spoiled food in the refrigerator. He's lost 15 pounds.

Medical review: William has hypertension, high cholesterol, and osteoarthritis. He takes six medications but daughter suspects he's not taking them consistently—bottles have more pills than they should given refill dates. Recent labs showed slightly elevated liver enzymes.

Functional assessment: Activities of Daily Living (ADLs)—bathing, dressing, toileting, transferring, continence, feeding—William manages independently though hygiene has declined. Instrumental Activities of Daily Living (IADLs)—managing finances, medications, shopping, housekeeping, transportation—William is struggling significantly.

Formulation: William presents with both depression and mild cognitive impairment. The depression is clear from neurovegetative symptoms (sleep, appetite, energy), anhedonia, social withdrawal, and passive suicidal thinking (he mentions "I'd be better off dead" when pressed). The cognitive impairment is shown by MoCA score and functional problems (getting lost, unpaid bills, medication mismanagement).

The question is: Which came first? Is this depression causing cognitive problems (pseudodementia)? Is it dementia causing depression? Or both co-occurring?

Based on timeline (cognitive problems emerged after wife's death along with clear depressive symptoms) and type of cognitive problems (motivation and attention difficulties more than memory), you suspect primary depression with secondary cognitive effects.

Treatment plan:

- Start antidepressant medication (SSRI—safe for older adults)
- Individual therapy focusing on grief and depression
- Medication management assistance (pill organizer, daughter oversight)
- Social worker referral for meal delivery and housekeeping support
- Reassess cognition after treating depression (if pseudodementia, cognition will improve)
- Family meeting about level of support needed
- Possible adult day program for structure and socialization

Safety planning: William isn't imminently suicidal but has passive ideation and several risk factors (recent loss, isolation, depression, chronic pain). You address gun safety (William has firearms—daughter secures them temporarily), increase contact (daughter calls daily, therapy weekly), and provide crisis numbers.

Outcome: After six weeks of treatment, William's mood improves significantly. His appetite and sleep normalize. He starts playing golf again. Importantly, his cognition improves—MoCA score increases to 26, and functional problems largely resolve. This confirms that cognitive impairment was secondary to depression (pseudodementia), not primary dementia. With continued treatment and support, William maintains improvement.

Couples and Families

Assessing couples and families requires understanding relationship patterns, communication dynamics, and systemic interactions—not just individual symptoms. The identified patient's problems often reflect relationship dysfunction requiring systemic intervention.

Presenting problem often focuses on one person—"My husband is depressed" or "Our son is defiant." Your task is broadening perspective to relationship and family patterns. How does the "problem" function in the relationship? What patterns maintain it?

Relationship history provides context. How did the couple meet? What attracted them to each other? How has the relationship changed over time? What were high points? What were crises? How did they handle past problems? Understanding the relationship's trajectory helps explain current difficulties.

Communication patterns reveal relationship dynamics. You observe:

- **Who speaks first and most**? Often indicates power dynamics.
- **Do partners listen to each other**? Or interrupt, talk over, dismiss?

- **What's the emotional tone**? Contemptuous? Defensive? Warm? Distant?
- **Do they make eye contact**? Physical orientation to each other reveals connection or distance.
- **Can they express needs directly**? Or indirectly through criticism or complaints?

Gottman's Four Horsemen predict relationship demise:

1. **Criticism**: Attacking partner's character ("You're so selfish") not behavior ("I felt hurt when...")
2. **Contempt**: Disrespect, disgust, mockery, eye-rolling. Most toxic pattern.
3. **Defensiveness**: Refusing responsibility, making excuses, counter-attacking
4. **Stonewalling**: Withdrawing, shutting down, refusing to engage

Conflict patterns reveal much about relationship health:

- **Demand-withdraw**: One partner demands discussion/change, other withdraws. Creates escalating cycle—more demand leads to more withdrawal leads to more demand.
- **Pursue-distance**: One partner pursues connection/intimacy, other distances. Pursuer feels rejected; distancer feels suffocated.
- **Attack-defend**: One attacks, other defends, escalating conflict without resolution.

Family structure assessment examines boundaries, hierarchies, alignments, and coalitions. Healthy families have clear generational boundaries—parents are in charge, children are children. Problematic patterns include:

- **Enmeshment**: Overly involved, no privacy, no individual identity
- **Disengagement**: Disconnected, little emotional connection or support
- **Triangulation**: Two people pull in third to manage their tension
- **Parentification**: Child takes on parental role with siblings or parents

Family life cycle stage affects functioning. Couples adjusting to new baby face different challenges than couples launching adolescents or adjusting to empty nest. Problems often emerge during transitions—stuckness at one stage or difficulty adapting to new demands.

Cultural factors shape family values, roles, and communication. What's normative in one culture is problematic in another. Extended family involvement valued in some cultures might be labeled "enmeshed" by therapists from other backgrounds. You assess within cultural context, not imposing your cultural norms.

Case Example: Couple Assessment - James and Maria

James and Maria, married 12 years with two children (ages 8 and 10), enter therapy. Maria scheduled the appointment, saying "James is depressed and won't get help." James attends reluctantly.

Initial session observation: Maria speaks first and dominates the conversation. She describes James's problems: he's withdrawn, irritable, drinks too much, doesn't help with kids. James sits with arms crossed, looking away. When he speaks, Maria interrupts with corrections and criticisms.

Presenting problem exploration: You ask each partner to describe the problem from their perspective without interruption.

Maria: "James has changed. He used to be fun and engaged. Now he comes home, drinks beer, and zones out in front of TV. He's irritable with the kids. He barely talks to me. I feel like a single parent. I think he's depressed and needs medication."

James: "Maria is always on me about something—I don't do enough, I'm not involved enough, I'm not present enough. Nothing I do is right. I work 50 hours a week to provide for this family. When I come home, I want some peace, but she has a list of complaints. So yeah, I have a beer and try to relax. Maybe I would talk more if she wasn't always criticizing."

You notice the demand-withdraw pattern immediately. Maria demands engagement and change; James withdraws. Her demands increase; his withdrawal increases.

Relationship history: They met in college, married young. Early years were happy—they laughed together, enjoyed shared interests. Maria stopped working when their first child was born. James took on more financial pressure. Maria felt isolated at home. James felt unappreciated. The pattern developed gradually—Maria asking for more help, James feeling criticized, Maria feeling ignored, James withdrawing.

Communication observation: You ask them to discuss a recent disagreement. They immediately reenact dysfunctional patterns:

Maria: "You were supposed to pick up Tommy from practice Tuesday but forgot."
James: "I didn't forget. I was stuck at work."
Maria: "You could have called. You always do this. You never follow through."
James: "Here we go again. Nothing I do is good enough." (crosses arms, looks away)
Maria: "Don't shut down! This is exactly what you do! You withdraw and leave me to handle everything alone."

The pattern is clear: Maria criticizes, James becomes defensive and withdraws, Maria pursues more intensely, James stonewalls. Both are stuck.

Individual assessment: You meet with each separately to assess for individual mental health problems.

James: Shows some depressive symptoms—low mood, decreased energy, anhedonia, increased alcohol use (4-5 beers nightly, up from 1-2 a year ago). But his depression seems reactive to relationship problems, not primary Major Depressive Disorder. The drinking is concerning but not yet Alcohol Use Disorder—no significant consequences, no tolerance or withdrawal. It's self-medication for relationship stress.

Maria: Shows anxiety symptoms—worry, tension, irritability, sleep problems. She feels overwhelmed by sole responsibility for home and children. She's lonely—James is physically present but emotionally absent. She's angry and resentful. Her pursuing and criticizing, while understandable, push James further away.

Formulation: This couple has developed a pursue-demand/withdraw-distance cycle that's maintained by each person's response to the other. Maria feels alone and pursues James for connection, but her pursuing comes out as criticism. James experiences the criticism as attack and withdraws to protect himself. His withdrawal confirms Maria's fears of abandonment and increases her pursuing. The cycle intensifies over time.

Neither partner is "the problem." They're stuck in a pattern where each person's attempted solution (Maria pursuing, James withdrawing) makes the problem worse. Both have individual symptoms (James's depression and drinking, Maria's anxiety) but these are secondary to relationship dysfunction.

Treatment plan:

- Couple therapy focusing on changing communication and breaking the pursue-withdraw cycle
- Teach each partner to recognize the pattern when it starts
- Help Maria express needs without criticism—using "I" statements, describing feelings not attacking character
- Help James stay engaged even when feeling criticized—responding instead of withdrawing
- Rebuild emotional connection through structured positive interactions
- Address individual symptoms (James's drinking, Maria's anxiety) as they relate to relationship dynamics
- Possible individual therapy for James if depression doesn't improve with relationship work

Interventions: You interrupt the pattern in session. When Maria begins criticizing, you intervene: "Maria, I hear that you're feeling alone and want more connection with James. Can you tell him that directly—what you want, not what he's doing wrong?"

Maria (hesitantly): "I miss you. I want to feel like we're a team again. I want to talk and laugh like we used to."

This is vulnerability, not criticism. You ask James to respond.

James (surprised, softening): "I miss that too. I don't want to fight. I just feel like I can't do anything right, so I shut down."

This is the beginning of change—getting underneath the criticism-withdrawal cycle to the vulnerable needs and feelings beneath. Treatment continues helping them communicate these needs without triggering the dysfunctional pattern.

Family assessment considers how the entire family system functions. You might meet with whole family, observe parent-child interactions, and assess how family patterns contribute to the identified patient's problems.

Presenting problem in family context: A child is acting out. But observation reveals parents are in conflict about discipline. One is strict, the other permissive. The child has learned to play them against each other. Parents' conflict gets expressed through battles over the child's behavior. The child's acting out serves a function—it unites the parents (against the child) and distracts from marital problems.

Family roles may be rigid and problematic. One child is "the good one," another "the problem." A parent confides in a child about adult issues (parentification). Siblings compete for parental approval. You identify these patterns and help families develop healthier dynamics.

Crisis Situations

Crisis assessment requires immediate evaluation of safety, rapid decision-making about intervention level, and quick action to stabilize the situation. Standard comprehensive assessment isn't possible or appropriate during crisis.

Crisis defined: A crisis is a time-limited, intense emotional response to a hazardous event that exceeds the person's usual coping resources. The person is in disequilibrium—normal functioning is disrupted. Crisis intervention goal is stabilization and return to pre-crisis functioning, not comprehensive treatment.

Immediate safety assessment comes first. Is the person dangerous to self or others right now? Do they need hospitalization? This overrides everything else. You assess:

- Suicidal ideation, intent, plan, means
- Homicidal ideation, intent, plan, means, access to victim
- Ability to care for self (eating, hygiene, basic functioning)
- Judgment and decision-making capacity
- Substance intoxication or withdrawal
- Psychotic symptoms affecting reality testing

ABC model provides structure for crisis assessment:

A - Antecedents: What led to this crisis? What's the precipitating event? Understanding triggers helps with intervention.

B - Behavior: What's the person doing now? How are they functioning? What symptoms are present? Observable behavior provides concrete information.

C - Consequences: What are results of the behavior? What happens if you don't intervene? What's at risk? Understanding consequences guides intervention level.

Crisis intervention principles:

- **Immediate**: Act now, don't wait
- **Proximal**: Intervene where the crisis is occurring when possible
- **Time-limited**: Crisis intervention is brief, focused on stabilization
- **Focused on current crisis**: Don't do psychotherapy or address longstanding problems
- **Action-oriented**: Provide concrete help and direction
- **Goal of return to baseline**: Restore pre-crisis functioning

Support mobilization activates resources:

- Family and friends who can provide support
- Community resources (crisis lines, mobile crisis teams, emergency services)
- Existing providers (therapist, psychiatrist, case manager)
- Natural supports (church, neighbors, coworkers)

Crisis intervention isn't therapy—it's stabilization. Once stabilized, the person may need ongoing treatment, but during crisis you focus on immediate safety and coping.

Involuntary hospitalization becomes necessary when:

- Person is imminent danger to self (active suicide plan with intent)
- Person is imminent danger to others (credible homicidal threat)
- Person is gravely disabled (can't meet basic needs due to mental illness)

You initiate emergency detention when less restrictive options won't ensure safety. This isn't punitive—it's protection. Most people experiencing psychiatric emergencies aren't dangerous, but when they are, hospitalization saves lives.

Mobile crisis teams provide assessment and intervention in the community—at home, school, or wherever crisis occurs. They can assess whether hospitalization is needed or whether crisis can be managed with intensive community support. When available, mobile crisis prevents unnecessary emergency room visits and hospitalizations.

Case Example: Crisis Assessment - Kevin

You receive a crisis call about Kevin, a 28-year-old man. His girlfriend called 911 after he sent her a text: "I can't do this anymore. I'm sorry. Goodbye." Police transported Kevin to the emergency room, where you're conducting psychiatric evaluation.

Immediate safety assessment: Kevin is tearful, agitated, but cooperative. He reports suicidal thoughts: "I want to die. I can't handle this pain anymore."

You ask specific questions:

- "Do you have a plan for how you would kill yourself?" "I was going to shoot myself. I have a gun at home."
- "When were you planning to do this?" "Tonight. I was going to do it when I got home."
- "What stopped you?" "My girlfriend figured it out and called 911. I'm glad she did. I'm scared of what I might do."
- "Are you having thoughts of hurting anyone else?" "No, just myself."

Kevin presents **imminent suicide risk**: specific plan, high-lethality means (gun), intent to act tonight, no alternative safety strategies. This requires immediate intervention—hospitalization.

Crisis assessment: You assess briefly what led to this:

Antecedent: Kevin was laid off from his job two weeks ago. His father died by suicide when Kevin was 16. Kevin's been depressed for months but the job loss triggered acute crisis. He drank heavily last night, which increased impulsivity and worsened mood.

Behavior: Kevin is having active suicidal thoughts with plan and intent. He's tearful, hopeless, and sees no alternatives. He hasn't been eating or sleeping. He's been drinking daily.

Consequences: Without intervention, Kevin is at high risk of suicide attempt tonight. He has means (gun), plan, intent, and opportunity.

Decision: Kevin needs voluntary or involuntary psychiatric hospitalization. You explain: "Kevin, I understand you're in terrible pain right now. The good news is this pain can be treated. But you're not safe to go home tonight. You need to be in the hospital where we can keep you safe and start treatment."

Kevin agrees to voluntary admission. If he'd refused, you would initiate involuntary hold based on imminent danger to self.

Crisis intervention: While arranging admission, you provide immediate support:

- Validate his pain: "You're going through something very difficult. The job loss and your father's suicide make this especially hard."
- Install hope: "This pain feels permanent right now, but it's not. Depression is treatable. This crisis will pass."
- Remove means: "Your girlfriend is securing the gun. It won't be accessible when you leave the hospital."
- Mobilize support: "Your girlfriend is here and wants to help. We're also contacting your sister."

Hospital admission: Kevin is admitted to inpatient psychiatric unit. Treatment includes medication for depression, safety monitoring, therapy processing current crisis and grief about father's suicide, and discharge planning with outpatient follow-up.

Outcome: After five days, Kevin's acute crisis resolves. Suicidal ideation decreases significantly with medication and support. He develops safety plan and engages with outpatient treatment. Crisis intervention and hospitalization likely saved his life.

Practice Questions

1. When assessing children, you should:

A. Only interview the child
B. Gather information from multiple sources
C. Rely solely on parent report
D. Use only standardized tests

2. Play-based assessment is useful because:

A. It's fun
B. Children communicate through play when verbal skills are limited
C. It replaces verbal assessment
D. It's faster than interviews

3. Depression in children often presents as:

A. Sadness only
B. Irritability and behavioral problems
C. The same as adult depression
D. Always mild

4. The Child Behavior Checklist (CBCL) assesses:

A. Intelligence
B. Internalizing and externalizing problems
C. Only ADHD
D. Academic achievement

5. When assessing adolescents, confidentiality:

A. Is absolute
B. Requires balancing teen privacy with parent rights and safety
C. Means telling parents everything
D. Doesn't matter

6. Increased risk-taking in adolescence results from:

A. Poor judgment
B. Brain development with reward systems maturing faster than impulse control
C. Bad parenting
D. Peer pressure only

7. Depression in older adults often presents with:

A. Clear reports of sadness
B. Somatic complaints and cognitive concerns
C. The same symptoms as younger adults
D. No symptoms

8. The Mini-Mental State Examination (MMSE) screens for:

A. Depression
B. Anxiety
C. Cognitive impairment
D. Personality disorders

9. Pseudodementia refers to:

A. Faking cognitive problems
B. Cognitive problems from depression that resolve with treatment
C. Early Alzheimer's disease
D. Normal aging

10. Elder abuse includes:

A. Only physical abuse
B. Physical, emotional, financial, and neglect
C. Only neglect
D. Nothing measurable

11. Polypharmacy in older adults:

A. Is always beneficial
B. Increases risk of side effects and interactions
C. Should be encouraged
D. Doesn't affect mental status

12. When assessing couples, you should observe:

A. Only what they report
B. Communication patterns and interactions
C. Only individual symptoms
D. Nothing beyond verbal content

13. Gottman's "Four Horsemen" that predict relationship problems are:

A. Communication, trust, intimacy, commitment
B. Criticism, contempt, defensiveness, stonewalling
C. Love, respect, honesty, loyalty
D. Anger, sadness, fear, joy

14. The demand-withdraw pattern involves:

A. Equal communication
B. One partner demanding discussion while other withdraws
C. Both partners communicating clearly
D. No specific pattern

15. Contempt in relationships is characterized by:

A. Healthy disagreement
B. Disrespect, mockery, and disgust
C. Temporary anger
D. Normal conflict

16. In family assessment, enmeshment refers to:

A. Close, healthy relationships
B. Overly involved relationships with no privacy or boundaries
C. Distant relationships
D. Normal family closeness

17. Parentification occurs when:

A. Parents act like parents
B. Children take on parental responsibilities
C. Families have clear boundaries
D. Parents are involved

18. In crisis assessment, immediate priority is:

A. Complete history
B. Safety evaluation
C. Insurance verification
D. Detailed diagnosis

19. Crisis intervention is:

A. Long-term therapy
B. Time-limited, focused on stabilization
C. Comprehensive treatment
D. Unnecessary

20. Involuntary hospitalization is appropriate when:

A. Person refuses outpatient treatment
B. Person is imminent danger to self or others
C. Family requests it
D. Therapist is frustrated

21. Collateral information from teachers helps assess:

A. Only intelligence
B. School functioning and peer relationships
C. Nothing useful
D. Only academic problems

22. The Montreal Cognitive Assessment (MoCA) is more sensitive than MMSE for detecting:

A. Depression
B. Anxiety
C. Mild cognitive impairment
D. Personality changes

23. When a child's behavior differs significantly at school versus home, this suggests:

A. The child is manipulative
B. Environmental factors affecting behavior
C. Nothing meaningful
D. Always pathology

24. Adolescents' focus on peer relationships over parents is:

A. Abnormal
B. Developmentally normal identity work
C. Signs of family problems
D. Always concerning

25. Capacity assessment evaluates:

A. Intelligence
B. Ability to make specific decisions
C. Overall competence
D. Likeability

26. In couple therapy, triangulation occurs when:

A. Three people communicate openly
B. Two people pull in third to manage their tension
C. Couples have children
D. Families are healthy

27. Grief in older adults:

A. Is always pathological
B. Is normal but can become complicated requiring treatment
C. Never requires treatment
D. Doesn't occur

28. Mobile crisis teams:

A. Only work in hospitals
B. Provide assessment and intervention in community
C. Are unnecessary
D. Only transport to hospitals

29. Activities of Daily Living (ADLs) include:

A. Managing finances and shopping
B. Bathing, dressing, toileting, feeding
C. Only walking
D. Cognitive tasks

30. Instrumental Activities of Daily Living (IADLs) include:

A. Only personal hygiene
B. Managing finances, medications, housekeeping
C. Only eating
D. Physical mobility only

31. Trauma assessment in children requires:

A. Immediate detailed questioning
B. Age-appropriate language and creating safety
C. Confronting the child
D. Only talking to parents

32. When parents disagree about discipline:

A. One parent is always right
B. Children may act out and play parents against each other
C. It has no impact
D. Children always benefit

33. Stonewalling in relationships means:

A. Healthy boundaries
B. Withdrawing and refusing to engage
C. Active listening
D. Clear communication

34. Older adults who attempt suicide:

A. Are less likely to complete
B. Are more likely to complete due to lethal means and serious intent
C. Never complete
D. Are just seeking attention

35. The ABC model of crisis assessment examines:

A. Always Be Caring
B. Antecedents, Behavior, Consequences
C. Assessment, Baseline, Comparison
D. Nothing specific

36. Medication review in older adults is critical because:

A. All medications are dangerous
B. Multiple medications increase side effects and interactions
C. Older adults don't need medications
D. It's not actually important

37. A child drawing violent or disturbing pictures:

A. Always indicates abuse
B. May indicate trauma but requires further assessment
C. Is always normal
D. Should be ignored

38. Pursue-distance pattern in couples involves:

A. Both seeking connection equally
B. One pursuing intimacy while other distances
C. Healthy communication
D. No specific dynamic

39. Assessing suicide risk in older adults requires:

A. Assuming they're not serious
B. Direct, careful questioning
C. Avoiding the topic
D. Only asking once

40. Crisis intervention goals include:

A. Solving all longstanding problems
B. Stabilization and return to baseline
C. Long-term therapy
D. Complete personality change

41. When children regress after trauma:

A. It indicates developmental delay
B. It's a common trauma response
C. It should be punished
D. It's manipulative

42. Family life cycle transitions:

A. Have no impact
B. Often trigger problems as families adjust
C. Are always smooth
D. Only affect adults

43. Capacity is:

A. All-or-nothing
B. Decision-specific and can fluctuate
C. Permanent once lost
D. The same as intelligence

44. Multiple informants in child assessment:

A. Create confusion
B. Provide different perspectives revealing full picture
C. Are unnecessary
D. Always agree

45. Somatic complaints in older adults with depression:

A. Are always medical problems
B. May be depression presenting atypically
C. Should be ignored
D. Never require medical evaluation

46. During crisis, assessment should be:

A. Comprehensive as always
B. Focused on immediate safety
C. Delayed until later
D. Unnecessary

47. Disengagement in families refers to:

A. Healthy independence
B. Disconnection with little emotional support
C. Normal boundaries
D. Temporary distance

48. Anticholinergic medications in older adults can cause:

A. No problems
B. Confusion and cognitive impairment
C. Better memory
D. Increased energy

49. When assessing families, cultural factors:

A. Don't matter
B. Shape values, roles, and what's normative
C. Are the same across families
D. Should be ignored

50. A crisis is defined as:

A. Any problem
B. Time-limited intense response exceeding usual coping
C. Chronic difficulty
D. Minor stressor

Answer Key with Detailed Explanations

1. B. Gather information from multiple sources
Child assessment requires multiple informants—child, parents, teachers—because children may not recognize or report problems, and behavior varies across contexts. Each perspective reveals different aspects. Parents know history and home behavior. Teachers report academic and peer functioning. The child provides their subjective experience. Discrepancies between sources are clinically meaningful.

2. B. Children communicate through play when verbal skills are limited
Young children lack verbal skills and abstract thinking to articulate internal experiences. Play provides a natural medium for communication—children reenact experiences, express emotions, and reveal themes through play. A child who can't verbalize trauma might show it through aggressive play or reenact scenarios with dolls. Play observation reveals information not accessible through interview.

3. B. Irritability and behavioral problems
Depression in children often presents differently than in adults. Rather than clearly reporting sadness, children may show irritability, behavioral problems, social withdrawal, declining school performance, and somatic complaints. Parents often bring children for "behavior problems" without recognizing underlying depression. Understanding atypical presentations prevents misdiagnosis.

4. B. Internalizing and externalizing problems
The CBCL assesses both internalizing problems (anxiety, depression, somatic complaints, withdrawal) and externalizing problems (aggression, rule-breaking, attention problems). Parents and teachers complete versions appropriate to their context. It provides standardized measurement of broad behavioral and emotional functioning, helping identify problem areas requiring assessment and intervention.

5. B. Requires balancing teen privacy with parent rights and safety
Adolescent confidentiality requires balancing competing needs: teen's need for privacy to discuss sensitive issues, parents' right to information about their minor child, and safety requirements. You explain upfront what's private and what must be shared (danger to self or others, abuse). You encourage teens to include parents appropriately while respecting developmental need for some privacy.

6. B. Brain development with reward systems maturing faster than impulse control
Adolescent risk-taking results from uneven brain development—the reward system (especially for social rewards) develops rapidly during adolescence while the prefrontal cortex (impulse control, judgment) develops more slowly. Teens understand risks but weight rewards differently. This isn't poor judgment or bad parenting—it's normal neurodevelopment. Understanding this prevents pathologizing normal adolescence.

7. B. Somatic complaints and cognitive concerns
Depression in older adults often presents atypically with somatic complaints (pain, fatigue, gastrointestinal problems), cognitive concerns ("I think I have dementia"), irritability, or social withdrawal rather than clearly reported sadness. Traditional screening might miss these presentations. Asking about sleep, appetite, energy, interest, and social engagement—not just "Are you depressed?"—improves detection.

8. C. Cognitive impairment
The MMSE briefly screens cognitive functioning, assessing orientation, registration, attention/calculation, recall, and language. It doesn't diagnose specific causes but identifies cognitive impairment requiring further evaluation. Scores 24-30 suggest normal cognition, 18-23 mild impairment, 0-17 severe impairment. Used in older adults to screen for dementia or delirium and track cognitive changes.

9. B. Cognitive problems from depression that resolve with treatment
Pseudodementia refers to cognitive impairment caused by depression that improves when depression is treated. Depression can cause poor concentration, memory problems, and difficulty with complex tasks that mimic dementia. True dementia is progressive and doesn't resolve with mood treatment. Distinguishing these requires careful assessment and sometimes trial of depression treatment with cognitive reassessment.

10. B. Physical, emotional, financial, and neglect
Elder abuse encompasses physical abuse (hitting, restraining), emotional abuse (threats, humiliation), financial exploitation (stealing money, coercion), sexual abuse, and neglect (failure to provide care, abandonment). It's common but underreported. Social workers screen routinely, recognize warning signs (unexplained injuries, fearfulness, poor hygiene, unpaid bills despite adequate income), and report as mandated reporters.

11. B. Increases risk of side effects and interactions
Polypharmacy (taking multiple medications) is common in older adults who average 7-8 medications. More medications mean increased risk of side effects, drug interactions, confusion about regimens, and falls. Some medications interact to cause psychiatric symptoms. Comprehensive medication review identifies problematic medications, interactions, and adherence issues affecting mental status.

12. B. Communication patterns and interactions
Couple assessment requires observing how partners communicate and interact, not just what they report. You observe: who speaks first and most, whether they listen or interrupt, emotional tone, nonverbal behavior (eye contact, body orientation), whether they express needs directly or through criticism. These observations reveal relationship dynamics that partners may not describe accurately.

13. B. Criticism, contempt, defensiveness, stonewalling

Gottman identified four communication patterns that predict relationship failure: criticism (attacking character not behavior), contempt (disrespect, disgust, mockery—most toxic), defensiveness (refusing responsibility, counter-attacking), and stonewalling (withdrawing, refusing to engage). Presence of these "four horsemen"—especially contempt—predicts divorce with high accuracy. Identifying these patterns guides intervention.

14. B. One partner demanding discussion while other withdraws

Demand-withdraw pattern involves one partner pursuing discussion or change while the other withdraws and avoids. This creates escalating cycle—more demand triggers more withdrawal triggers more demand. Often the demanding partner feels unheard and pursues harder; the withdrawing partner feels attacked and distances more. Both partners' responses maintain the problematic cycle.

15. B. Disrespect, mockery, and disgust

Contempt is the most toxic of Gottman's Four Horsemen. It involves treating partner with disrespect, mockery, sarcasm, disgust, or superiority—eye-rolling, name-calling, hostile humor. Contempt communicates "I'm better than you" and destroys the respect and admiration necessary for relationship health. Presence of contempt strongly predicts relationship failure.

16. B. Overly involved relationships with no privacy or boundaries

Enmeshment describes overly involved family relationships with diffuse boundaries—everyone knows everything about everyone, little privacy, difficulty with individual identity separate from family. Members are overly reactive to each other's moods and problems. This prevents healthy individuation. It differs from normal closeness by interfering with autonomy and individual development.

17. B. Children take on parental responsibilities

Parentification occurs when children carry adult responsibilities—emotionally caring for parents, managing household tasks, parenting younger siblings. This role reversal interferes with normal child development. The child's needs go unmet while meeting others' needs. This can create competence but at the cost of childhood and creates later difficulties with boundaries and self-care.

18. B. Safety evaluation

During crisis, immediate priority is safety assessment—is the person dangerous to self or others right now? This overrides everything else including detailed history, diagnosis, or insurance. You assess suicidal/homicidal risk, ability to care for self, judgment, reality testing. Safety evaluation determines intervention level (outpatient support vs. hospitalization). Comprehensive assessment comes after stabilization.

19. B. Time-limited, focused on stabilization

Crisis intervention is brief, focused intervention aimed at stabilizing the situation and returning the person to pre-crisis functioning. It's not long-term therapy or comprehensive treatment. Goals are immediate: ensure safety, reduce symptoms, restore coping, mobilize supports. Once stabilized, the person may need ongoing treatment, but crisis intervention itself is time-limited and focused on current crisis.

20. B. Person is imminent danger to self or others
Involuntary hospitalization is appropriate when the person is imminent danger to self (active suicide plan with intent), imminent danger to others (credible homicidal threat), or gravely disabled (can't meet basic needs due to mental illness). This isn't punishment—it's protection. It requires specific dangerousness criteria, not just family preference or refusing treatment. It's used only when less restrictive options won't ensure safety.

21. B. School functioning and peer relationships
Teacher reports provide information about academic functioning, behavior in classroom, attention and concentration, peer relationships, and any concerning changes. Teachers observe children in structured settings with peers—different from home context. Their perspective reveals how the child functions outside family, identifies learning problems, and provides comparison to developmental norms.

22. C. Mild cognitive impairment
The MoCA (Montreal Cognitive Assessment) is more sensitive than MMSE for detecting mild cognitive impairment—subtle changes that might not show on MMSE. It includes more challenging tasks assessing executive function, abstraction, and complex attention. Cutoff is 26/30 (versus MMSE's 24/30). Used increasingly in older adults to detect early cognitive changes requiring monitoring or intervention.

23. B. Environmental factors affecting behavior
When children behave significantly differently across contexts (fine at school but problematic at home, or vice versa), this suggests environmental factors—not inherent pathology or manipulation. The child adapts to different demands and relationships in different settings. Understanding what's different about each environment guides intervention. Perhaps home has inconsistent discipline, or school has bullying problems.

24. B. Developmentally normal identity work
Adolescents' focus on peer relationships is developmentally normal and necessary for identity formation. Teens need to establish identity separate from family—this happens through peer relationships. Peer opinions matter intensely not because teens don't love parents but because peers help answer "Who am I among people like me?" This isn't rejection of parents—it's normal development.

25. B. Ability to make specific decisions
Capacity assessment evaluates ability to make specific decisions—medical treatment, financial management, living arrangements. It's decision-specific (someone might have capacity for some decisions but not others) and can fluctuate (confusion might worsen at night or during illness). Legal competency is determined by courts, but clinicians provide input about capacity for specific decisions.

26. B. Two people pull in third to manage their tension
Triangulation occurs when two people pull a third person into their relationship to manage anxiety or tension between them. Parents in marital conflict focus on child's behavior instead of addressing their relationship. Two siblings pull in parent to mediate. The triangle reduces immediate tension but prevents resolution between the original two and burdens the third person.

27. B. Is normal but can become complicated requiring treatment
Grief is normal response to loss—older adults face multiple losses of loved ones, health, independence, roles. Normal grief includes emotional pain, yearning, preoccupation with deceased, but gradually improves. Complicated grief persists unchanged for many months or includes specific features (intense guilt, identity confusion, suicidal ideation). Major depression can develop following loss. Normal grief doesn't require treatment, but complicated grief and depression do.

28. B. Provide assessment and intervention in community
Mobile crisis teams provide psychiatric assessment and crisis intervention in community settings—at home, school, or wherever crisis occurs. They assess whether hospitalization is needed or whether crisis can be managed with community support. When available, mobile crisis prevents unnecessary emergency room visits and hospitalizations, assesses in person's natural environment, and provides immediate intervention.

29. B. Bathing, dressing, toileting, feeding
Activities of Daily Living (ADLs) are basic self-care tasks: bathing, dressing, toileting, transferring (moving from bed to chair), continence, and feeding. These are fundamental functions necessary for independent living. Assessment of ADLs indicates level of physical dependence and need for assistance. Problems with ADLs suggest significant physical or cognitive impairment.

30. B. Managing finances, medications, housekeeping
Instrumental Activities of Daily Living (IADLs) are more complex tasks necessary for independent living: managing finances, taking medications correctly, shopping, housekeeping, food preparation, telephone use, and transportation. IADLs require more cognitive function than ADLs. Problems with IADLs emerge earlier in cognitive decline than problems with basic ADLs.

31. B. Age-appropriate language and creating safety
Trauma assessment in children requires creating safety, using age-appropriate language, and respecting the child's pace. Children may not have words for traumatic experiences. They may not understand what happened. They may be afraid to tell. You don't push too hard too soon (can re-traumatize). You watch for behavioral indicators in play, look for trauma-related symptoms, and create conditions where child can disclose when ready.

32. B. Children may act out and play parents against each other
When parents disagree about discipline, children learn to play parents against each other, testing limits with the more permissive parent and avoiding the stricter one. Parental conflict often gets expressed through battles over child's behavior. The child's acting out may serve function of uniting parents (against child) or distracting from marital problems. Consistent discipline requires parental agreement.

33. B. Withdrawing and refusing to engage
Stonewalling is withdrawing from interaction, shutting down, refusing to engage in conversation. The person might turn away, give one-word answers, or leave the room. Stonewalling protects the withdrawing partner from feeling overwhelmed but leaves the other partner feeling abandoned and increases their pursuing. It's one of Gottman's Four Horsemen predicting relationship failure.

34. B. Are more likely to complete due to lethal means and serious intent
Older adults who attempt suicide are more likely to complete than younger people because they use more lethal means (especially firearms), have more serious intent (less ambivalence), and are more socially isolated (less likely to be discovered). Suicide attempts in older adults aren't attention-seeking—they're deadly serious. Risk assessment must be thorough, and intervention must be immediate.

35. B. Antecedents, Behavior, Consequences
The ABC model structures crisis assessment: Antecedents (what led to crisis, precipitating events), Behavior (what person is doing now, current functioning and symptoms), Consequences (what happens if you don't intervene, what's at risk). This framework ensures you understand the crisis context, assess current status, and evaluate need for intervention.

36. B. Multiple medications increase side effects and interactions
Comprehensive medication review in older adults is critical because they take multiple medications (polypharmacy) increasing risk of side effects, drug interactions, and confusion. Many medications affect mental status—anticholinergics cause confusion, steroids affect mood, beta-blockers contribute to depression. You can't assess mental health without knowing what medications might be contributing to symptoms.

37. B. May indicate trauma but requires further assessment
Violent or disturbing drawings may indicate trauma but don't automatically confirm abuse—further assessment is needed. Children process experiences through play and art. Disturbing content warrants careful exploration but must be interpreted within context of child's overall functioning, history, and other information. Single drawings don't diagnose—they're one piece of assessment data requiring integration with other information.

38. B. One pursuing intimacy while other distances
Pursue-distance pattern involves one partner pursuing connection, intimacy, or communication while the other partner distances and withdraws. The pursuer feels rejected and pursues harder; the distancer feels suffocated and distances more. This creates escalating cycle. Often reflects attachment style differences—anxious attachment (fears abandonment, pursues) and avoidant attachment (fears engulfment, distances).

39. B. Direct, careful questioning
Suicide risk assessment in older adults requires direct, careful questioning just as with any age group. Ask specifically about thoughts of death, suicidal ideation, plans, intent, and means. Don't assume older adults aren't serious or avoid the topic out of discomfort. Older adults are at high risk—especially older white men—and deserve thorough assessment and intervention.

40. B. Stabilization and return to baseline
Crisis intervention goals are stabilization and return to pre-crisis functioning—not solving longstanding problems, providing long-term therapy, or comprehensive treatment. Focus is immediate: ensure safety, reduce acute symptoms, restore coping, mobilize supports. Once stabilized, ongoing treatment may address underlying problems, but crisis intervention itself is time-limited and focused on current crisis.

41. B. It's a common trauma response
Regression—loss of previously achieved developmental skills—is common after trauma. A toilet-trained child might start wetting again. A verbal child might become less communicative. This represents stress response and attempts to cope with overwhelming experiences. It's not developmental delay, manipulation, or behavior requiring punishment. With support and trauma treatment, children typically return to previous functioning.

42. B. Often trigger problems as families adjust
Family life cycle transitions—birth of child, children starting school, adolescence, launching children, retirement, aging—often trigger problems as families struggle to adapt to new demands. Families can get stuck at transitions, unable to modify roles and patterns to fit new stage. Problems emerging during transitions often reflect difficulty adjusting, not just individual pathology.

43. B. Decision-specific and can fluctuate
Capacity is decision-specific (someone might have capacity for simple decisions but not complex ones) and can fluctuate (confusion might worsen at night or during illness, improve with treatment). It's not all-or-nothing or permanent once lost. Legal competency is court determination, but clinicians assess capacity for specific decisions at specific times. Capacity assessment considers understanding, reasoning, appreciation of consequences, and ability to express choice.

44. B. Provide different perspectives revealing full picture (continued)
Multiple informants provide different perspectives that together reveal full picture of child's functioning. Discrepancies between reports are common and clinically meaningful—why does child behave differently at school versus home? What's different about those environments? No single informant has complete picture. Integration of multiple perspectives allows comprehensive understanding and more accurate assessment.

45. B. May be depression presenting atypically
Somatic complaints (pain, fatigue, gastrointestinal problems) in older adults may be depression presenting atypically, not just medical problems. Older adults often express emotional distress through physical symptoms. However, somatic complaints also warrant medical evaluation to rule out actual physical illness. The key is considering both possibilities—assessing for depression while ensuring medical conditions are evaluated and treated.

46. B. Focused on immediate safety
During crisis, assessment must be focused on immediate safety, not comprehensive as in routine clinical evaluation. You assess: Is person dangerous to self or others? Can they care for basic needs? What triggered this crisis? What's needed now for stabilization? Detailed history, comprehensive diagnosis, and long-term treatment planning come after immediate crisis is managed. Safety first, comprehensive assessment later.

47. B. Disconnection with little emotional support
Disengagement describes family relationships characterized by disconnection, emotional distance, and little support or involvement. Family members are isolated from each other, don't know what's happening in each other's lives, and don't provide emotional support. This differs from healthy

independence (which maintains connection) by representing lack of connection and support that families need to function well.

48. B. Confusion and cognitive impairment
Anticholinergic medications (many antihistamines, some antidepressants, bladder control medications, sleeping pills) can cause confusion, memory problems, and cognitive impairment in older adults. These effects are often mistaken for dementia. The anticholinergic burden from multiple medications compounds effects. Medication review identifying and reducing anticholinergic medications often improves cognition dramatically.

49. B. Shape values, roles, and what's normative
Cultural factors profoundly shape family values, roles, gender expectations, parenting practices, and what's considered normative versus problematic. Extended family involvement valued in some cultures might be labeled "enmeshed" by therapists from other backgrounds. Hierarchical structure normative in some cultures might be seen as problematic by therapists valuing egalitarian relationships. You assess families within their cultural context, not imposing your cultural norms.

50. B. Time-limited intense response exceeding usual coping
A crisis is time-limited (not chronic difficulty), involves intense emotional response (not just normal stress), and exceeds the person's usual coping resources (they can't handle it with typical strategies). The person experiences disequilibrium—normal functioning is disrupted. Crisis represents breakdown of usual coping when faced with hazardous event. Crisis intervention helps restore equilibrium and functioning.

Final Reflections

Special populations—children, adolescents, older adults, couples, families, people in crisis—require adapted assessment approaches while maintaining core clinical skills. You adjust your methods to developmental stages, relationship contexts, and crisis situations, but fundamental principles remain consistent: gather comprehensive information, understand the person in context, formulate clearly, and plan intervention appropriately.

Children teach you to look beyond words to behavior, play, and multiple perspectives. They remind you that problems don't exist in isolation—they're embedded in families and schools. Effective intervention addresses systems, not just individual children.

Adolescents teach you to distinguish normal development from pathology. Risk-taking, peer focus, parent conflict—these aren't always problems. They're often necessary developmental work. Your job is supporting healthy development while intervening when things go off track.

Older adults teach you that aging and pathology differ. Depression isn't normal aging. Neither is dementia. Both warrant assessment and treatment. Older adults also teach you about resilience—people who've survived decades of life bring wisdom and strength even when facing losses and challenges.

Couples and families teach you about systems—how individuals affect each other, how patterns maintain problems, how changing interactions changes individuals. The identified patient's problems often reflect relationship dysfunction. Effective intervention addresses patterns, not just individuals.

Crisis situations teach you to act quickly, prioritize safety, and stabilize before comprehensively treating. You learn what's essential assessment versus what can wait. You develop skills for rapid decision-making under pressure.

Each population has unique characteristics requiring specific knowledge and skills. But all share one thing: they're human beings seeking help during difficult times. Your expertise matters, but so does your humanity—your ability to connect, to understand, to provide hope and help when people need it most.

Essential Understanding for Practice

- Child assessment requires multiple informants because children may not recognize problems and behavior varies across contexts
- Play-based assessment provides communication medium when children lack verbal skills to articulate internal experiences
- Depression in children often presents as irritability and behavioral problems rather than clearly reported sadness
- Adolescent risk-taking results from brain development with reward systems maturing faster than impulse control systems
- Adolescent focus on peers is developmentally normal identity work, not rejection of parents or sign of family problems
- Depression in older adults often presents atypically with somatic complaints, cognitive concerns, or irritability rather than sadness
- Cognitive screening (MMSE, MoCA) distinguishes depression from dementia, with pseudodementia improving when depression is treated
- Polypharmacy in older adults increases risk of side effects, interactions, and mental status changes requiring comprehensive medication review
- Elder abuse includes physical, emotional, financial exploitation, and neglect—social workers screen routinely and report as mandated
- Couple assessment observes communication patterns and interactions, not just what partners report verbally
- Gottman's Four Horsemen (criticism, contempt, defensiveness, stonewalling) predict relationship failure with contempt most toxic
- Family assessment examines boundaries, hierarchies, roles, and patterns with enmeshment and disengagement representing problematic extremes

- Crisis assessment prioritizes immediate safety evaluation over comprehensive assessment, focusing on stabilization and return to baseline
- Involuntary hospitalization is appropriate when person is imminent danger to self or others or gravely disabled due to mental illness
- Cultural factors shape what's normative in families—assessment must occur within cultural context, not imposing therapist's cultural norms

Chapter 9: Therapeutic Modalities

Every client who enters therapy asks the same fundamental question, spoken or unspoken: Can you help me? Your answer comes not through words but through skillful application of therapeutic approaches that match their needs. The techniques matter—evidence shows certain interventions work better for specific problems. But technique without relationship fails. Relationship without technique meanders. Effective therapy integrates both.

You need a toolbox of approaches, not allegiance to one theory. The cognitive-behavioral therapist who can't recognize when a client needs trauma processing misses opportunities. The psychodynamic therapist who dismisses behavioral interventions leaves clients without concrete skills. The eclectic therapist who applies techniques randomly without coherent framework confuses more than helps. You must know multiple approaches deeply enough to use them skillfully and wisely enough to know when each fits.

Cognitive-Behavioral Therapy

Cognitive-Behavioral Therapy rests on a simple premise: thoughts, feelings, and behaviors interact. Change one element and others follow. A person who thinks "I'm worthless" feels depressed and withdraws from others. Withdrawal reduces positive experiences, confirming the thought "I'm worthless," deepening depression. CBT interrupts these cycles through systematic intervention.

Cognitive model proposes that psychological distress results not from situations themselves but from interpretations of situations. Two people lose jobs. One thinks "This is temporary—I'll find something better" and feels disappointed but hopeful. Another thinks "I'm a failure—I'll never succeed" and becomes depressed. The situation is identical; interpretations differ; emotional responses differ.

Automatic thoughts are immediate interpretations that flash through consciousness in specific situations. They're called automatic because they occur spontaneously without deliberate reasoning. A person walks past coworkers who are laughing. Automatic thought: "They're laughing at me." Emotion: embarrassment, anger. Behavior: avoidance. Most people don't question automatic thoughts—they accept them as facts.

Cognitive distortions are systematic errors in thinking that maintain psychological problems. Common distortions include:

All-or-nothing thinking: Seeing things in black-and-white categories. "If I'm not perfect, I'm a complete failure." No middle ground exists.

Overgeneralization: Drawing broad conclusions from single events. One rejection means "No one will ever love me." One mistake means "I always mess up."

Mental filter: Focusing exclusively on negatives while ignoring positives. Receiving 99 positive comments and one criticism, the person dwells on the criticism.

Discounting the positive: Transforming positive experiences into negatives. "They only said that to be nice—it doesn't count."

Jumping to conclusions: Making negative interpretations without evidence. **Mind reading**: "She thinks I'm stupid." **Fortune telling**: "This will definitely turn out badly."

Magnification and minimization: Exaggerating negatives or minimizing positives. Small mistakes become catastrophes; achievements become insignificant.

Emotional reasoning: Assuming feelings reflect reality. "I feel stupid, therefore I am stupid."

Should statements: Rigid rules about how things must be. "I should be able to handle this." "People should be fair." These create guilt (when directed at self) or anger (when directed at others).

Labeling: Attaching global labels based on specific behaviors. "I made a mistake" becomes "I'm a loser."

Personalization: Taking responsibility for events outside your control. "The project failed because of me" when multiple factors contributed.

Thought records are the primary tool for cognitive work. The client identifies:

1. **Situation**: What happened? Where? When? With whom?
2. **Automatic thoughts**: What went through your mind?
3. **Emotions**: What did you feel? How intense (0-100)?
4. **Evidence supporting the thought**: What makes you think this is true?
5. **Evidence against the thought**: What suggests this might not be completely true?
6. **Alternative thoughts**: What's a more balanced way to view this situation?
7. **Outcome**: How do you feel now? What will you do?

This process makes thinking visible and subject to examination. Initially, you complete thought records in session, modeling the process. Clients practice between sessions, bringing completed records to discuss.

Behavioral experiments test beliefs through action. A socially anxious client believes "If I speak up in meetings, everyone will think I'm stupid." You design experiment: speak once in next meeting, observe reactions. Results typically disconfirm catastrophic predictions—people respond neutrally or positively. Behavioral experiments provide evidence that words alone can't provide.

Behavioral activation treats depression by increasing engagement in meaningful activities. Depression causes withdrawal, which reduces positive experiences and opportunities for mastery, which worsens mood. The cycle deepens until the person barely functions.

You help clients identify activities that historically provided pleasure or accomplishment. You create activity schedules—planning specific activities at specific times. Initially, clients won't feel like doing activities. "When I feel better, I'll do more" maintains depression. The principle is "Do first, feel better later"—action precedes motivation.

Activities are rated for pleasure (P) and mastery (M) on 0-10 scales. This shows connections between activity and mood that clients often don't recognize. Clients discover that even small activities—taking a walk, calling a friend, cooking a meal—improve mood temporarily. Accumulating these small improvements creates sustained change.

Graded task assignment breaks overwhelming tasks into manageable steps. A depressed client thinks "I need to clean the entire house" and feels overwhelmed, does nothing. You break it down: "Today, wash three dishes." Tomorrow, a bit more. Each completed step provides mastery experience and contradicts thoughts like "I can't do anything."

Case Example: CBT for Depression - Rachel

Rachel, 38, presents with Major Depression. She reports feeling worthless, hopeless, and exhausted. She's been calling in sick to work and avoiding friends. Her automatic thoughts include "I'm a failure," "Nothing will ever get better," and "I'm letting everyone down."

Session 1-2: Assessment and psychoeducation

You explain the cognitive model: thoughts affect feelings and behaviors. You provide depression psychoeducation—it's common, treatable, not weakness. You introduce thought records as homework.

Session 3: First thought record review

Rachel brings a completed thought record:

Situation: Received email from friend suggesting lunch
Automatic thought: "She's just being nice. She doesn't really want to see me."
Emotion: Sad (70/100)
Behavior: Didn't respond to email

You work through evidence:

- **Supporting thought**: "Sometimes people are just polite"
- **Against thought**: "She specifically suggested next Tuesday and asked about my schedule—that's not just being polite. She's reached out multiple times. We've been friends for years."

Alternative thought: "She genuinely wants to see me. She's been a consistent friend who's reached out repeatedly."

Outcome: Sad (40/100). Decided to respond to email and accept lunch invitation.

This demonstrates the process. Rachel sees how examining evidence changes emotional intensity and behavior.

Sessions 4-6: Behavioral activation

Rachel's activity level is minimal—work, home, sleep. She's dropped all previously enjoyed activities. You create activity schedule together:

Monday: 15-minute walk after work
Tuesday: Lunch with friend
Wednesday: Cook a real meal (not takeout)
Thursday: Call sister
Friday: 15-minute walk
Weekend: One activity outside the house each day

Rachel tracks activities and rates mood before and after. She notices mood improves slightly after activities, even when she didn't feel like doing them beforehand. This demonstrates that action can precede motivation.

Sessions 7-10: Core belief work

Rachel's automatic thoughts connect to underlying core belief: "I'm inadequate." This belief developed through childhood experiences with critical parents who emphasized achievement over effort.

You help Rachel identify evidence against this belief:

- Successful career in demanding field
- Multiple meaningful friendships maintained over years
- Helped sister through difficult divorce
- Volunteers at animal shelter
- Manages household and finances independently

The belief "I'm inadequate" doesn't match reality. You develop alternative belief: "I'm competent in many areas. I have strengths and weaknesses like everyone."

Sessions 11-12: Relapse prevention

Rachel's depression has improved significantly—PHQ-9 dropped from 22 to 8. You prepare for termination and potential future episodes:

Warning signs: Sleep disruption, withdrawing from friends, increased negative thinking
Coping strategies: Resume thought records, ensure regular activity, reach out for support
Action plan: If symptoms worsen for two weeks, contact you for booster session

Outcome: Rachel terminates with significant improvement maintained at six-month follow-up. She reports using cognitive skills when negative thoughts arise and maintaining activity level even when mood dips temporarily.

Dialectical Behavior Therapy

Dialectical Behavior Therapy was developed by Marsha Linehan for individuals with Borderline Personality Disorder, particularly those with chronic suicidal behavior and self-harm. DBT recognizes that these individuals experience emotions more intensely, return to baseline more slowly, and lack skills for managing overwhelming emotional states. The treatment teaches concrete skills while validating the person's experience.

Dialectical philosophy underlies the approach. A dialectic is synthesis of opposites. DBT holds multiple truths simultaneously: You're doing the best you can AND you need to try harder. Your feelings are valid AND you need to change behaviors. Life is painful AND worth living. This both-and thinking replaces either-or thinking common in BPD.

Biosocial theory explains BPD development. Biological vulnerability to emotion dysregulation (intense emotions, slow return to baseline) combines with invalidating environment (emotions dismissed, minimized, or punished). The person never learns to identify, tolerate, or regulate emotions. They develop problematic coping strategies—self-harm provides relief, suicidal behavior brings attention, emotional outbursts get needs met temporarily.

DBT structure includes multiple components:

Individual therapy (weekly, 50-90 minutes) addresses motivation, applies skills to specific situations, reduces therapy-interfering behaviors (missing sessions, not completing homework, violating agreements), and manages crises. The therapist conducts chain analysis of problematic behaviors and helps apply skills.

Skills training group (weekly, 2-2.5 hours) teaches four skill modules systematically. This is psychoeducational, not process group. Members learn and practice specific skills.

Phone coaching (brief calls between sessions) provides in-the-moment coaching for applying skills during crises. This isn't therapy—it's brief consultation helping the client use skills they've learned.

Consultation team supports therapists working with this challenging population. DBT recognizes therapist burnout risk and provides structured support.

Four skill modules form the core of DBT:

Mindfulness skills teach observing and describing present moment experience without judgment. Skills include:

Observe: Notice internal and external experiences without trying to change them—thoughts, emotions, sensations, sights, sounds.

Describe: Put words to experiences using facts, not judgments. "My heart is racing" not "I'm having a panic attack." "I'm having the thought that I'm worthless" not "I am worthless."

Participate: Engage fully in current activity without self-consciousness. Be present in this moment, not dwelling on past or worrying about future.

Wise mind: Integrate emotion mind (feelings dominate) and reasonable mind (logic dominates). Wise mind includes both emotion and reason, providing balanced perspective.

Distress tolerance skills help survive crises without making things worse. When emotions are overwhelming and you can't solve the problem immediately, distress tolerance bridges the gap:

STOP: Stop, Take a step back, Observe, Proceed mindfully. Prevents impulsive actions during crisis.

TIP: Temperature (cold water on face changes physiology), Intense exercise (burns energy), Paced breathing, Paired muscle relaxation. These regulate nervous system.

Distract: Activities (engage in task requiring attention), Contributing (help someone else), Comparisons (remember worse times), Emotions (create opposite emotion through activity), Pushing away (mentally push problem away temporarily), Thoughts (occupy mind with other thoughts), Sensations (intense sensation—holding ice, biting lemon).

Self-soothe: Use five senses—vision (beautiful images), hearing (soothing music), smell (pleasant scents), taste (favorite food), touch (soft blanket, warm bath).

ACCEPTS: Activities, Contributing, Comparisons, Emotions, Pushing away, Thoughts, Sensations (same as Distract, different acronym).

Emotion regulation skills help understand and modify emotions:

Identify and label emotions: Recognize what you're feeling. This seems simple but many people struggle to name emotions beyond "good" or "bad."

Understand the function: Emotions provide information and motivate action. Anger signals boundary violation and motivates assertion. Fear signals danger and motivates protection.

Check the facts: Does your emotional intensity fit the situation? Sometimes emotions are justified (real threat, actual loss). Sometimes they're disproportionate (small trigger, intense reaction).

Opposite action: When emotion doesn't fit facts or isn't serving you, act opposite to emotion's urge. Sad? Get active instead of withdrawing. Angry? Speak gently instead of attacking. Anxious? Approach instead of avoiding.

Build positive experiences: Short-term (daily pleasant activities) and long-term (work toward meaningful goals). Increasing positive experiences reduces vulnerability to negative emotions.

Build mastery: Do things that create sense of accomplishment. Competence feels good and builds self-efficacy.

PLEASE: Treat Physical illness, balance Eating, avoid mood-Altering substances, balance Sleep, get Exercise. Physical health affects emotional vulnerability.

Interpersonal effectiveness skills help get needs met while maintaining relationships and self-respect:

DEAR MAN (asking for what you need):

- **D**escribe situation using facts
- **E**xpress feelings and opinions

- **A**ssert by asking clearly for what you want
- **R**einforce by explaining positive effects
- Stay **M**indful, don't get distracted
- Appear **C**onfident even if you don't feel it
- **N**egotiate, be willing to compromise

GIVE (maintaining relationships):

- Be **G**entle, no attacks or threats
- Act **I**nterested, listen
- **V**alidate the other person's feelings
- Use an **E**asy manner, be light-hearted when appropriate

FAST (maintaining self-respect):

- Be **F**air to self and others
- No **A**pologies when not warranted
- **S**tick to your values
- Be **T**ruthful

Chain analysis examines sequences leading to problematic behaviors. For self-harm episode:

Vulnerability factors: Baseline conditions making problem behavior more likely (poor sleep, skipped meals, high stress week)

Prompting event: Specific trigger (boyfriend cancelled plans)

Links in chain: Thoughts, feelings, sensations, actions between trigger and target behavior:

- Thought: "He doesn't care about me"
- Feeling: Hurt, then anger
- Thought: "I'm unlovable"
- Feeling: Intense emotional pain
- Urge: Cut to release pain
- Action: Went to bathroom, got razor
- Thought: "This will make it stop"
- Action: Cut arm
- Feeling: Temporary relief

Target behavior: Self-harm (cutting)

Consequences: Temporary emotional relief, then shame and guilt, hiding injury from others, boyfriend upset when he found out

Intervention points: Where could skills have interrupted the chain?

- After prompting event: Use mindfulness to observe feelings without acting
- During intense emotion: Use TIP skills to regulate physiology
- During urge: Use distress tolerance—hold ice instead of cutting
- After thought "This will make it stop": Challenge thought—cutting provides only temporary relief and creates new problems

Chain analysis makes the process visible, identifies intervention points, and guides skill application for future situations.

Case Example: DBT for Borderline Personality Disorder - Marcus

Marcus, 25, has BPD with chronic suicidal ideation, self-harm through cutting, unstable relationships, and emotional volatility. He's been hospitalized three times for suicide attempts. Previous therapies failed—he'd escalate, therapists would become frustrated, he'd feel abandoned and quit or get terminated.

Comprehensive DBT treatment:

Individual therapy: Weekly sessions focus on reducing life-threatening behaviors (suicide attempts, self-harm), therapy-interfering behaviors (missing sessions, late arrivals), and quality-of-life interfering behaviors (substance use, relationship conflicts). You use chain analysis when Marcus self-harms and teach skills application.

Skills group: Weekly 2.5-hour group teaches modules sequentially over six months, then repeats. Marcus learns mindfulness, distress tolerance, emotion regulation, and interpersonal effectiveness. Group provides structured teaching and practice.

Phone coaching: Marcus can call between sessions for brief (10-15 minute) coaching on applying skills. He calls during urges to self-harm; you coach him through using skills instead.

Month 1-2: Frequent crises

Marcus calls multiple times weekly with urges to self-harm or suicidal thoughts. You coach distress tolerance skills: "Use TIP—splash cold water on your face. That changes your physiology. Then use ACCEPTS—can you distract yourself for 15 minutes? What activities could occupy your attention?"

Initially, Marcus sometimes uses skills successfully, sometimes self-harms. You don't punish self-harm but do chain analysis understanding what happened and how to intervene differently next time.

Month 3-4: Skill building

Marcus begins recognizing emotional patterns. He identifies vulnerability factors: poor sleep and skipping meals increase emotional reactivity. He starts PLEASE skills—regular sleep schedule, eating three meals daily, avoiding alcohol. His baseline emotional state improves.

He practices opposite action when sad: instead of staying in bed, he forces himself to shower and take a walk. Initially he's skeptical ("This won't work"), but notices small mood improvements. Accumulated small improvements create change.

Month 5-6: Relationship work

Marcus's relationships are chaotic—intense, idealize-then-devalue pattern. He learns interpersonal effectiveness skills. When boyfriend is late, instead of exploding ("You don't care about me!") or withdrawing, Marcus uses DEAR MAN:

Describe: "You were 30 minutes late picking me up."
Express: "I felt hurt and worried."
Assert: "I need you to call if you're running late."
Reinforce: "When you communicate, I feel respected and our relationship is stronger."

Boyfriend responds positively. Marcus experiences getting needs met through effective communication instead of emotional outbursts.

Month 7-12: Consolidation

Self-harm decreases dramatically—from multiple times weekly to once monthly to stopping entirely for several months. Suicidal ideation becomes less frequent and intense. Marcus still has emotional ups and downs but manages them with skills.

Relationship stabilizes. Work attendance improves. Marcus completes skills training group and joins second cycle for repetition and reinforcement. After one year, he's functioning at higher level than ever before—maintaining relationship and employment, managing emotions, not self-harming.

DBT didn't eliminate BPD or create perfect emotional stability. But it gave Marcus tools for managing intense emotions and achieving life worth living. That's the goal—not perfection, but a life the person wants to live.

Trauma-Informed Care

Trauma-informed care isn't a specific therapy technique—it's an approach recognizing the widespread impact of trauma and integrating this understanding into all aspects of service delivery. You assume trauma history is common and organize services to avoid re-traumatization while supporting recovery.

Core principles guide trauma-informed practice:

Safety: Physical and emotional safety is paramount. The environment is safe—comfortable, private, predictable. Emotional safety means the person doesn't feel judged, coerced, or threatened. Without safety, healing can't occur.

Trustworthiness and transparency: You explain what you're doing and why. You follow through on commitments. You acknowledge limitations honestly. Trust develops through consistent, predictable behavior over time.

Peer support: Connection with others who've experienced similar trauma provides validation, hope, and practical strategies. Mutual support groups, peer specialists, and trauma survivor networks support recovery.

Collaboration and mutuality: You work with the client, not on them. Power differentials are reduced where possible. Decisions are made jointly. The person's voice and choice are respected.

Empowerment, voice, and choice: Treatment emphasizes strengths, builds on capacities, and supports the person in making choices. You recognize that trauma involved powerlessness—recovery requires reclaiming power over one's life.

Cultural, historical, and gender issues: You recognize how culture, history, and gender shape trauma experiences and recovery. Historical trauma (slavery, genocide, colonization) affects entire communities across generations. Gender affects trauma types (women experience more sexual violence, men more combat exposure) and responses.

Trauma responses are adaptations, not pathology. Hypervigilance kept the person safe in dangerous environments. Emotional numbing protected against overwhelming pain. Dissociation allowed survival during unbearable experiences. These strategies made sense given circumstances—they just no longer serve well in current life.

You reframe symptoms: "You're not broken—you developed survival strategies that worked in terrible circumstances. Those strategies are creating problems now, and we can develop new ones. But the strategies themselves weren't the problem—the trauma was."

Avoiding re-traumatization requires constant attention:

Avoid power struggles: Coercion, force, and power assertion recreate trauma dynamics. You offer choices, respect autonomy, and work collaboratively.

Provide control: Let clients control aspects of therapy—where to sit, pace of discussion, topics to address. Control over small things begins restoring sense of agency.

Respect boundaries: Don't push too hard too fast. Clients control what they discuss and when. Premature exploration of trauma can re-traumatize.

Explain procedures: Surprise and unpredictability feel threatening. Explain what will happen, why, and what the person can expect.

Address power dynamics: Acknowledge that you hold power as therapist. Work to minimize harmful effects while maintaining therapeutic structure.

Believe clients: Trust clients' accounts of their experiences. Disbelief re-traumatizes.

Recognize triggers: Help clients identify trauma triggers (situations, sensations, emotions that activate trauma memories). Develop strategies for managing triggered states.

Phase-based trauma treatment progresses through stages:

Phase 1: Safety and stabilization

Before processing trauma, establish safety and build coping skills. For someone in active domestic violence, first priority is safety planning—not trauma processing. For someone using substances to cope, address substance use first. For someone with severe emotion dysregulation, build regulation skills first.

This phase includes: establishing safety (physical, emotional, relational), developing coping skills (emotion regulation, distress tolerance, grounding), creating support systems, stabilizing life circumstances (housing, income, basic needs).

Some clients remain in Phase 1 indefinitely. That's acceptable. If life remains unstable or coping skills remain inadequate, processing trauma may destabilize rather than help.

Phase 2: Processing traumatic memories

Once stable with adequate skills, clients can process traumatic memories through evidence-based trauma therapies: Prolonged Exposure, Cognitive Processing Therapy, or EMDR. Processing involves confronting trauma memories (which naturally evokes distress), making sense of what happened, and integrating experiences so they no longer dominate consciousness.

Not all trauma survivors need or want trauma processing. Some achieve good functioning through Phase 1 work alone. Processing is offered, not mandated.

Phase 3: Integration and reconnection

After processing trauma, work focuses on building the life the person wants—developing meaningful relationships, pursuing goals and values, reconnecting with community. Trauma no longer defines identity. The person is a survivor who experienced trauma, not a trauma victim whose identity is consumed by trauma.

Case Example: Trauma-Informed Care - Sophia

Sophia, 32, enters therapy for depression and anxiety. Initial assessment reveals extensive trauma history: childhood sexual abuse by uncle, adolescent dating violence, adult sexual assault, and recent car accident.

Trauma-informed approach from first contact:

Intake forms: Rather than asking "Have you been abused?" (which implies judgment), forms ask "Have you experienced physical, sexual, or emotional harm?" and "What experiences have affected your life?"

Office environment: Waiting room has comfortable seating, pleasant lighting, magazines, and water available. Sophia can see exit clearly—she's not trapped. Therapy room has two doors, and you ask Sophia where she'd like to sit, ensuring she feels safe.

First session: You explain confidentiality clearly, including limits. You ask permission before taking notes. You explain what therapy involves and what Sophia can expect. This transparency builds trust.

Building safety (Sessions 1-8):

Sophia's life is chaotic—unstable housing, limited income, few supports. Before addressing trauma, you work on stabilization:

- Connect Sophia with housing assistance and financial resources
- Help her identify and develop support systems
- Teach grounding techniques for managing flashbacks
- Develop emotion regulation and distress tolerance skills
- Address substance use (Sophia drinks to sleep and numb flashbacks)

You explain: "Trauma processing is important, but we need to build your foundation first. You need stable ground to stand on before we dig into difficult memories."

Skills development (Sessions 9-16):

You teach specific skills for managing trauma responses:

Grounding: When flashbacks occur, Sophia learns to ground herself in present moment—naming five things she sees, four things she hears, three things she can touch, two things she smells, one thing she tastes. This pulls her out of past into present.

Containment: Sophia imagines placing traumatic memories in a safe container (box with lock) so they don't overwhelm her outside of therapy. She can open the container during sessions with support, then close it again after.

Self-soothing: Sophia develops list of activities that provide comfort without harm—hot bath, weighted blanket, calling supportive friend, listening to calming music, petting her cat.

Body awareness: Trauma is stored in the body. Sophia learns to notice body sensations without being overwhelmed—recognizing tension, pain, or numbness as information, not danger.

Trauma processing (Sessions 17-30):

Once Sophia is stable with good skills, you begin Cognitive Processing Therapy. Sophia writes about her traumatic experiences and examines stuck points—problematic beliefs developed from trauma:

Stuck point: "The abuse was my fault" (common belief among childhood sexual abuse survivors)

Evidence for: "I didn't tell anyone" "I didn't fight back" "Sometimes my body responded"

Evidence against: "I was a child—adults are responsible for protecting children, not the reverse" "Children don't have power to stop adult abuse" "Physical response doesn't indicate consent or desire" "He used his authority and my trust to manipulate me"

Alternative belief: "The abuse was not my fault. My uncle was responsible for his actions. I was a child doing the best I could in a situation I didn't understand or have power to stop."

Through repeated examination, Sophia's beliefs shift. Guilt decreases. Self-blame reduces. She develops more balanced understanding of her experiences.

Integration (Sessions 31-40):

Sophia's trauma symptoms have decreased significantly. She no longer has daily flashbacks. Nightmares are occasional rather than nightly. She can discuss trauma without being overwhelmed. Now focus shifts to building the life she wants:

- Sophia returns to school, pursuing degree she'd abandoned
- She develops healthier relationships, recognizing red flags that previously drew her to unsafe partners
- She volunteers at crisis center, finding meaning in helping others
- She reconnects with family members who were supportive
- She pursues hobbies she'd neglected—painting, hiking

Trauma is part of Sophia's history but no longer defines her present. She's building a future not determined by her past.

Motivational Interviewing

Motivational Interviewing addresses the fundamental problem that people want to change and don't want to change simultaneously. This ambivalence is normal, not resistance. MI helps people explore their ambivalence and resolve it in the direction of change.

Spirit of MI underlies all techniques:

Partnership: You work with the client, not on them. You're collaborators, not expert-and-patient. The client is the expert on their own life.

Acceptance: You accept the person as they are, including their ambivalence. Acceptance includes absolute worth (unconditional positive regard), accurate empathy (understanding the client's perspective), autonomy support (respecting the client's right to choose), and affirmation (recognizing and acknowledging strengths).

Compassion: You actively promote the client's welfare, prioritizing their needs.

Evocation: Motivation comes from within the client, not from you. Your job is drawing out the person's own reasons for change, not imposing yours.

Core skills create the foundation:

Open-ended questions: Ask questions that require more than yes/no answers. "What concerns you about your drinking?" not "Are you concerned about your drinking?" Open questions explore thoughts, feelings, and motivations.

Affirmations: Recognize and acknowledge strengths, efforts, and positive qualities. "You've managed to stay sober for three days despite intense cravings—that takes real strength." Affirmations build self-efficacy and rapport.

Reflections: Mirror back what the client says, showing understanding and encouraging further exploration. Reflections should outnumber questions in good MI. Types of reflections:

Simple reflection: Repeat or rephrase what was said. Client: "I know I drink too much." Reflection: "You're aware your drinking is excessive."

Complex reflection: Add meaning or continue the paragraph. Client: "I know I drink too much." Reflection: "You're concerned about how much you drink, and you're not sure if you're ready to change."

Amplified reflection: Exaggerate slightly to evoke the other side of ambivalence. Client: "I can quit whenever I want." Reflection: "So drinking isn't really a problem at all for you." (Often evokes: "Well, I didn't say that...")

Double-sided reflection: Acknowledge both sides of ambivalence. "On one hand, you enjoy drinking and it helps you relax. On the other hand, you're worried about your health and your wife is threatening to leave."

Summarizing: Periodically summarize what's been discussed, gathering information and preparing to move forward. Summaries can emphasize change talk (statements favoring change).

Change talk is any self-expressed argument for change. You listen for and reinforce change talk:

DARN: Preparatory change talk

- **D**esire: "I want to quit"
- **A**bility: "I think I could do it"
- **R**easons: "My health is suffering"
- **N**eed: "I have to change"

CAT: Mobilizing change talk (stronger)

- **C**ommitment: "I will quit"
- **A**ctivation: "I'm ready to start"
- **T**aking steps: "I've already cut back"

You use OARS skills to elicit and strengthen change talk. You selectively reinforce change talk while gently redirecting sustain talk (statements favoring status quo).

Sustain talk is any self-expressed argument against change. "I don't really drink that much" or "I can handle it" or "Quitting would be too hard." You don't argue with sustain talk—that increases it. Instead, you reflect it without emphasis and ask questions that might evoke change talk.

Client: "Quitting would be impossible. All my friends drink."

Poor response: "You could find new friends" (generates resistance)

Good response: "Your social life revolves around drinking. That would make change challenging. What might help you manage the social aspect?" (acknowledges concern, opens exploration)

Rolling with resistance: When clients express resistance, you don't confront or argue. You roll with it—acknowledge it, explore it, sometimes amplify it slightly to evoke the other side.

Client: "I don't have a drinking problem. You're overreacting."

Poor response: "You've had three DUIs and your liver enzymes are elevated. That's a problem." (arguing increases resistance)

Good response: "You don't see your drinking as problematic, and here I am suggesting you need to change. That must be frustrating. Help me understand your perspective." (acknowledges frustration, invites collaboration)

Developing discrepancy: Help clients see the gap between current behavior and important values or goals. When behavior conflicts with values, motivation for change increases.

"You mentioned your family is the most important thing in your life. You also said your drinking is causing problems with your wife and kids. How do you make sense of that?"

This isn't confrontation—it's helping the client recognize their own discrepancy. The discomfort of cognitive dissonance motivates change.

Stages of change inform MI approach:

Precontemplation: Not considering change. MI helps build awareness and concern.

Contemplation: Ambivalent about change. MI helps resolve ambivalence toward change.

Preparation: Deciding to change and planning. MI helps strengthen commitment and develop plan.

Action: Actively changing. MI supports action and builds self-efficacy.

Maintenance: Sustaining change. MI supports maintaining motivation and managing lapses.

You match intervention to stage. Pushing action with someone in precontemplation generates resistance. Exploring ambivalence with someone ready for action wastes time.

Case Example: Motivational Interviewing for Substance Use - David

David, 42, was mandated to therapy after second DUI. He's defensive and minimizes his drinking. "I just had bad luck. Everyone drinks and drives occasionally."

Poor approach (generates resistance):

Therapist: "You have a serious alcohol problem. You need to stop drinking."
David: "I don't have a problem. I just made some mistakes."
Therapist: "Two DUIs aren't mistakes—they're a pattern. Your drinking is out of control."
David: "You don't understand. I have a stressful job. I need to unwind."
Therapist: "That's just an excuse. You need to take responsibility."

This confrontational approach increases David's defensiveness. He argues harder for drinking. Resistance intensifies.

MI approach:

Session 1: Engagement and evocation

You: "You're here because the court required it after your second DUI. That must be frustrating."

David: "Yeah, it's ridiculous. I wasn't even that drunk."

You: "From your perspective, this feels like an overreaction. Help me understand what happened."

David explains the arrests—stressful day, had a few drinks, got pulled over. Bad luck.

You: "Sounds like you see these as unfortunate circumstances rather than signs of a drinking problem."

David: "Exactly. I drink like everyone else."

You: "You drink about the same as your friends and coworkers. At the same time, you're here facing serious consequences. What are your thoughts about that?"

David (pausing): "Well, I guess most people don't get two DUIs."

You: "So even though you don't see yourself as different from others in how much you drink, you're experiencing consequences others aren't. What do you make of that?"

David: "I don't know. Maybe I've been unlucky. Or maybe..." (trails off)

You: "Maybe...?"

David: "Maybe I've been drinking more than I realized. My wife says I drink every night. I guess I do."

This is change talk—David questioning his own minimization. You reinforce it.

You: "You're starting to wonder if your drinking might be more than you've been telling yourself. What concerns you about that?"

Session 2: Exploring ambivalence

You use decisional balance—exploring both sides:

What do you like about drinking?

- Relaxes me after stressful days
- Helps me sleep
- Social—my friends all drink
- Enjoy the taste of good wine

What concerns you about drinking?

- Legal problems—DUIs, license suspension, fines
- Wife is upset, threatens divorce
- Sometimes I drink more than I intend
- Health—doctor said liver enzymes elevated
- Missing my kids' events because I'm too drunk
- Spending a lot of money

You reflect: "So drinking serves important functions for you—relaxation, sleep, socializing. And at the same time, it's creating serious problems with the law, your marriage, your health, and your relationship with your kids."

David: "Yeah. I guess when you lay it out like that, the problems outweigh the benefits."

This is change talk. You amplify it.

You: "The costs have started to outweigh the benefits for you. What matters most to you as you think about this?"

David: "My kids. I don't want to be the dad who's always drunk. My dad was an alcoholic, and it sucked. I swore I'd be different."

You: "Your kids matter enormously to you, and you don't want them to experience what you experienced with your father. How does your current drinking fit with the father you want to be?"

David (distressed): "It doesn't. I'm becoming what I swore I wouldn't be."

Developing discrepancy—David sees the gap between his values (being a good father) and his behavior (drinking heavily). This discomfort motivates change.

Session 3: Planning

David has moved to preparation stage. He's decided to quit drinking. Now you help him plan.

You: "You've decided to stop drinking. That's a significant decision. What's your plan?"

David outlines plan—quit cold turkey, avoid bars, tell friends he's not drinking.

You: "Those are good starts. What obstacles might you encounter?"

David identifies challenges—social pressure, stress, sleep problems, cravings.

You: "How might you handle those obstacles?"

Together you develop detailed plan: social strategies (suggest non-drinking activities, be honest about not drinking), stress management (exercise, therapy, mindfulness), sleep hygiene (establish routine, try medication if needed), managing cravings (call sponsor, use delay tactics, remind yourself of reasons for quitting).

You: "On a scale of 0-10, how confident are you that you can succeed with this plan?"

David: "Maybe a 6?"

You: "Six is pretty good. What makes it a 6 and not a 4?"

David: "I'm motivated. I'm scared of losing my family. I've made a commitment."

You: "Those are powerful reasons. What would it take to get from 6 to 7 or 8?"

David: "Maybe having more support? Like AA or something?"

You: "Would you be willing to try an AA meeting?"

David: "Yeah, I think I should."

Outcome: David attends AA, establishes sobriety, and maintains it. MI helped him move from defensive denial to motivated change by evoking his own reasons for change rather than imposing yours.

Practice Questions

1. In CBT, automatic thoughts are:

A. Always accurate
B. Immediate interpretations that occur spontaneously
C. Only negative
D. Easy to identify

2. All-or-nothing thinking is:

A. Healthy
B. Seeing things in black-and-white categories
C. Rare
D. Only in schizophrenia

3. Thought records help clients:

A. Avoid thinking
B. Examine evidence for and against automatic thoughts
C. Only think positively
D. Stop having thoughts

4. Behavioral activation treats depression by:

A. Analyzing childhood
B. Increasing meaningful activities
C. Avoiding difficult situations
D. Only using medication

5. The principle "Do first, feel better later" means:

A. Ignore feelings
B. Action can precede motivation
C. Never rest
D. Feelings don't matter

6. DBT was originally developed for:

A. Depression
B. Anxiety
C. Borderline Personality Disorder
D. Psychosis

7. Dialectical thinking involves:

A. Either-or choices
B. Holding multiple truths simultaneously
C. Avoiding conflict
D. One correct answer

8. DBT includes which skill modules:

A. Only mindfulness
B. Mindfulness, distress tolerance, emotion regulation, interpersonal effectiveness
C. Only medication management
D. No specific skills

9. Wise mind integrates:

A. Only emotion
B. Only logic
C. Emotion mind and reasonable mind
D. Neither emotion nor logic

10. Distress tolerance skills help:

A. Eliminate all distress
B. Survive crises without making things worse
C. Avoid all problems
D. Never feel upset

11. Chain analysis in DBT examines:

A. Nothing useful
B. Sequence from trigger through actions to consequence
C. Only the target behavior
D. Past childhood

12. Trauma-informed care emphasizes:

A. Immediate trauma processing
B. Safety, trustworthiness, collaboration, empowerment
C. Confrontation
D. Power assertion

13. Phase-based trauma treatment begins with:

A. Trauma processing
B. Safety and stabilization
C. Medication
D. Hospitalization

14. Grounding techniques help:

A. Avoid reality
B. Orient to present moment during flashbacks
C. Eliminate memories
D. Cause dissociation

15. Trauma processing should occur:

A. Immediately
B. After establishing safety and skills
C. Never
D. Without preparation

16. Motivational Interviewing addresses:

A. Only addiction
B. Ambivalence about change
C. Psychosis
D. Dementia

17. The spirit of MI includes:

A. Confrontation
B. Partnership, acceptance, compassion, evocation
C. Authority
D. Diagnosis

18. Change talk includes:

A. Arguments against change
B. Self-expressed arguments for change
C. Therapist's reasons
D. Only actions

19. Rolling with resistance means:

A. Arguing harder
B. Acknowledging resistance without confrontation
C. Giving up
D. Forcing change

20. Developing discrepancy involves:

A. Arguing with the client
B. Helping clients see gap between behavior and values
C. Creating guilt
D. Avoiding values

21. OARS skills include:

A. Only questions
B. Open-ended questions, Affirmations, Reflections, Summaries
C. Confrontation
D. Medication

22. In CBT, behavioral experiments:

A. Are unnecessary
B. Test beliefs through action
C. Only involve thinking
D. Are dangerous

23. Cognitive distortions are:

A. Always accurate
B. Systematic errors in thinking
C. Signs of psychosis
D. Untreatable

24. Opposite action in DBT means:

A. Acting impulsively
B. Acting opposite to emotion's urge when emotion doesn't fit facts
C. Never feeling emotions
D. Avoiding action

25. DEAR MAN is used for:

A. Meditation
B. Asking for what you need
C. Avoiding people
D. Suppressing emotions

26. Mindfulness involves:

A. Never thinking
B. Observing present moment without judgment
C. Controlling thoughts
D. Only positive thoughts

27. When traumatic memories are processed successfully:

A. They're erased completely
B. They're integrated and no longer dominate consciousness
C. They become more intrusive
D. Nothing changes

28. Containment techniques help:

A. Avoid memories completely
B. Mentally place traumatic memories in safe container temporarily
C. Eliminate memories
D. Create new memories

29. Sustain talk is:

A. Helpful for change
B. Arguments against change
C. Same as change talk
D. Ignored completely

30. Amplified reflection:

A. Agrees with client completely
B. Exaggerates slightly to evoke the other side of ambivalence
C. Argues
D. Changes the subject

31. Graded task assignment:

A. Makes tasks harder
B. Breaks overwhelming tasks into manageable steps
C. Avoids all tasks
D. Requires perfection

32. TIP skills in DBT regulate:

A. Nothing
B. Nervous system through Temperature, Intense exercise, Paced breathing
C. Only thoughts
D. Only behaviors

33. Emotional reasoning is:

A. Logical thinking
B. Assuming feelings reflect reality
C. Healthy
D. Rare

34. Should statements create:

A. Motivation
B. Guilt or anger
C. Joy
D. Nothing

35. The evocation principle in MI means:

A. Telling clients what to do
B. Drawing out client's own reasons for change
C. Avoiding discussion
D. Imposing solutions

36. GIVE skills maintain:

A. Distance
B. Relationships
C. Anger
D. Avoidance

37. Trauma symptoms are:

A. Weakness
B. Adaptations that made sense given circumstances
C. Untreatable
D. Imaginary

38. Fortune telling is:

A. Predicting accurately
B. Jumping to negative conclusions about future
C. Planning
D. Hope

39. FAST skills maintain:

A. Speed
B. Self-respect
C. Relationships
D. Avoidance

40. Complex reflection:

A. Repeats exactly what was said
B. Adds meaning or continues the paragraph
C. Changes the subject
D. Argues

41. Behavioral activation activity schedules:

A. Overwhelm clients
B. Plan specific activities at specific times
C. Are optional
D. Don't affect mood

42. Personalization involves:

A. Healthy self-reflection
B. Taking responsibility for events outside your control
C. Accountability
D. Self-care

43. The contemplation stage involves:

A. Not considering change
B. Ambivalence about change
C. Actively changing
D. Maintaining change

44. Biosocial theory explains BPD through:

A. Only biology
B. Biological emotion dysregulation plus invalidating environment
C. Only environment
D. Random causes

45. Magnification:

A. Is realistic
B. Exaggerates negatives
C. Minimizes negatives
D. Has no impact

46. Double-sided reflection:

A. Ignores ambivalence
B. Acknowledges both sides of ambivalence
C. Takes sides
D. Argues

47. PLEASE skills reduce:

A. Nothing
B. Vulnerability to negative emotions through physical health
C. Happiness
D. Energy

48. Discounting the positive:

A. Is realistic
B. Transforms positive experiences into negatives
C. Is healthy
D. Never happens

49. Building mastery involves:

A. Becoming perfect
B. Doing things that create sense of accomplishment
C. Avoiding challenges
D. Only thinking

50. Mental filter:

A. Sees both positive and negative
B. Focuses exclusively on negatives while ignoring positives
C. Is balanced
D. Is rare

51. Phone coaching in DBT:

A. Replaces therapy
B. Provides brief in-the-moment skill coaching
C. Is unlimited
D. Isn't part of DBT

52. Overgeneralization:

A. Is accurate
B. Draws broad conclusions from single events
C. Is specific
D. Is healthy

53. ACCEPTS skills:

A. Accept defeat
B. Distract during crisis through Activities, Contributing, Comparisons, etc.
C. Avoid everything
D. Cause problems

54. Core beliefs:

A. Are situation-specific
B. Are fundamental assumptions about self, others, world
C. Change easily
D. Don't affect emotions

55. Therapy-interfering behaviors in DBT include:

A. Only violence
B. Missing sessions, not completing homework, violating agreements
C. Asking questions
D. Using skills

56. Labeling:

A. Is specific
B. Attaches global labels based on specific behaviors
C. Is helpful
D. Never occurs

57. Autonomy support in MI:

A. Forcing change
B. Respecting client's right to choose
C. Making decisions for client
D. Avoiding discussion

58. Self-soothing uses:

A. Harmful behaviors
B. Five senses to provide comfort
C. Avoidance
D. Substances

59. Jumping to conclusions includes:

A. Careful evaluation
B. Mind reading and fortune telling
C. Evidence-based thinking
D. Slow processing

60. Observe skill in mindfulness:

A. Judges everything
B. Notices experiences without trying to change them
C. Avoids present
D. Only focuses on negatives

61. Wisdom about biological vulnerabilities in DBT means:

A. Blaming biology
B. Understanding that some people experience emotions more intensely
C. Ignoring biology
D. Biology determines everything

62. Activity ratings in behavioral activation:

A. Are unnecessary
B. Track pleasure and mastery to show activity-mood connection
C. Cause depression
D. Only track negatives

63. Invalidating environment:

A. Validates all emotions
B. Dismisses, minimizes, or punishes emotions
C. Is helpful
D. Doesn't affect development

64. Describe skill in mindfulness:

A. Judges
B. Puts words to experiences using facts
C. Avoids language
D. Uses only judgments

65. Re-traumatization occurs when:

A. Trauma is discussed
B. Practices recreate trauma dynamics like powerlessness
C. Help is provided
D. Safety is prioritized

66. Affirmations in MI:

A. Are insincere
B. Recognize strengths and efforts
C. Focus only on problems
D. Are unnecessary

67. Participate skill means:

A. Watching from outside
B. Engaging fully in current activity
C. Avoiding activity
D. Multi-tasking

68. Emotion mind:

A. Integrates emotion and logic
B. Emotions dominate thinking
C. Ignores emotions
D. Is always best

69. Evidence for thoughts in CBT:

A. Isn't examined
B. Is evaluated objectively
C. Is assumed accurate
D. Doesn't matter

70. Reasonable mind:

A. Integrates emotion and logic
B. Logic dominates, emotions minimized
C. Has no logic
D. Is always best

71. STOP skill in DBT:

A. Stops all activity permanently
B. Stop, Take step back, Observe, Proceed mindfully
C. Just stops thinking
D. Causes problems

72. Partnership in MI means:

A. Therapist decides everything
B. Working with client, not on them
C. Client has no say
D. No structure

73. Alternative thoughts in CBT:

A. Are forced positive thinking
B. Are more balanced interpretations considering all evidence
C. Ignore problems
D. Are always positive

74. Building positive experiences in DBT:

A. Is impossible
B. Reduces vulnerability to negative emotions
C. Causes problems
D. Only involves thinking

75. Commitment language in change talk:

A. Is weak
B. Indicates strong intent to change
C. Doesn't predict behavior
D. Is discouraged

Answer Key with Detailed Explanations

1. B. Immediate interpretations that occur spontaneously
Automatic thoughts are immediate interpretations that flash through consciousness in specific situations without deliberate reasoning. They're called "automatic" because they occur spontaneously. They aren't always accurate, aren't always negative (though negative ones cause problems), and many people don't naturally identify them without training. CBT teaches clients to recognize automatic thoughts so they can be examined.

2. B. Seeing things in black-and-white categories
All-or-nothing thinking is a cognitive distortion where things are seen in black-and-white categories with no middle ground. "If I'm not perfect, I'm a complete failure" or "If someone doesn't like me, I'm totally unlovable." This distortion is common, unhealthy, and maintains depression and anxiety. It's not limited to schizophrenia—it occurs across many conditions and in non-clinical populations.

3. B. Examine evidence for and against automatic thoughts
Thought records help clients examine evidence for and against automatic thoughts, identify cognitive distortions, and develop more balanced alternative thoughts. This process makes thinking visible and subject to examination. It doesn't avoid thinking, force positive thinking, or stop thoughts—it helps evaluate thoughts objectively and develop realistic alternatives when thoughts are biased.

4. B. Increasing meaningful activities
Behavioral activation treats depression by increasing engagement in activities that provide pleasure or mastery. Depression causes withdrawal, which reduces positive experiences, which worsens mood. Scheduling and completing activities—even before you feel motivated—breaks this cycle. The activity-mood connection becomes clear through tracking. This isn't analyzing childhood, avoiding difficulties, or only using medication—it's systematic behavioral intervention.

5. B. Action can precede motivation
"Do first, feel better later" means that action can precede motivation rather than waiting to feel motivated before acting. Depressed people often think "When I feel better, I'll do more." Behavioral activation reverses this: "Do more, then you'll feel better." Accumulated small actions improve mood. This doesn't mean ignoring feelings or never resting—it means using behavior change to drive mood change.

6. C. Borderline Personality Disorder
DBT was specifically developed by Marsha Linehan for Borderline Personality Disorder, particularly for individuals with chronic suicidal behavior and self-harm. It addresses emotion dysregulation core to BPD. While DBT is now used for other conditions involving emotion dysregulation, it was originally designed for and has strongest evidence for BPD.

7. B. Holding multiple truths simultaneously
Dialectical thinking holds multiple truths simultaneously, synthesizing apparent opposites. "You're doing the best you can AND you need to try harder." Both truths exist. This both-and thinking replaces either-or thinking common in BPD. It's not avoiding conflict or having one correct answer—it's recognizing that seemingly contradictory truths can coexist.

8. B. Mindfulness, distress tolerance, emotion regulation, interpersonal effectiveness
DBT teaches four skill modules: mindfulness (observing present without judgment), distress tolerance (surviving crises without making things worse), emotion regulation (understanding and modifying emotions), and interpersonal effectiveness (getting needs met while maintaining relationships and self-respect). These skills are taught systematically in group format with individual therapy applying skills to specific situations.

9. C. Emotion mind and reasonable mind
Wise mind integrates emotion mind (where feelings dominate) and reasonable mind (where logic dominates). It includes both emotion and reason, providing balanced perspective. Neither pure emotion nor pure logic is optimal—wise mind brings both together. A decision made in wise mind considers both feelings and facts, leading to choices that are both emotionally satisfying and practically sound.

10. B. Survive crises without making things worse
Distress tolerance skills help survive crises without engaging in behaviors that make things worse (self-harm, substance use, impulsive destructive actions). The goal isn't eliminating distress—it's getting through intense moments without adding to problems. Once the crisis passes, the person can use other skills or solve problems. Distress tolerance bridges the gap between crisis and effective action.

11. B. Sequence from trigger through actions to consequence
Chain analysis examines the sequence of events leading to problematic behavior: vulnerability factors (baseline conditions), prompting event (trigger), links in chain (thoughts, feelings, actions), target behavior, and consequences. This detailed analysis identifies intervention points—places where skills could have interrupted the chain. It's about understanding so the client can make different choices, not blame.

12. B. Safety, trustworthiness, collaboration, empowerment
Trauma-informed care emphasizes safety (physical and emotional), trustworthiness and transparency (explaining what you're doing, following through), collaboration and mutuality (working with not on clients), empowerment voice and choice (supporting autonomy), and cultural sensitivity. It doesn't emphasize immediate trauma processing, confrontation, or power assertion—these can re-traumatize.

13. B. Safety and stabilization
Phase-based trauma treatment begins with safety and stabilization—establishing physical and emotional safety, building coping skills, creating support systems, stabilizing life circumstances. Before processing trauma memories, the person needs stable foundation and adequate skills. Processing traumatic memories when the person is unstable or lacks skills can destabilize rather than help.

14. B. Orient to present moment during flashbacks
Grounding techniques help orient to present moment during flashbacks or dissociation. Examples: name five things you see, four you hear, three you touch, two you smell, one you taste. This pulls attention from past traumatic memory into present reality. It doesn't avoid reality, eliminate memories, or cause dissociation—it interrupts dissociation and reconnects to present.

15. B. After establishing safety and skills
Trauma processing should occur after establishing safety and developing adequate coping skills. Processing trauma memories evokes distress—the person needs skills for managing that distress and stable life circumstances to contain the work. Processing trauma immediately without preparation can overwhelm and destabilize. Some people never process trauma formally but achieve good functioning through safety and stabilization alone.

16. B. Ambivalence about change
Motivational Interviewing addresses ambivalence about change—the normal human experience of wanting to change and not wanting to change simultaneously. While originally developed for addiction, MI is used for any behavior change where ambivalence exists. It's not for psychosis, dementia, or conditions where ambivalence isn't the primary issue.

17. B. Partnership, acceptance, compassion, evocation
The spirit of MI includes partnership (collaborative, not expert-patient), acceptance (unconditional positive regard, empathy, autonomy support, affirmation), compassion (actively promoting client welfare), and evocation (drawing out client's own motivation rather than imposing external motivation). It's not about confrontation, authority, or diagnosis—it's about respectful collaboration supporting change.

18. B. Self-expressed arguments for change
Change talk is any self-expressed argument for change—statements the client makes favoring change. Examples: "I want to quit," "I need to change," "I'm ready to start." Change talk predicts actual behavior change. MI practitioners listen for change talk, reinforce it through reflection and questions, and strengthen it. Change talk comes from the client, not the therapist.

19. B. Acknowledging resistance without confrontation
Rolling with resistance means acknowledging resistance without confronting or arguing. When clients express resistance, you don't fight it—you reflect it, explore it, sometimes amplify it slightly to evoke the other side of ambivalence. Arguing increases resistance. Rolling with it reduces resistance and opens exploration. It's not giving up or forcing change—it's working with resistance skillfully.

20. B. Helping clients see gap between behavior and values

Developing discrepancy means helping clients see the gap between current behavior and important values or goals. When people recognize that their behavior conflicts with deeply held values, motivation for change increases. This isn't arguing or creating guilt—it's helping clients articulate their own discrepancy. The discomfort of cognitive dissonance (behavior doesn't match values) motivates change.

21. B. Open-ended questions, Affirmations, Reflections, Summaries

OARS skills are the foundation of MI: Open-ended questions (require more than yes/no), Affirmations (recognize strengths and efforts), Reflections (mirror back what client says), and Summaries (gather and emphasize important content). These skills create collaborative conversation that evokes and strengthens change talk. They don't include confrontation or medication—those aren't MI techniques.

22. B. Test beliefs through action

Behavioral experiments test beliefs through action, providing evidence that words alone can't provide. A socially anxious client believes "If I speak up, everyone will think I'm stupid." You design experiment: speak once in next meeting, observe reactions. Results typically disconfirm catastrophic predictions—people respond neutrally or positively. Experiments aren't unnecessary or dangerous—they're evidence-gathering that challenges beliefs.

23. B. Systematic errors in thinking

Cognitive distortions are systematic, predictable errors in thinking that maintain psychological problems: all-or-nothing thinking, overgeneralization, mental filter, jumping to conclusions, emotional reasoning, labeling, personalization. They're not accurate, not signs of psychosis, and are treatable—CBT specifically targets and modifies these thinking patterns. Everyone has some cognitive distortions; problems arise when they're pervasive and rigid.

24. B. Acting opposite to emotion's urge when emotion doesn't fit facts

Opposite action means acting opposite to emotion's urge when the emotion doesn't fit the facts or isn't serving you well. Sad? Get active instead of withdrawing. Angry unjustifiably? Speak gently instead of attacking. Anxious about safe situation? Approach instead of avoiding. It's not acting impulsively, never feeling emotions, or avoiding action—it's using behavior to modify emotions.

25. B. Asking for what you need

DEAR MAN is an interpersonal effectiveness skill for asking for what you need: Describe situation, Express feelings, Assert by asking clearly, Reinforce positive effects, stay Mindful, appear Confident, Negotiate. This structured approach helps people ask for needs directly and effectively, particularly important for those who struggle with assertion or fear rejection.

26. B. Observing present moment without judgment

Mindfulness involves observing present moment experience—thoughts, emotions, sensations, surroundings—without judgment, without trying to change or avoid it. It's not never thinking, controlling thoughts, or only positive thoughts. It's awareness and acceptance of whatever is happening right now. This reduces suffering that comes from fighting reality or being lost in past/future.

27. B. They're integrated and no longer dominate consciousness
When traumatic memories are successfully processed, they're integrated into the person's life narrative and no longer dominate consciousness. Memories don't disappear—they're still accessible but no longer intrusive, overwhelming, or central to identity. Processing doesn't erase memories or make them more intrusive—it changes their emotional intensity and meaning so the person isn't controlled by them.

28. B. Mentally place traumatic memories in safe container temporarily
Containment techniques help clients mentally place traumatic memories in a safe container (imagined box with lock, safe, vault) so memories don't overwhelm them outside of therapy. The person can open the container during sessions with support, then close it after. It's temporary management, not avoiding or eliminating memories or creating new ones—it's creating psychological distance when needed.

29. B. Arguments against change
Sustain talk is self-expressed arguments against change—statements favoring the status quo. "I don't drink that much," "Quitting would be too hard," "I can handle it." Sustain talk is normal part of ambivalence, not something to argue with or ignore completely. MI practitioners acknowledge sustain talk without emphasis while evoking change talk more actively.

30. B. Exaggerates slightly to evoke the other side of ambivalence
Amplified reflection exaggerates the client's statement slightly, often evoking the other side of ambivalence. Client: "I can quit whenever I want." Reflection: "So drinking isn't really a problem at all for you." This often evokes: "Well, I didn't say that..." bringing out ambivalence. It's strategic, not arguing or agreeing completely—it gently pushes to evoke change talk.

31. B. Breaks overwhelming tasks into manageable steps
Graded task assignment breaks overwhelming tasks into small, manageable steps. A depressed client thinks "I need to clean the entire house" and feels overwhelmed, does nothing. You break it down: today, wash three dishes. Each completed step provides mastery experience and contradicts thoughts like "I can't do anything." It doesn't make tasks harder, avoid them, or require perfection—it makes change achievable.

32. B. Nervous system through Temperature, Intense exercise, Paced breathing
TIP skills regulate the nervous system during intense emotion: Temperature (cold water on face changes physiology), Intense exercise (burns energy), Paced breathing (slows breathing to calm), and sometimes Paired muscle relaxation. These physiological interventions calm the autonomic nervous system, reducing emotional intensity. They're not just about thoughts or behaviors—they're about changing body state.

33. B. Assuming feelings reflect reality
Emotional reasoning is assuming that feelings reflect reality: "I feel stupid, therefore I am stupid." "I feel like a failure, therefore I am a failure." Feelings are real and valid, but they don't always reflect objective reality. This distortion is common and creates problems—people base conclusions on feelings rather than evidence. It's not logical, healthy, or rare—it's a cognitive distortion requiring challenge.

34. B. Guilt or anger
Should statements create guilt when directed at self ("I should be able to handle this") and anger when directed at others ("They should treat me fairly"). These rigid rules about how things must be set up disappointment and distress when reality doesn't match expectations. Flexible preferences ("I'd prefer...") are healthier than rigid demands ("must," "should," "have to").

35. B. Drawing out client's own reasons for change
Evocation means drawing out the client's own reasons for change rather than imposing external motivation. The therapist doesn't lecture about why the client should change—the therapist asks questions that help the client articulate their own reasons. Motivation that comes from within is stronger and more sustainable than motivation imposed from outside.

36. B. Relationships
GIVE skills maintain relationships during interpersonal interactions: be Gentle (no attacks), act Interested (listen), Validate the other person, use an Easy manner (be light-hearted when appropriate). These skills help maintain positive relationships even during difficult conversations or conflicts. They don't maintain distance, anger, or avoidance—they maintain connection.

37. B. Adaptations that made sense given circumstances
Trauma symptoms are adaptations that made sense given circumstances, not weakness, untreatable conditions, or imaginary problems. Hypervigilance kept the person safe in danger. Dissociation allowed survival during unbearable experiences. Emotional numbing protected against overwhelming pain. These strategies worked in traumatic contexts—they just no longer serve well in current safety. Reframing symptoms as adaptations reduces shame and guides treatment.

38. B. Jumping to negative conclusions about future
Fortune telling is a cognitive distortion involving negative predictions about the future without evidence: "This will definitely turn out badly," "I'll never succeed," "They'll reject me for sure." It's not accurate prediction or healthy planning—it's catastrophizing about future events that haven't happened. These predictions increase anxiety and become self-fulfilling as people avoid situations or don't try hard.

39. B. Self-respect
FAST skills maintain self-respect during interpersonal interactions: be Fair to self and others, No Apologies when not warranted, Stick to your values, be Truthful. These skills help maintain dignity and self-respect even when asking for needs or maintaining relationships. They don't maintain speed, relationships (that's GIVE), or avoidance—they maintain self-respect.

40. B. Adds meaning or continues the paragraph
Complex reflection adds meaning or continues what the client said, showing deeper understanding. Client: "I know I drink too much." Simple reflection: "You're aware your drinking is excessive." Complex reflection: "You're concerned about how much you drink, and you're not sure if you're ready to change." Complex reflections deepen conversation and demonstrate understanding beyond surface content.

41. B. Plan specific activities at specific times
Activity schedules in behavioral activation plan specific activities at specific times—not vague intentions but concrete plans. "Monday 6 PM: 15-minute walk" not "Exercise sometime this week." Specific planning increases follow-through. Schedules don't overwhelm clients if activities are appropriately sized. They're essential not optional—structure prevents default to inactivity. Activity affects mood—tracking shows this connection.

42. B. Taking responsibility for events outside your control
Personalization is taking responsibility for events outside your control: "The project failed because of me" when multiple factors contributed, "My child struggled because I'm a bad parent" when genetics and environment both play roles. Some accountability is healthy, but personalization involves excessive self-blame for things beyond your control or influence. It creates guilt and maintains depression.

43. B. Ambivalence about change
The contemplation stage (from Stages of Change model) involves ambivalence—the person sees the problem and is considering change but isn't yet ready to act. They're weighing pros and cons, uncertain. Precontemplation means not considering change. Preparation means ready to change soon. Action means actively changing. Maintenance means sustaining change. MI in contemplation stage helps resolve ambivalence toward change.

44. B. Biological emotion dysregulation plus invalidating environment
Biosocial theory (Linehan's explanation of BPD development) proposes that biological vulnerability to emotion dysregulation (intense emotions, slow return to baseline) combines with invalidating environment (emotions dismissed, minimized, punished). Neither alone causes BPD—the interaction creates the disorder. The person never learns to identify, tolerate, or regulate emotions and develops problematic coping strategies. Understanding this reduces blame and guides treatment.

45. B. Exaggerates negatives
Magnification is exaggerating the importance or severity of negatives: making mountains out of molehills, turning small mistakes into catastrophes. "I made one error on the report—I'm going to get fired." This cognitive distortion is paired with minimization (shrinking positives). Together they maintain depression and anxiety by making negative events seem enormous and positive events insignificant.

46. B. Acknowledges both sides of ambivalence
Double-sided reflection acknowledges both sides of the client's ambivalence: "On one hand, you enjoy drinking and it helps you relax. On the other hand, you're worried about your health and your wife is threatening to leave." This shows you understand the complexity of their experience. It doesn't ignore ambivalence, take sides, or argue—it reflects the full picture including competing motivations.

47. B. Vulnerability to negative emotions through physical health
PLEASE skills reduce vulnerability to negative emotions by maintaining physical health: treat Physical illness, balance Eating, avoid mood-Altering substances, balance Sleep, get Exercise. Physical health affects emotional health. Poor sleep, irregular eating, substance use, sedentary

lifestyle, and untreated illness all increase emotional vulnerability. PLEASE skills create physical foundation supporting emotional stability.

48. B. Transforms positive experiences into negatives
Discounting the positive transforms positive experiences into negatives: "They only said that to be nice—it doesn't really count." "I got the promotion but only because my boss felt sorry for me." This distortion prevents people from experiencing positive events fully and maintains negative beliefs about self. It's not realistic or healthy—it's a cognitive distortion requiring challenge through examining evidence.

49. B. Doing things that create sense of accomplishment
Building mastery involves doing things that create a sense of accomplishment or competence—learning new skills, completing challenging tasks, achieving goals. Mastery experiences feel good, build self-efficacy, and counter depression. This isn't becoming perfect or only thinking—it's taking action that demonstrates competence. Even small mastery experiences (learning to cook a new dish, fixing something broken) provide psychological benefits.

50. B. Focuses exclusively on negatives while ignoring positives
Mental filter focuses exclusively on negatives while filtering out positives—like looking through dark glasses that only let negative information through. A person receives 99 positive comments and one criticism, dwells on the criticism and forgets the positives. This distortion maintains depression by preventing positive experiences from registering. It's not balanced, rare, or seeing both sides—it's biased negative attention.

51. B. Provides brief in-the-moment skill coaching
Phone coaching in DBT provides brief (typically 10-15 minutes) in-the-moment coaching for applying skills during crises. The client calls when experiencing urges to self-harm or intense emotions, and the therapist coaches them through using skills. It doesn't replace therapy, isn't unlimited (clear boundaries exist), and is a core DBT component—it extends skills training into real-world crises.

52. B. Draws broad conclusions from single events
Overgeneralization draws sweeping, broad conclusions from single events: one rejection means "No one will ever love me," one mistake means "I always mess everything up," one bad experience means "This will never work." The words "always," "never," "everyone," and "no one" signal overgeneralization. This distortion maintains hopelessness by making negative events seem like permanent, pervasive patterns.

53. B. Distract during crisis through Activities, Contributing, Comparisons, etc.
ACCEPTS is a distress tolerance skill using distraction during crisis: Activities (engage in task requiring attention), Contributing (help someone), Comparisons (remember worse times or compare to others with bigger problems), Emotions (create opposite emotion), Pushing away (mentally distance from problem), Thoughts (occupy mind with other thoughts), Sensations (intense sensations like holding ice). Distraction helps survive crisis moments without harmful actions.

54. B. Are fundamental assumptions about self, others, world
Core beliefs are fundamental assumptions developed early in life that shape how we see ourselves, others, and the world: "I'm competent/inadequate," "People are trustworthy/untrustworthy," "The world is safe/dangerous." They're not situation-specific—they're broad, pervasive views. They don't change easily but can be modified with sustained work. Core beliefs generate automatic thoughts and drive emotional responses.

55. B. Missing sessions, not completing homework, violating agreements
Therapy-interfering behaviors in DBT are behaviors that interfere with treatment progress: missing sessions without calling, arriving very late, not completing homework, violating therapy agreements (calling excessively, showing up intoxicated), attacking or threatening therapist. These behaviors are addressed directly in treatment—not ignored or leading to termination—because they block progress. The goal is reducing these behaviors so therapy can work.

56. B. Attaches global labels based on specific behaviors
Labeling attaches global labels to self or others based on specific behaviors: "I made a mistake" becomes "I'm a loser." "He forgot my birthday" becomes "He's a terrible person." Labels are absolute, extreme, and overgeneralized. They're not specific, helpful, or rare—they're cognitive distortions that maintain negative self-concept and relationship problems. Describing specific behaviors ("I made an error") is more accurate and less damaging than global labels.

57. B. Respecting client's right to choose
Autonomy support in MI means respecting the client's right to make their own choices, including the choice not to change. You don't force, coerce, or make decisions for the client. You provide information, explore options, and support the client's decision-making—but ultimately, the choice is theirs. This isn't avoiding discussion or forcing change—it's genuine respect for autonomy, which paradoxically often facilitates change.

58. B. Five senses to provide comfort
Self-soothing in distress tolerance uses the five senses to provide comfort: vision (beautiful images, art), hearing (soothing music), smell (pleasant scents, aromatherapy), taste (favorite food, tea), touch (soft blanket, warm bath, pet an animal). These sensory experiences provide comfort without harmful behaviors. They're not harmful, about avoidance, or using substances—they're healthy ways to self-soothe during distress.

59. B. Mind reading and fortune telling
Jumping to conclusions includes two specific types: mind reading (assuming you know what others think: "She thinks I'm stupid") and fortune telling (predicting negative future: "This will definitely fail"). Both involve negative interpretations without evidence. They're not careful evaluation, evidence-based thinking, or slow processing—they're quick, automatic negative assumptions that maintain anxiety and depression.

60. A. Notices experiences without trying to change them
The observe skill in mindfulness means noticing internal and external experiences without trying to change, judge, or push them away—just watching thoughts, emotions, sensations, sights, and sounds

as they arise and pass. It's not judging, avoiding present, or only focusing on negatives—it's open awareness of whatever is happening. Observation creates space between experience and reaction.

61. B. Understanding that some people experience emotions more intensely
DBT's biosocial theory recognizes that some people have biological vulnerability to emotion dysregulation—they experience emotions more intensely, reach peak more quickly, and return to baseline more slowly. This isn't blaming biology or saying biology determines everything—it's acknowledging biological factors that, combined with environmental factors, create problems. Understanding this reduces self-blame and normalizes experiences.

62. B. Track pleasure and mastery to show activity-mood connection
Activity ratings in behavioral activation track pleasure (P) and mastery (M) for each activity on 0-10 scales. This shows the connection between activity and mood that clients often don't recognize. Data reveals that certain activities improve mood, even if the client didn't expect it. Ratings aren't unnecessary, don't cause depression, and don't only track negatives—they objectively demonstrate the activity-mood relationship.

63. B. Dismisses, minimizes, or punishes emotions
An invalidating environment dismisses, minimizes, or punishes emotional experiences: "You're too sensitive," "Stop crying," "That's not a real problem," "You shouldn't feel that way." Emotions are treated as wrong, excessive, or manipulative. This prevents learning to identify, tolerate, and regulate emotions. It doesn't validate all emotions, isn't helpful, and does affect development—it's a risk factor for emotion dysregulation problems.

64. B. Puts words to experiences using facts
The describe skill in mindfulness means putting words to experiences using objective facts rather than judgments or interpretations: "My heart is racing" not "I'm having a panic attack," "I'm having the thought that I'm worthless" not "I am worthless." Description creates distance between experience and interpretation. It doesn't judge, avoid language, or use only judgments—it uses factual, objective language.

65. B. Practices recreate trauma dynamics like powerlessness
Re-traumatization occurs when helping practices recreate trauma dynamics: powerlessness (forced treatment, no choices), boundary violations, broken trust, coercion, punitive responses. Examples: restraints, isolation, forced medication, disbelief, power assertion. It's not about discussing trauma or providing help—it's about practices that repeat traumatic experiences. Trauma-informed care specifically works to avoid re-traumatization by prioritizing safety, choice, and trustworthiness.

66. B. Recognize strengths and efforts
Affirmations in MI recognize and acknowledge the client's strengths, efforts, positive qualities, and past successes: "You've managed to stay sober for three days despite intense cravings—that takes real strength." Affirmations aren't insincere flattery, don't only focus on problems, and aren't unnecessary—they build self-efficacy, strengthen alliance, and support change by recognizing existing capacities.

67. B. Engaging fully in current activity
The participate skill means engaging fully in current activity without self-consciousness—being absorbed in what you're doing, not watching yourself from outside. It's the opposite of constant self-monitoring. Participation creates flow states where you're immersed in the present. It's not watching from outside, avoiding activity, or multi-tasking—it's complete engagement with present moment.

68. B. Emotions dominate thinking
Emotion mind is when emotions dominate thinking and decision-making. Facts and consequences take a backseat to feelings. Someone in emotion mind acts impulsively based on intense feeling without considering consequences. It's not integration of emotion and logic (that's wise mind), doesn't ignore emotions, and isn't always best—effective functioning requires balance between emotion mind, reasonable mind, and wise mind.

69. B. Is evaluated objectively
In CBT, evidence for thoughts is evaluated objectively—examining facts supporting and contradicting automatic thoughts. This isn't assumed accurate, isn't ignored, and does matter greatly. The cognitive restructuring process specifically examines evidence to determine whether thoughts are accurate, distorted, or partially true. Objective evaluation of evidence is central to cognitive therapy.

70. B. Logic dominates, emotions minimized
Reasonable mind is when logic dominates and emotions are minimized or ignored. Facts, logic, and rational analysis guide decisions without considering feelings. Someone in pure reasonable mind might make technically correct decisions that feel wrong or violate values. It's not integration (that's wise mind), doesn't have no logic, and isn't always best—balance is needed.

71. B. Stop, Take step back, Observe, Proceed mindfully
STOP skill in DBT helps interrupt impulsive reactions: Stop (freeze, don't react immediately), Take a step back (create space physically or mentally), Observe (notice what's happening internally and externally), Proceed mindfully (choose response considering goals and values). It doesn't stop all activity permanently, just stop thinking, or cause problems—it creates pause between stimulus and response allowing mindful choice.

72. B. Working with client, not on them
Partnership in MI means working with the client as collaborators, not expert working on patient. Both bring expertise—client knows their life, therapist knows about change processes. Decisions are made jointly. Power differentials are reduced where possible. It's not therapist deciding everything, client having no say, or no structure—it's collaborative structure respecting both parties' contributions.

73. B. Are more balanced interpretations considering all evidence
Alternative thoughts in CBT are more balanced interpretations that consider all evidence—not forced positive thinking, not ignoring problems, not always positive. They're realistic appraisals based on evidence. Automatic thought: "I'm a complete failure." Alternative thought: "I didn't succeed at this task, but I've succeeded at many others. This doesn't define me completely." Alternative thoughts are balanced and evidence-based.

74. B. Reduces vulnerability to negative emotions
Building positive experiences in DBT reduces vulnerability to negative emotions. When life includes positive experiences—pleasant activities, meaningful relationships, accomplishments—the person is less vulnerable to depression and overwhelming negative emotions. This isn't impossible, doesn't cause problems, and isn't only thinking—it's actively creating positive experiences through planned activities and working toward meaningful goals.

75. B. Indicates strong intent to change
Commitment language in change talk indicates strong intent to change: "I will quit," "I'm going to start," "I promise I'll change." This is stronger than desire ("I want to") or ability ("I could"). Commitment language predicts actual behavior change more strongly than other forms of change talk. It's not weak, does predict behavior, and is encouraged—MI practitioners listen for and reinforce commitment language.

Where This Takes You

Therapeutic modalities provide structure for change. CBT shows how thoughts, feelings, and behaviors interact—changing one changes others. DBT recognizes that some people feel emotions more intensely and need specific skills for regulation. Trauma-informed care creates safety allowing healing from experiences that taught the world is dangerous. Motivational interviewing respects ambivalence and evokes internal motivation rather than imposing external pressure.

You don't need to be expert in every approach, but you need foundational competence in multiple modalities. You recognize which approach fits which problem. You adapt flexibly when one approach isn't working. You integrate techniques thoughtfully rather than applying them randomly.

The techniques matter—research shows what works. But technique without relationship fails. You can apply CBT perfectly, but if the client doesn't trust you, doesn't feel understood, doesn't believe you care, the techniques won't help. The relationship provides the context where techniques can work.

You're learning tools. Use them wisely. Use them well. Use them in service of helping people build lives worth living.

Core Understanding for Your Practice

- CBT addresses the interaction between thoughts, feelings, and behaviors with automatic thoughts as immediate interpretations subject to examination
- Cognitive distortions are systematic thinking errors including all-or-nothing thinking, overgeneralization, mental filter, and emotional reasoning
- Behavioral activation treats depression by increasing meaningful activities, demonstrating that action can precede motivation
- Thought records examine evidence for and against automatic thoughts, identifying distortions and developing balanced alternatives
- DBT was developed for BPD, teaching mindfulness, distress tolerance, emotion regulation, and interpersonal effectiveness skills

- Dialectical thinking holds multiple truths simultaneously, synthesizing apparent opposites with both-and rather than either-or logic
- Wise mind integrates emotion mind and reasonable mind, providing balanced perspective including both feelings and logic
- Chain analysis in DBT examines sequences from trigger through actions to consequences, identifying intervention points
- Trauma-informed care prioritizes safety, trustworthiness, collaboration, empowerment, and avoiding re-traumatization
- Phase-based trauma treatment begins with safety and stabilization before processing traumatic memories
- Motivational Interviewing addresses ambivalence through partnership, acceptance, compassion, and evocation of internal motivation
- OARS skills (Open-ended questions, Affirmations, Reflections, Summaries) create collaborative conversation evoking change talk
- Change talk is self-expressed arguments for change that predict actual behavior change and should be reinforced
- Rolling with resistance means acknowledging without confronting, reducing rather than increasing resistance
- Effective therapy integrates evidence-based techniques with strong therapeutic relationship—neither alone is sufficient

Chapter 10: Clinical Interventions by Problem Area

Mental health problems come in patterns. Depression looks different from anxiety, which looks different from trauma, which looks different from addiction. Each problem requires specific understanding and targeted intervention. You can't treat everything the same way and expect good results.

This doesn't mean every person with depression gets identical treatment. Two people with depression may need different approaches based on contributing factors, co-occurring problems, strengths, and circumstances. But understanding problem-specific interventions provides foundation for individualizing treatment.

Depression and Suicidal Ideation

Depression steals energy, hope, and the ability to imagine a better future. People describe it as living under a heavy blanket, moving through thick fog, being trapped in a pit with no way out. The cognitive triad of depression—negative views of self, world, and future—maintains the problem even when circumstances improve.

Assessment priorities include severity, duration, precipitants, contributing factors, functional impact, suicide risk, and co-occurring conditions. Depression ranges from mild (functioning continues with effort) to severe (can barely get out of bed). Chronic depression (persistent for years) differs from episodic depression (discrete episodes with recovery between).

Contributing factors guide intervention:

Biological: Genetic vulnerability, medical conditions (hypothyroidism, chronic pain, neurological conditions), hormonal changes (postpartum, menopause), medication side effects, substance use, sleep problems.

Psychological: Negative thinking patterns, perfectionism, rumination, trauma history, learned helplessness, low self-esteem.

Social: Isolation, relationship problems, financial stress, work problems, lack of social support, major losses.

Cognitive-behavioral interventions form the foundation:

Behavioral activation increases engagement in activities providing pleasure or mastery. You create activity schedule with specific planned activities. The client tracks mood before and after activities, demonstrating the activity-mood connection. Even when the client doesn't feel like it, completing activities improves mood. Accumulated small improvements create sustained change.

Cognitive restructuring addresses negative thinking. You teach thought records, help identify cognitive distortions, examine evidence for and against thoughts, and develop balanced alternatives. Common depressive thoughts: "I'm worthless," "Nothing will ever get better," "I always mess everything up," "Everyone would be better off without me."

Problem-solving helps address real problems contributing to depression. Depression impairs problem-solving ability—people feel overwhelmed and helpless. You break problems into manageable pieces, brainstorm solutions, evaluate options, implement solutions, and assess results. Success experiences counter helplessness.

Medication treats moderate to severe depression effectively. SSRIs (selective serotonin reuptake inhibitors) and SNRIs (serotonin-norepinephrine reuptake inhibitors) are first-line treatments. They take 4-6 weeks for full effect. You collaborate with prescribers, help clients understand medications, manage side effects, and maintain adherence. Combined medication and therapy works better than either alone for moderate to severe depression.

Interpersonal therapy addresses relationship problems contributing to depression. Depression often involves grief (loss of important relationship), role disputes (conflicts with significant others), role transitions (life changes like retirement, divorce), or interpersonal deficits (social isolation, difficulty forming relationships). IPT helps resolve these issues, which alleviates depression.

Behavioral experiments test depressive beliefs. A client believes "If I try to do anything, I'll fail." You design experiment: attempt a small task, observe results. Usually the person succeeds or at least doesn't experience catastrophic failure. Evidence contradicts the belief.

Pleasant event scheduling specifically targets anhedonia (inability to experience pleasure). Even if activities aren't initially pleasurable, engaging in them begins reactivating reward systems. Over time, capacity for pleasure returns.

Suicidal ideation requires careful, ongoing assessment. Many depressed people think about death or suicide. You assess frequency, intensity, intent, plan, means, protective factors, and history. Suicidal thoughts exist on continuum from passive ("I wish I wouldn't wake up") to active ("I plan to kill myself tomorrow").

Safety planning for suicidal clients includes:

1. **Warning signs**: What tells you a crisis is developing?
2. **Internal coping strategies**: What can you do yourself?
3. **Social supports**: Who can you talk to?
4. **Family members who can help**: Who can you contact for support?
5. **Professional contacts**: Who can you call in crisis?
6. **Means restriction**: How do you make the environment safer?

Clients keep written copies accessible. You review and update plans regularly. Safety planning doesn't prevent all suicides, but it provides structure for managing crises.

Case Example: Depression Treatment - Patricia

Patricia, 52, presents with Major Depression following job loss. She's been unemployed for four months, spending most days in bed. Her PHQ-9 score is 21 (severe). She reports feeling worthless, hopeless, and like a burden to her family. She has passive suicidal ideation ("I wish I would just disappear") but no plan or intent.

Initial sessions: Safety and engagement

You assess suicide risk carefully. Patricia has thoughts but no plan, strong protective factors (family, religious beliefs), and willingness to commit to safety. You develop safety plan and contract for safety.

You provide psychoeducation about depression—it's common, treatable, caused by multiple factors, not weakness or character flaw. Patricia's been blaming herself for being depressed ("I should be able to handle this"). Understanding depression as illness reduces self-blame.

Behavioral activation (weeks 1-4)

Patricia's activity level is minimal. She stays in bed until afternoon, does minimal housework, rarely leaves home. You create activity schedule starting small:

Week 1:

- Get out of bed by 10 AM daily
- Shower and dress four days
- One 10-minute walk

Patricia resists: "I don't have energy for this." You explain: "I know you're exhausted. Depression causes that. But we've found that increasing activity actually increases energy. It seems backward, but it works. Let's try it as an experiment."

Patricia completes most scheduled activities. Tracking shows mood improves slightly after activities (from 2/10 to 4/10), even when she didn't feel like doing them. This demonstrates the principle that action precedes motivation.

Week 2-4: Gradually increase activities. Add cooking meals, calling friends, applying for jobs online. Patricia notices mood improving with increased activity. PHQ-9 drops to 17.

Cognitive restructuring (weeks 5-8)

Patricia's thinking is pervasively negative:

- "I'm a failure" (lost job, unemployed four months)
- "I'll never find another job" (ageism, economy, long unemployment)

- "My family would be better off without me" (burdening them financially and emotionally)

You work through thought records:

Thought: "I'm a failure"
Evidence for: Lost job, unemployed four months, draining savings
Evidence against: Worked successfully for 25 years, received promotions and positive reviews, laid off due to company downsizing not performance, raised successful children, maintained 30-year marriage
Alternative: "I lost my job due to circumstances beyond my control. I'm experiencing a difficult period, but that doesn't make me a failure as a person. I have many successes in my life."

Patricia's beliefs begin shifting. She recognizes that losing a job doesn't define her worth, that unemployment is situational not permanent, that her catastrophic predictions aren't facts.

Problem-solving (weeks 9-12)

Real problems require real solutions. Patricia needs employment. Depression has impaired her problem-solving—she's felt overwhelmed and hopeless. You break it down:

Problem: Need income
Brainstorm solutions: Full-time job, part-time job, temporary work, freelance consulting, early retirement
Evaluate: Full-time in her field seems unlikely given age discrimination. Part-time or consulting more realistic. Early retirement possible but would reduce lifetime income.
Implement: Patricia updates resume, contacts former colleagues about consulting opportunities, applies for part-time positions, explores early retirement calculations.

Within two weeks, Patricia has two consulting projects. This success counters helplessness and provides hope.

Medication consultation (week 6)

Patricia's depression is severe. You refer for medication evaluation. She starts SSRI. Combined with therapy, she shows steady improvement. PHQ-9 drops to 8 by week 12.

Relapse prevention (weeks 13-16)

Patricia's functioning has improved dramatically. She has consulting work providing income and structure. Mood is stable. Suicidal thoughts are gone. You prepare for termination:

Warning signs: Sleep disruption, withdrawing from family, negative thinking increasing, activity level dropping
Coping strategies: Resume thought records, maintain activity schedule, problem-solve rather than ruminate, reach out for support
Action plan: If symptoms return and last two weeks, contact for booster session

Patricia terminates therapy having learned skills for managing depression. Six-month follow-up shows maintained improvement.

Anxiety and Panic

Anxiety is normal—it alerts us to danger and motivates protective action. Anxiety disorders occur when this system misfires—triggering intense alarm when no real danger exists or maintaining anxiety long after danger has passed. The person knows rationally they're safe but can't turn off the anxiety response.

Types of anxiety problems each require somewhat different interventions:

Generalized Anxiety Disorder involves chronic, excessive worry about multiple areas—health, finances, work, family, world events. The person recognizes worry is excessive but can't control it. Physical symptoms accompany mental worry: muscle tension, fatigue, sleep problems, irritability.

Panic Disorder involves recurrent unexpected panic attacks plus persistent worry about future attacks. Panic attacks are abrupt surges of intense fear with physical symptoms: racing heart, sweating, trembling, shortness of breath, chest pain, nausea, dizziness, fear of dying or losing control. They peak within minutes and are terrifying.

Social Anxiety Disorder involves intense fear of social situations where the person might be scrutinized. They fear acting in ways that will be negatively evaluated—showing anxiety symptoms, saying something embarrassing, being judged. Anxiety is out of proportion to actual threat.

Specific Phobias involve marked fear of specific objects or situations—flying, heights, animals, blood, enclosed spaces. The phobic object almost always provokes fear, is avoided or endured with intense distress.

Assessment priorities include specific anxiety type, triggers, safety behaviors (subtle avoidance maintaining anxiety), functional impact, and co-occurring problems (particularly depression and substance use).

Cognitive-behavioral treatment is first-line intervention:

Psychoeducation about anxiety helps clients understand:

- Anxiety is a normal response to perceived threat
- The fight-or-flight response causes physical symptoms
- Anxiety isn't dangerous—uncomfortable but not harmful
- Avoidance maintains anxiety by preventing learning
- Exposure helps anxiety decrease naturally

Cognitive restructuring challenges anxious thoughts:

Catastrophic thinking: "If I panic on the plane, I'll lose control and go crazy." You examine evidence—has this ever happened? What's the actual likelihood? What would really occur?

Probability overestimation: "I'll definitely fail the presentation." You evaluate realistic probability based on evidence, not feeling.

Intolerance of uncertainty: "I need to know for certain it will be okay." You help clients tolerate uncertainty, recognizing that certainty is often impossible and attempting to achieve it maintains anxiety.

Exposure therapy is the most effective anxiety intervention. Exposure involves gradually and repeatedly facing feared situations while learning that:

1. Anxiety decreases naturally without escape (habituation)
2. Feared catastrophic outcomes don't occur
3. You can tolerate anxiety
4. The situation is safe or manageable

Exposure hierarchy lists feared situations from least to most anxiety-provoking (0-100 scale). Treatment starts with moderate items (50-60 range), practices until anxiety decreases by at least 50%, then progresses to harder items.

Exposure must be:

- **Graduated**: Start easier, progress to harder
- **Prolonged**: Stay in situation long enough for anxiety to decrease (usually 30-60 minutes)
- **Repeated**: Practice multiple times until fear decreases substantially
- **Without safety behaviors**: No subtle avoidance preventing full confrontation

Interoceptive exposure for panic disorder involves deliberately inducing feared physical sensations to learn they're not dangerous:

- Hyperventilation (dizziness, tingling)
- Spinning (dizziness)
- Chest breathing (breathlessness)
- Running in place (racing heart)
- Staring at light then reading (vision changes)

Initially terrifying, clients learn these sensations are uncomfortable but not dangerous. Fear of panic symptoms decreases.

Relaxation training helps manage anxiety symptoms:

Diaphragmatic breathing: Slow, deep breathing activates parasympathetic nervous system, reducing physiological arousal. In through nose (count to 4), hold (count to 4), out through mouth (count to 6).

Progressive muscle relaxation: Systematically tense then release muscle groups, teaching recognition of tension and ability to release it.

Mindfulness: Observing anxiety without judgment or struggle often reduces intensity. Fighting anxiety amplifies it; accepting it paradoxically reduces it.

Worry time: For GAD, schedule specific 30-minute "worry time" daily. When worry arises outside this time, postpone it to worry time. This contains worry rather than having it intrude constantly.

Medication treats anxiety effectively but isn't first-line treatment alone. SSRIs treat anxiety disorders long-term. Benzodiazepines provide rapid relief but risk dependence and withdrawal. Beta-blockers reduce physical symptoms (racing heart, trembling) for performance anxiety.

Case Example: Social Anxiety Treatment - Marcus

Marcus, 28, has severe social anxiety. He avoids meetings at work, turns down promotions requiring public speaking, and has no social life outside his long-term girlfriend. He fears people will think he's stupid or boring. Even casual conversations trigger intense anxiety.

Assessment and psychoeducation (sessions 1-2)

Marcus rates social anxiety 8/10 in severity. It started in adolescence but worsened after he froze during a presentation in college. He's avoided public speaking since.

You explain the social anxiety cycle:

1. Anticipate social situation
2. Predict catastrophe ("They'll think I'm stupid")
3. Experience intense anxiety (racing heart, sweating, shaking)
4. Use safety behaviors (avoid eye contact, speak minimally, leave early)
5. Feel relief from escaping
6. Belief strengthens ("See, I can't handle social situations")

Avoidance and safety behaviors prevent learning that social situations are safe and that anxiety decreases naturally. Treatment will break this cycle through exposure.

Creating exposure hierarchy (session 3)

You and Marcus create hierarchy of feared situations rated 0-100:

- 30: Brief conversation with grocery store cashier
- 40: Longer conversation with neighbor
- 50: Lunch with one coworker
- 60: Small group conversation (3-4 people)
- 70: Speak up once in team meeting

- 80: Present briefly (5 minutes) in meeting
- 90: Give longer presentation (15 minutes)
- 95: Present to unfamiliar audience

Beginning exposure (sessions 4-12)

You start at 40-50 level. Marcus's first exposure: have lunch with coworker, stay the full hour, participate in conversation without safety behaviors (no rehearsing everything beforehand, no monitoring himself constantly for signs of anxiety, no avoiding eye contact).

Before exposure, Marcus predicts catastrophe: anxiety will be unbearable (100/100), he'll freeze and have nothing to say, coworker will think he's weird, he'll have to leave early.

Marcus completes exposure. Reality: initial anxiety was 85/100, peaked at 90/100 around 15 minutes, then gradually decreased to 40/100 by end of lunch. He didn't freeze—he had some awkward moments but so did coworker. Conversation flowed reasonably well. Coworker suggested lunch again next week.

This experience contradicts Marcus's predictions. Anxiety was high but decreased without escape. He didn't freeze. Coworker didn't judge him negatively. The situation was manageable.

Repeated exposure (sessions 5-12)

Marcus repeats similar exposures—lunches with different coworkers, conversations with neighbors, small group interactions. Each time, anxiety peaks then decreases. Each time, catastrophic predictions don't come true. The pattern becomes clear: anxiety is uncomfortable but temporary and manageable.

By session 12, Marcus can attend small social gatherings with manageable anxiety (30-40/100). He's speaking up in team meetings occasionally. The breakthrough: he volunteered to give a brief update in a meeting (5 minutes). Anxiety was high (80/100) initially but he completed it. Feedback was positive. No one thought he was stupid.

Cognitive work throughout

You challenge anxious thoughts:

Thought: "Everyone will think I'm stupid"
Evidence for: I feel stupid, I sometimes stumble over words
Evidence against: Coworkers have said I'm knowledgeable, I've been promoted twice, everyone stumbles over words sometimes, I'm focusing on myself more than others are
Alternative: "Some people might notice if I'm nervous, but most are focused on themselves. Even if I'm not perfectly articulate, that doesn't mean people think I'm stupid. I have genuine expertise to offer."

Eliminating safety behaviors

Marcus's safety behaviors include:

- Rehearsing everything he'll say
- Constantly monitoring himself for anxiety signs
- Avoiding eye contact
- Speaking very little
- Leaving situations early

You help Marcus drop these behaviors during exposures. Initially this increases anxiety, but it allows full confrontation with fear and natural anxiety reduction.

Outcome (session 16)

Marcus has made dramatic progress. Social anxiety is 3/10. He attends social events, speaks up at work, just gave a 15-minute presentation with manageable anxiety. He accepted a promotion requiring occasional presentations. He's dating more confidently. Exposure therapy worked—gradually facing fears in a systematic way allowed him to learn that social situations are manageable and that he's more capable than he believed.

Trauma and PTSD

Trauma shatters assumptions about safety, control, and predictability. Someone who experienced life-threatening danger, witnessed violence, or was violated sexually can't just "get over it." The brain's alarm system remains activated long after danger has passed. Memories intrude unbidden. Triggers activate full-blown fight-or-flight response. The world no longer feels safe.

PTSD symptoms cluster into four categories:

Intrusion: Unwanted memories, nightmares, flashbacks, intense distress at reminders, physiological reactions to cues. The trauma keeps coming back uninvited.

Avoidance: Avoiding thoughts, feelings, conversations about trauma; avoiding people, places, activities that are reminders. Avoidance provides temporary relief but maintains PTSD by preventing processing.

Negative alterations in cognitions and mood: Can't remember parts of trauma, negative beliefs ("I'm permanently damaged," "The world is completely dangerous," "I can't trust anyone"), persistent negative emotions, inability to experience positive emotions, feeling detached from others.

Alterations in arousal and reactivity: Hypervigilance, exaggerated startle, irritability and anger, reckless behavior, concentration problems, sleep disturbance. The nervous system stays in threat mode.

Assessment priorities include trauma history, current symptoms across all four clusters, functional impact, co-occurring problems (depression, substance use), social support, and safety (current violence, suicidal ideation).

Phase-based treatment progresses through stages:

Phase 1: Safety and stabilization

Before processing trauma, establish safety. For someone in active domestic violence, safety planning and potentially leaving the relationship comes first. For someone using substances to cope, address substance use. For someone with severe emotion dysregulation, build regulation skills.

This phase includes:

- Ensuring physical safety
- Developing emotion regulation and distress tolerance skills
- Creating support systems
- Psychoeducation about trauma and PTSD
- Establishing therapeutic relationship
- Teaching grounding and containment techniques

Some clients remain in Phase 1 for extended periods or permanently. That's acceptable if it results in improved functioning.

Phase 2: Processing traumatic memories

Once stable, clients can process trauma through evidence-based treatments:

Prolonged Exposure (PE) involves:

Imaginal exposure: Repeatedly recounting the trauma in detail during sessions, typically 30-45 minutes. Recorded so client listens daily between sessions. Initially intensely distressing, emotional intensity decreases across repetitions. Memories are processed and integrated rather than remaining fragmented and overwhelming.

In vivo exposure: Gradually approaching trauma-related situations that are safe but avoided. A car accident survivor might avoid driving, riding in cars, accident location. Graduated exposure to these situations allows learning they're safe and reduces avoidance.

PE helps organize traumatic memories, reduce emotional intensity, and decrease avoidance. Clients learn they can handle trauma memories without being overwhelmed.

Cognitive Processing Therapy (CPT) focuses on how trauma affected beliefs. Clients identify "stuck points"—problematic beliefs like "It was my fault," "I should have done something different," "I can never trust anyone," "The world is completely dangerous."

Through Socratic questioning and written exercises, clients examine evidence for and against stuck points, consider alternative interpretations, and develop more balanced beliefs. Changing trauma-related beliefs reduces PTSD symptoms.

EMDR (Eye Movement Desensitization and Reprocessing) involves recalling traumatic memories while engaging in bilateral stimulation (eye movements, alternating hand taps, alternating sounds).

The bilateral stimulation is thought to facilitate reprocessing of memories. EMDR includes preparation, desensitization, installation of positive beliefs, and body scan.

All three approaches have strong evidence. Choice depends on client preference, therapist training, and clinical considerations.

Phase 3: Integration and reconnection

After processing trauma, focus shifts to building meaningful life. This might include:

- Developing healthy relationships
- Pursuing education or career goals
- Reconnecting with community and activities
- Finding meaning and purpose
- Consolidating treatment gains
- Preparing for potential future challenges

Medication helps PTSD symptoms but doesn't replace trauma-focused psychotherapy. SSRIs reduce overall symptoms. Prazosin reduces nightmares. Medication combined with therapy works better than either alone.

Case Example: PTSD Treatment - Sarah

Sarah, 29, was sexually assaulted two years ago. She has intrusive memories, nightmares, hypervigilance, avoids dating and situations resembling the assault location, feels disconnected from friends, and experiences intense shame and self-blame. She meets full PTSD criteria.

Phase 1: Stabilization (sessions 1-8)

Sarah is safe currently—the perpetrator was prosecuted and imprisoned. But she's emotionally unstable—intense emotions overwhelm her, she dissociates frequently, she's been drinking heavily to cope.

You don't jump into trauma processing. First, you build foundation:

Sessions 1-3: Safety and psychoeducation

- Explain PTSD symptoms as normal responses to abnormal events
- Teach grounding techniques for managing flashbacks (5-4-3-2-1: name five things you see, four you hear, three you touch, two you smell, one you taste)
- Develop crisis management plan
- Build therapeutic relationship

Sessions 4-6: Skills building

- Teach emotion regulation skills (identifying emotions, understanding their function, distress tolerance)
- Address substance use (Sarah agrees to stop drinking, attends AA)
- Teach containment (imagining placing traumatic memories in locked box so they don't overwhelm her outside sessions)

Sessions 7-8: Preparation for processing

- Explain trauma processing
- Sarah decides on Cognitive Processing Therapy—the structured, cognitive focus appeals to her
- You establish that Sarah has adequate skills and stability for processing

Phase 2: Trauma processing with CPT (sessions 9-20)

Sarah writes about her assault and how it's affected her beliefs about safety, trust, power/control, esteem, and intimacy.

Stuck points identified:

- "It was my fault—I shouldn't have gone to that party"
- "I should have fought harder"
- "I'm damaged goods—no one will want me now"
- "I can't trust my judgment about people"
- "The world is completely dangerous"

You work through each stuck point:

Stuck point: "It was my fault"

Questions to consider:

- Who is responsible for assault—the person who chose to assault or the person who attended a party?
- Would you blame your best friend if she were assaulted at a party?
- Does attending a party give someone the right to assault you?
- What percentage of people at parties get assaulted? (Showing that attending parties doesn't normally result in assault—the perpetrator's choice caused the assault)

Through repeated examination, Sarah's belief shifts: "The assault was not my fault. Attending a party is normal behavior. The perpetrator chose to assault me. He's responsible for his actions, not me."

Stuck point: "I'm damaged goods"

Questions:

- Does experiencing trauma permanently damage someone?
- Do you view other trauma survivors as damaged?
- What evidence do you have that you're fundamentally changed in negative ways?
- What strengths have you shown since the assault?

Sarah recognizes: "The assault was terrible, but it doesn't define who I am. I'm not damaged—I'm a person who experienced trauma and is recovering. I have many positive qualities that didn't disappear because of the assault."

Sessions 9-20: Work through all stuck points systematically. Sarah's beliefs gradually shift from extreme, rigid, self-blaming to more balanced, realistic, compassionate.

Phase 3: Integration (sessions 21-24)

Sarah's PTSD symptoms have decreased dramatically. She still has occasional intrusive memories but they're brief and manageable. Nightmares are rare. She's no longer hypervigilant. She's dating someone new. She's reconnected with friends.

Now you focus on moving forward:

- Building healthy relationship skills
- Continuing personal growth
- Finding meaning (Sarah volunteers at rape crisis center, finding purpose in helping others)
- Relapse prevention

Sarah terminates therapy having processed trauma, changed trauma-related beliefs, and built a life not controlled by the assault. Follow-up shows maintained gains.

Practice Questions (Continuing with questions 76-100 for this chapter)

76. Behavioral activation for depression involves:

A. Only thinking about activities
B. Scheduling and completing meaningful activities
C. Avoiding difficult tasks
D. Only talking about feelings

77. The cognitive triad of depression includes negative views of:

A. Only self
B. Self, world, and future
C. Only relationships
D. Only the past

78. Pleasant event scheduling targets:

A. Anxiety
B. Anhedonia (inability to experience pleasure)
C. Anger
D. Psychosis

79. Safety planning for suicidal clients includes:

A. Just hospitalization
B. Warning signs, coping strategies, supports, professional contacts, means restriction
C. Only medication
D. Avoiding all discussion

80. In anxiety treatment, safety behaviors:

A. Help reduce anxiety
B. Are subtle avoidance maintaining anxiety
C. Should be encouraged
D. Don't matter

81. Exposure therapy must be:

A. Brief and one-time
B. Graduated, prolonged, repeated, without safety behaviors
C. Only imaginal
D. Avoided

82. Interoceptive exposure involves:

A. Avoiding all physical sensations
B. Deliberately inducing feared physical sensations to learn they're not dangerous
C. Only medication
D. Ignoring symptoms

83. The social anxiety cycle includes:

A. Only thoughts
B. Anticipation, catastrophic predictions, anxiety, safety behaviors, relief, belief strengthening
C. No specific pattern
D. Random events

84. Worry time for GAD involves:

A. Worrying constantly
B. Scheduling specific daily time for worry, postponing worry outside that time
C. Eliminating all worry
D. Medication only

85. PTSD intrusion symptoms include:

A. Only avoidance
B. Unwanted memories, nightmares, flashbacks
C. Only negative thoughts
D. No specific symptoms

86. Phase 1 of trauma treatment focuses on:

A. Immediate trauma processing
B. Safety and stabilization
C. Only medication
D. Forcing memories

87. Prolonged Exposure involves:

A. Avoiding trauma memories
B. Repeatedly recounting trauma and approaching safe but avoided situations
C. Only medication
D. Ignoring symptoms

88. Cognitive Processing Therapy focuses on:

A. Only memories
B. How trauma affected beliefs and examining stuck points
C. Avoiding cognition
D. Only behavior

89. Stuck points in CPT are:

A. Helpful beliefs
B. Problematic beliefs developed from trauma
C. Accurate thoughts
D. Unchangeable

90. Grounding techniques help:

A. Increase dissociation
B. Orient to present during flashbacks
C. Avoid reality
D. Eliminate memories

91. Exposure hierarchy lists:

A. Random situations
B. Feared situations from least to most anxiety-provoking
C. Only easy situations
D. Only impossible situations

92. Habituation means:

A. Anxiety increases over time
B. Anxiety decreases naturally with sustained exposure
C. Anxiety stays constant
D. Avoidance works

93. Catastrophic thinking in anxiety involves:

A. Realistic assessment
B. Predicting worst possible outcomes
C. Balanced thinking
D. Positive expectations

94. Avoidance maintains PTSD by:

A. Helping process trauma
B. Preventing processing and learning that reminders are safe
C. Reducing symptoms
D. Curing PTSD

95. The purpose of imaginal exposure is:

A. Creating new trauma
B. Processing traumatic memories through repeated recounting
C. Avoiding memories
D. Imagination exercises

96. Hypervigilance in PTSD means:

A. Relaxation
B. Constant scanning for threat
C. Appropriate caution
D. Sleepiness

97. Problem-solving for depression helps:

A. Avoid all problems
B. Address real problems contributing to depression
C. Only think about problems
D. Create more problems

98. Intolerance of uncertainty in anxiety involves:

A. Accepting uncertainty
B. Needing absolute certainty and inability to tolerate ambiguity
C. Healthy caution
D. Flexibility

99. In vivo exposure means:

A. Only imagined exposure
B. Real-life exposure to feared situations
C. Avoiding situations
D. Virtual reality only

100. Containment techniques help:

A. Eliminate all trauma memories
B. Mentally place traumatic memories in safe container temporarily
C. Avoid all thoughts
D. Create new memories

Answer Key with Detailed Explanations (Questions 76-100)

76. B. Scheduling and completing meaningful activities
Behavioral activation involves scheduling specific meaningful activities that provide pleasure or mastery, then completing them even when motivation is low. It's not just thinking about or talking about activities—it's actual behavioral engagement. The activity-mood connection is tracked to demonstrate that action can precede motivation and that increased activity improves mood.

77. B. Self, world, and future
The cognitive triad of depression describes negative views of self ("I'm worthless"), world ("Everything is terrible"), and future ("Nothing will ever get better"). This three-part negative perspective maintains depression by creating hopelessness. CBT challenges these negative views across all three domains through examining evidence and developing more balanced perspectives.

78. B. Anhedonia (inability to experience pleasure)
Pleasant event scheduling specifically targets anhedonia—the inability to experience pleasure that's common in depression. Even if activities aren't initially pleasurable, engaging in them begins reactivating reward systems and rebuilding capacity for pleasure. Over time, with repeated engagement in pleasant activities, the ability to experience pleasure returns.

79. B. Warning signs, coping strategies, supports, professional contacts, means restriction
Comprehensive safety planning includes: identifying warning signs of crisis, internal coping strategies (what I can do myself), social supports (people to talk to), family who can help, professional contacts (therapist, crisis line, emergency services), and making environment safe (means restriction). This provides structure for managing suicidal crises. It's not just hospitalization or medication—it's multilayered prevention.

80. B. Are subtle avoidance maintaining anxiety
Safety behaviors are subtle forms of avoidance that prevent full confrontation with feared situations and maintain anxiety. Examples: gripping steering wheel tightly (thinking this prevents accidents), constantly monitoring yourself for anxiety signs, avoiding eye contact, leaving situations early. Safety behaviors prevent learning that situations are safe and that anxiety decreases naturally. Effective exposure eliminates safety behaviors.

81. B. Graduated, prolonged, repeated, without safety behaviors
Effective exposure therapy must be: graduated (starting easier, progressing to harder), prolonged (staying long enough for anxiety to decrease, typically 30-60 minutes), repeated (practicing multiple times), and without safety behaviors (no subtle avoidance). Brief, one-time, or partial exposures are less effective. All four elements are necessary for optimal results.

82. B. Deliberately inducing feared physical sensations to learn they're not dangerous
Interoceptive exposure deliberately induces feared physical sensations (hyperventilation for dizziness, running for racing heart, spinning for disorientation) to help clients learn these sensations are uncomfortable but not dangerous. This is particularly useful for panic disorder where fear of physical sensations maintains panic. Through repeated exposure, fear of the sensations themselves decreases.

83. B. Anticipation, catastrophic predictions, anxiety, safety behaviors, relief, belief strengthening
The social anxiety cycle involves: anticipating social situation, predicting catastrophe ("They'll think I'm stupid"), experiencing intense anxiety, using safety behaviors to cope, feeling relief from escaping, and having beliefs strengthened by the experience ("See, I can't handle it"). Treatment breaks this cycle through exposure without safety behaviors, allowing new learning.

84. B. Scheduling specific daily time for worry, postponing worry outside that time
Worry time for GAD involves scheduling a specific 30-minute period daily dedicated to worry. When worry arises outside this time, the person postpones it to worry time. This contains and limits worry rather than having it intrude throughout the day. It doesn't eliminate worry or involve worrying constantly—it structures and contains it.

85. B. Unwanted memories, nightmares, flashbacks
PTSD intrusion symptoms include recurrent unwanted memories, distressing dreams/nightmares, dissociative reactions (flashbacks), intense psychological distress at trauma cues, and physiological reactions to reminders. These represent trauma memories intruding into consciousness against the person's will. Avoidance is a separate symptom cluster. Intrusion specifically describes unwanted recurrence of trauma content.

86. B. Safety and stabilization
Phase 1 of phase-based trauma treatment focuses on establishing safety (physical and emotional), building coping skills, creating support systems, and stabilizing life circumstances. This must occur before trauma processing because processing evokes distress—the person needs foundation and skills to manage that distress. Immediate trauma processing without stabilization can overwhelm and destabilize.

87. B. Repeatedly recounting trauma and approaching safe but avoided situations
Prolonged Exposure involves imaginal exposure (repeatedly recounting trauma in detail during sessions and listening to recordings between sessions) and in vivo exposure (gradually approaching trauma-related situations that are safe but avoided). Through repeated confrontation, emotional intensity decreases, memories are organized and integrated, and avoidance reduces. It's not avoiding, only using medication, or ignoring symptoms—it's systematic processing through exposure.

88. B. How trauma affected beliefs and examining stuck points
Cognitive Processing Therapy focuses specifically on how trauma affected beliefs about safety, trust, power/control, esteem, and intimacy. Clients identify stuck points—problematic beliefs like "It was my fault" or "I can't trust anyone"—and examine evidence for and against them through Socratic questioning and written exercises. Changing trauma-related beliefs reduces PTSD symptoms. It's not avoiding cognition or only focusing on memory or behavior—it's cognitive restructuring of trauma-related beliefs.

89. B. Problematic beliefs developed from trauma
Stuck points are problematic beliefs that developed from or were reinforced by trauma: "It was my fault," "I should have done something different," "The world is completely dangerous," "I can never trust anyone." These beliefs maintain PTSD symptoms and interfere with functioning. They're not helpful, accurate, or unchangeable—they're targets for modification through examining evidence and developing balanced alternatives.

90. B. Orient to present during flashbacks
Grounding techniques help orient to present moment during flashbacks or dissociation: name five things you see, four you hear, three you can touch, two you smell, one you taste. This pulls attention from past traumatic memory into present reality. It doesn't increase dissociation, avoid reality, or eliminate memories—it interrupts dissociation and flashbacks by reconnecting to present.

91. B. Feared situations from least to most anxiety-provoking
Exposure hierarchy is a list of feared situations ranked from least to most anxiety-provoking, typically rated 0-100. Treatment usually starts with moderate items (50-60 range), practices until anxiety decreases significantly, then progresses to harder items. The hierarchy isn't random, only easy, or only impossible—it's systematic progression from manageable to more challenging fears.

92. B. Anxiety decreases naturally with sustained exposure
Habituation is the natural decrease in anxiety that occurs with sustained exposure to feared stimuli. When someone stays in a feared situation without escaping, anxiety initially increases then gradually decreases—usually within 30-60 minutes. This teaches that anxiety is temporary and that escape isn't necessary. Habituation is the mechanism underlying exposure therapy's effectiveness.

93. B. Predicting worst possible outcomes
Catastrophic thinking predicts worst possible outcomes without evidence: "If I panic on the plane, I'll lose control and go crazy," "If I make a mistake, I'll be fired and lose everything." These catastrophic predictions maintain anxiety by making situations seem more dangerous than they are. Treatment involves examining evidence for predictions and developing realistic alternatives.

94. B. Preventing processing and learning that reminders are safe
Avoidance maintains PTSD by preventing processing of traumatic memories and preventing learning that trauma reminders are safe. When someone avoids, they never learn that: they can handle trauma memories without being overwhelmed, reminders won't cause the trauma to recur, anxiety about reminders decreases with exposure. Avoidance provides temporary relief but maintains long-term symptoms by blocking new learning.

95. B. Processing traumatic memories through repeated recounting
The purpose of imaginal exposure (in Prolonged Exposure therapy) is processing traumatic memories by repeatedly recounting the trauma in detail during therapy sessions. Through repetition, emotional intensity decreases, memories become organized rather than fragmented, and the person learns they can handle remembering without being overwhelmed. It's not creating new trauma, avoiding memories, or just imagination exercises—it's systematic memory processing.

96. B. Constant scanning for threat
Hypervigilance in PTSD means constantly scanning the environment for potential threats, being always "on alert," checking surroundings repeatedly, inability to relax because of perceived need to watch for danger. The nervous system remains in threat-detection mode even in safe environments. It's not relaxation, appropriate caution, or sleepiness—it's exhausting, excessive vigilance driven by trauma.

97. B. Address real problems contributing to depression
Problem-solving in depression treatment addresses real problems contributing to depression: unemployment, financial stress, relationship conflicts, health problems. Depression impairs problem-solving ability—people feel overwhelmed and helpless. Treatment breaks problems into manageable pieces, brainstorms solutions, evaluates options, implements solutions, and assesses results. Success experiences counter learned helplessness. It's not avoiding, only thinking about, or creating problems—it's actively solving them.

98. B. Needing absolute certainty and inability to tolerate ambiguity
Intolerance of uncertainty involves needing absolute certainty about outcomes and inability to tolerate ambiguity: "I need to know for certain it will be okay," "What if something bad happens?" This maintains anxiety because certainty is often impossible—attempting to achieve it through excessive checking, reassurance-seeking, or avoidance creates more anxiety. Treatment involves building tolerance for uncertainty through exposure to ambiguous situations.

99. B. Real-life exposure to feared situations
In vivo exposure means real-life (not imagined or virtual) exposure to feared situations. For someone with driving phobia, this means actually driving (not just imagining driving). For social anxiety, it means actual social interactions. In vivo exposure is typically graduated—starting with easier situations and progressing to harder ones—but it involves real-world practice in feared situations.

100. B. Mentally place traumatic memories in safe container temporarily
Containment techniques help clients mentally place traumatic memories in an imagined safe container (box with lock, safe, vault) so memories don't overwhelm them outside of therapy sessions. The person can "open" the container during sessions with support, then "close" it afterward. It's temporary management providing psychological distance, not eliminating memories, avoiding all thoughts, or creating new memories—it's a tool for managing intrusive memories between processing sessions.

Closing Thoughts

Clinical interventions work when they match the problem. Depression responds to behavioral activation and cognitive restructuring because withdrawal and negative thinking maintain depression.

Anxiety responds to exposure because avoidance maintains anxiety. Trauma responds to processing because unprocessed memories remain fragmented and overwhelming.

But matching intervention to problem isn't enough. You must implement interventions skillfully, adjust when progress stalls, attend to the therapeutic relationship, and individualize treatment to each person's unique circumstances.

The techniques in this chapter are tools. Learn them well. Practice them until they become second nature. But never forget that behind every diagnosis is a person suffering, hoping you can help. Your skill with techniques matters, but so does your compassion, your persistence, and your genuine care for the person sitting across from you.

Essential Clinical Knowledge

- Behavioral activation treats depression by increasing meaningful activities, demonstrating that action can precede motivation
- The cognitive triad of depression (negative views of self, world, future) maintains depression through hopeless perspective
- Safety planning for suicidal clients includes warning signs, coping strategies, supports, professional contacts, and means restriction
- Exposure therapy must be graduated, prolonged, repeated, and without safety behaviors to achieve habituation
- Safety behaviors are subtle avoidance that prevents full confrontation with fears and maintains anxiety
- The social anxiety cycle involves anticipation, catastrophic predictions, anxiety, safety behaviors, and belief strengthening
- Interoceptive exposure deliberately induces feared physical sensations to learn they're not dangerous
- Phase-based trauma treatment begins with safety and stabilization before processing traumatic memories
- Prolonged Exposure involves repeatedly recounting trauma and approaching safe but avoided situations
- Cognitive Processing Therapy focuses on examining and modifying stuck points—problematic trauma-related beliefs
- Grounding techniques orient to present moment during flashbacks by engaging all five senses
- Avoidance maintains PTSD by preventing processing and learning that reminders are safe
- Habituation is natural anxiety decrease with sustained exposure without escape

- Problem-solving for depression addresses real problems through systematic approach breaking them into manageable steps
- Effective treatment matches evidence-based interventions to specific problems while individualizing to each client's unique circumstances

Chapter 11: Group and Family Therapy

Something happens when people come together. A woman who's been struggling alone with depression discovers five others in the room feel exactly the same way. A teenager who's been convinced his family doesn't understand him hears his parents describe their own confusion and pain. A man who's been hiding his anxiety realizes he's not uniquely broken—others share his struggle.

Individual therapy provides the safety of one-on-one connection, the focused attention of a therapist dedicated to understanding you. But group and family therapy offer something individual work can't: the power of connection with others facing similar challenges, the opportunity to see your problems reflected in different mirrors, the chance to help others while helping yourself.

Groups and families are complex systems where everyone affects everyone else. Change one person and you change the system. Help one family member communicate differently and the whole family shifts. These modalities require different skills than individual therapy—you're orchestrating multiple relationships, managing group dynamics, tracking patterns across people, and facilitating change at the system level.

Group Therapy Techniques and Stages

Group therapy isn't individual therapy with more people in the room. It's a fundamentally different modality with unique therapeutic factors. Irvin Yalom identified these factors—the mechanisms through which groups create change. Understanding these factors helps you facilitate groups effectively.

Therapeutic factors in groups explain why groups work:

Universality: Members discover they're not alone—others share similar struggles, feelings, and experiences. This normalizes problems and reduces shame. The isolated person realizes "I'm not the only one" and feels immediate relief. Universality is particularly powerful early in group.

Altruism: Helping others feels good and builds self-esteem. Members who feel worthless discover they have something valuable to offer. The depressed person who offers support to another member experiences purpose and competence. Giving is as therapeutic as receiving.

Installation of hope: Seeing others improve creates hope for your own improvement. When a member who was severely depressed six months ago now functions well, newer members think "If she can get better, maybe I can too." Hope is particularly powerful when members are at different stages of recovery.

Imparting information: Groups provide education about problems and coping strategies. You teach skills, members share techniques that worked for them, and collective wisdom accumulates. Information reduces anxiety through understanding and provides concrete tools.

Corrective recapitulation of the primary family: Groups recreate family dynamics, allowing members to work through unresolved family issues in the safer group context. Someone who couldn't express anger to a parent might learn to express it appropriately with a group member who reminds them of that parent.

Development of socializing techniques: Groups are social laboratories where members learn interpersonal skills. Someone with social anxiety practices conversation. Someone who's aggressive learns to communicate without attacking. The group provides real-time feedback and opportunities for practicing new behaviors.

Imitative behavior: Members learn by observing others—how to express feelings appropriately, how to set boundaries, how to ask for support. Modeling is powerful learning mechanism. You model healthy communication, and members incorporate it.

Interpersonal learning: Groups reveal interpersonal patterns. The way someone acts in group reflects how they act in life. You help members recognize patterns ("You're doing with Sarah what you described doing with your sister"), understand impact on others, and try new behaviors. This real-time interpersonal work is uniquely powerful.

Group cohesiveness: Feeling accepted and valued by the group creates safety for taking risks. Cohesive groups feel like safe families—places where you can be yourself, express difficult feelings, and know you'll be supported. Cohesion is the group equivalent of therapeutic alliance in individual therapy.

Catharsis: Expressing intense emotions in supportive environment provides relief and helps process feelings. Catharsis alone isn't sufficient, but combined with interpersonal learning and cognitive understanding, it's therapeutic. The group provides safe container for emotional expression.

Existential factors: Groups confront existential realities—life is sometimes unfair, we're ultimately responsible for our lives, we're alone even when connected to others, life has no inherent meaning. Processing these realities in supportive context reduces existential anxiety.

Group stages describe predictable phases groups move through. Understanding stages helps you facilitate appropriately and not panic when conflict emerges.

Forming (Stage 1): Members are anxious and polite. They seek acceptance, test boundaries, and figure out group norms. Trust is low. Cohesion hasn't developed. Members look to you for guidance and structure.

Your role: Provide structure and safety. Establish clear norms (confidentiality, respect, attendance). Help members connect through universality. Encourage sharing. Model appropriate self-disclosure and feedback. Create safe environment where people can take small risks.

Common issues: Members wonder "Will I be accepted?" "Is this safe?" "What are the rules?" Some members are silent, others dominate. Conflict is avoided. Discussion stays surface-level. Members direct questions to you rather than engaging each other.

Storming (Stage 2): Conflict emerges. Members challenge you and each other. Subgroups form. Competition for attention increases. Some members want to leave. This stage is uncomfortable but necessary—working through conflict builds trust and cohesion.

Your role: Don't shut down conflict—facilitate it. Help members express disagreement respectfully. Interpret conflict as progress ("The group feels safe enough now to disagree"). Maintain boundaries and safety while allowing appropriate confrontation. Don't take challenges personally—they're part of development.

Common issues: Members challenge your leadership, disagree with your interventions, or question group's value. Subgroups and alliances form. Some members are scapegoated. Attendance becomes inconsistent. Members express frustration about lack of progress. You might feel attacked or inadequate.

Norming (Stage 3): Conflict resolves into cooperation. Cohesion develops. Trust increases. Members feel accepted and valued. The group develops its own identity and culture. Members interact more with each other and less exclusively with you. Productive work happens.

Your role: Step back and let the group work. Members should be supporting, challenging, and helping each other. You facilitate rather than direct. Point out group processes. Help members give and receive feedback. Encourage interpersonal risk-taking.

Common issues: The group might get too comfortable—avoiding difficult topics to maintain harmony. Some members might resist deeper work. Others might feel disappointed that problems persist. The initial honeymoon phase of cohesion can give way to frustration when change is harder than expected.

Performing (Stage 4): The group functions effectively. Members work deeply on problems. Feedback is direct but caring. The group self-manages to some extent. Therapeutic factors are maximized. This is the most productive phase.

Your role: Facilitate deep work. Help members explore patterns and try new behaviors. Point out here-and-now processes. Connect group interactions to outside life. Encourage interpersonal risk-taking and honest feedback. The group does much of the therapeutic work itself.

Common issues: Some members progress faster than others, creating tension. As termination approaches, anxiety increases. Members might regress or create crises to avoid ending.

Adjourning (Stage 5): The group prepares to end. Members process feelings about termination, review progress, say goodbye. Grief and loss are expected. This stage is particularly powerful—members practice healthy endings and separations.

Your role: Help members process termination feelings. Review learning and progress. Encourage members to articulate what they've gained. Facilitate goodbyes. Help members plan for maintaining gains. Don't rush this stage—working through termination is therapeutic.

Common issues: Members minimize the group's importance to avoid sadness. Others regress, creating crises to extend the group. Some leave prematurely to avoid goodbye. Anger at you for "abandoning" them might emerge.

Group composition affects dynamics and outcomes. Homogeneous groups (similar diagnoses or problems) are cohesive quickly and provide strong universality. Members immediately relate. But they might reinforce problematic perspectives and lack diverse viewpoints.

Heterogeneous groups (varied diagnoses and problems) take longer to develop cohesion but offer richer interpersonal learning. Diversity provides multiple perspectives and reduces risk of groupthink. Members learn from people different from themselves.

The right composition depends on group purpose. Support groups for specific issues (bereaved parents, cancer survivors, sexual assault survivors) benefit from homogeneity—shared experience creates immediate connection. Process groups focused on interpersonal learning benefit from heterogeneity—diversity enriches learning.

Group norms are explicit and implicit rules governing behavior. Establishing productive norms early is crucial:

Confidentiality: What's said in group stays in group. This isn't absolute—members can discuss their own material outside group, but they can't share others' content. You discuss limits (mandated reporting of abuse, danger to self or others).

Attendance and commitment: Members commit to attending regularly and arriving on time. Irregular attendance disrupts cohesion. You address attendance problems directly.

Participation: Everyone is encouraged to participate, but no one is forced. Silence is respected but gently explored. Members should share airtime—no one dominates.

Respect: Members treat each other with respect even when disagreeing. Personal attacks aren't allowed. Feedback should be direct but caring.

Here-and-now focus: While members discuss outside problems, the group also focuses on what's happening in the room right now. Current interactions reveal patterns.

Responsibility: Members take responsibility for their own progress. They set personal goals and work actively on them. The group supports but doesn't rescue.

Subgrouping and socializing: Outside friendships between members can undermine the group. Private conversations create secrets and alliances. You discourage socializing outside group or, if it occurs, require that it be brought into group discussion.

Leader tasks include multiple simultaneous responsibilities:

Creating and maintaining safety: Physical safety (no violence), emotional safety (respectful interaction), and confidentiality. Without safety, risk-taking won't occur.

Establishing and enforcing norms: You set initial norms and enforce them consistently. When someone arrives late repeatedly, you address it. When someone dominates, you redirect.

Facilitating interaction: You encourage members to talk to each other, not just to you. "Don't tell me—tell Sarah directly." You want members engaging with each other.

Managing group dynamics: You track what's happening at multiple levels—individual content, interpersonal processes, whole-group dynamics. You intervene when dynamics become problematic.

Activating therapeutic factors: You highlight universality ("Notice how three people described the same fear"), encourage altruism ("Your support of Tom was really helpful"), and point out interpersonal learning opportunities.

Working in the here-and-now: You focus attention on current interactions, not just outside problems. "Tom, you just criticized yourself for rambling. You do that a lot. Has anyone else noticed?"

Promoting self-disclosure: You model appropriate self-disclosure and encourage members to share. But you protect people from excessive disclosure before sufficient trust exists.

Linking: You connect members who share similarities or whose issues relate. "Mary, what Tom described sounds similar to what you said last week about your brother."

Supporting and confronting: You provide both support and challenge. Pure support feels good but doesn't create change. Pure confrontation feels attacking. The balance creates growth.

Case Example: Interpersonal Process Group - Codependency Issues

You're leading an interpersonal process group—eight members, mixed diagnoses, meeting weekly for 90 minutes. The group has been meeting for four months and is in norming stage, developing good cohesion.

Session excerpt:

Tom, 45, arrives 20 minutes late, apologizing profusely. This is his third late arrival in five weeks. The group has been discussing Rachel's difficulty setting boundaries with her adult children.

Tom: "Sorry I'm late. Traffic was terrible. What did I miss?"

You: "Tom, before we catch you up, I'd like the group to give you feedback about the late arrivals. This is the third time recently."

Tom (defensive): "I can't help traffic. I tried to get here on time."

Sarah: "Tom, I appreciate that traffic exists, but you always seem to have some reason you're late. I'm starting to feel like the group isn't a priority for you."

Tom: "That's not fair. I pay for this. I'm committed."

You: "Tom, I'm curious about something. Right now, Sarah gave you difficult feedback, and your response was to defend yourself. Does that pattern sound familiar? Do you do that in other relationships?"

Tom (pausing): "Yeah. My wife says I always have an excuse and never just own up to things."

You: "What would it be like to just acknowledge Sarah's feedback without defending?"

Tom (thinking): "Sarah, you're right. I have been late a lot. The group is important to me, but I guess I'm not showing that. I'm sorry."

Sarah: "Thank you. That feels different."

You: "Tom, what just happened? How did that feel?"

Tom: "Uncomfortable. But also kind of relieving. Defending is exhausting."

You: "And Sarah, how did Tom's acknowledgment feel compared to his initial defense?"

Sarah: "Much better. I felt heard. When he defended, I wanted to push harder. When he acknowledged it, I immediately softened."

You (to group): "This is such rich material. What Tom and Sarah just demonstrated is a common interpersonal cycle—one person gives feedback, the other defends, the first person pushes harder because they don't feel heard, the defender feels attacked and defends more. It escalates. But when someone drops the defense and just acknowledges, the cycle breaks. I'm wondering who else relates to this pattern?"

Rachel: "I do it constantly with my kids. They complain that I'm intrusive, I defend by saying I'm just trying to help, they get more upset. It never resolves."

Michael: "I'm on the other side. My partner does what Tom just did initially—defends everything. It makes me crazy. I just want acknowledgment."

You: "So we're seeing both sides of this dynamic represented in the room. Rachel and Tom relate to the defending side. Michael relates to Sarah's experience. This is perfect opportunity for learning. Let's practice."

You facilitate role-plays where members practice receiving feedback without defending, and giving feedback without attacking. The group discusses how these patterns developed (for Tom, a critical parent meant any feedback felt like attack, so he learned to defend automatically). Members connect group interactions to outside relationships and commit to trying new responses.

This session demonstrates multiple therapeutic factors: interpersonal learning (Tom sees his pattern), universality (others share the pattern), here-and-now focus (working with what's happening in the room), corrective emotional experience (Tom tries new response and it feels better), and cohesion (group supports Tom's risk-taking).

Specialized groups address specific populations or problems:

Psychoeducational groups teach information and skills. Examples: anger management, social skills training, parenting skills, illness education (diabetes management, cardiac rehabilitation). These are more structured with curriculum, homework, and specific skill practice. The leader teaches actively.

Support groups provide mutual support for people facing similar challenges. Examples: bereavement, chronic illness, addiction recovery (AA, NA), caregivers, trauma survivors. These emphasize universality, hope, and mutual aid. Structure is minimal, with members sharing experiences and supporting each other. Many are peer-led.

Therapy groups focus on psychological growth and symptom reduction through interpersonal learning. These are less structured than psychoeducational groups, with members setting individual goals. The leader facilitates interpersonal process. Examples: interpersonal process groups, groups for depression, groups for personality disorders.

Skills training groups teach specific skills systematically. Examples: DBT skills training (mindfulness, distress tolerance, emotion regulation, interpersonal effectiveness), CBT groups for anxiety, assertiveness training. Structured with specific curriculum, homework, and practice exercises.

Family Therapy Approaches

Families are systems—interconnected networks where each person affects all others. You can't understand individual problems without understanding the family context. A child's behavior problem might reflect parental conflict. An adult's depression might maintain family homeostasis. Family therapy addresses problems at the system level.

Family systems theory provides foundation for understanding families:

Circular causality: Family interactions are circular, not linear. A causes B causes C causes A. Dad criticizes, son withdraws, mom rescues son, dad feels undermined and criticizes more. You can enter the circle anywhere—it has no beginning. Interventions can target any part of the cycle.

Homeostasis: Families resist change to maintain stability. Even dysfunctional patterns are familiar and predictable. When one person changes, the system pushes back to restore equilibrium. A daughter gets better, and suddenly another child develops problems. Understanding homeostasis helps you anticipate and address resistance.

Triangulation: When tension exists between two people, they pull in a third to stabilize the relationship. Parents in marital conflict focus on a child's problems instead of addressing their relationship. The child's problems serve a function—reducing tension between the parents. The child becomes the "identified patient," but the real problem is the marriage.

Boundaries: Families need boundaries between subsystems. Clear boundaries allow connection while maintaining appropriate distance. Problems occur at extremes:

Enmeshment: Boundaries are too diffuse. Family members are overly involved in each other's lives with little privacy or individuality. Children can't develop autonomy. Problems in one person spread to all members.

Disengagement: Boundaries are too rigid. Family members are disconnected with little involvement or support. When someone has a problem, others don't notice or help.

Healthy families have clear boundaries—connected but allowing independence.

Family roles: Members develop roles that maintain family functioning. Common roles include:

Hero: The successful, responsible child who makes family look good. Achieves to compensate for family problems.

Scapegoat: The problem child who acts out. Blamed for family difficulties, this child's problems allow family to avoid addressing deeper issues.

Lost child: The quiet, invisible child who avoids attention. Adapts by becoming independent and self-sufficient.

Mascot: The family comedian who reduces tension through humor. Distracts from serious problems.

Roles develop to serve family needs, not individual needs. Therapy helps families abandon rigid roles.

Communication patterns reveal family functioning:

Direct vs. indirect: Healthy families communicate directly—"I'm upset with you." Dysfunctional families communicate indirectly—complaining to others, hinting, expecting mind-reading.

Clear vs. unclear: Clear communication specifies speaker, listener, and message. Unclear communication is vague about who's being addressed or what's meant.

Congruent vs. incongruent: Congruent communication aligns verbal and nonverbal messages. Incongruent communication sends contradictory messages—saying "I'm fine" while looking miserable.

Structural family therapy (Salvador Minuchin) focuses on family structure—organization, boundaries, and power hierarchies. The therapist assesses and restructures family organization.

Assessment involves understanding:

Boundaries: Are they clear, enmeshed, or disengaged? Between parents and children? Between siblings? Extended family?

Hierarchies: Do parents lead? Or does a child have inappropriate power? Are generational boundaries clear?

Alliances and coalitions: Are there inappropriate alliances (parent-child coalition against other parent)? Do parents present united front?

Interventions restructure the family:

Joining: The therapist connects with family, respecting their organization while positioning to influence it. You adapt to family style initially to gain credibility.

Reframing: Relabeling behavior to change its meaning. An "oppositional" teenager is reframed as "fiercely independent." An "overinvolved" mother is "deeply caring." Reframing reduces defensiveness and opens possibilities.

Enactment: Having family members interact with each other during session rather than talking to you about problems. "Don't tell me about the argument—show me. Have the argument here." This reveals actual patterns.

Boundary making: Strengthening weak boundaries or softening rigid ones. You might meet separately with parental subsystem to strengthen their alliance, or insist that parents discuss discipline directly instead of through the children.

Unbalancing: Temporarily siding with one person to destabilize homeostasis and create change. You might support a disempowered parent, challenging the family's usual pattern.

Strategic family therapy (Jay Haley, Cloe Madanes) focuses on solving specific problems through strategic interventions designed to change patterns maintaining problems.

Assessment identifies:

The problem: Specifically defined in behavioral terms. "Our son is defiant" becomes "When we ask him to do chores, he refuses and argues."

The sequence: What happens before, during, and after the problem behavior? What maintains it?

The function: What purpose does the problem serve in family system? A child's anxiety might keep parents united. An adult's depression might allow them to avoid life responsibilities.

Interventions use directives—tasks assigned to family:

Direct: Straightforward assignments. "This week, spend 30 minutes daily in one-on-one time with your son doing an activity he chooses."

Paradoxical: Prescribing the symptom to create change through resistance. Tell a couple who argues constantly to schedule two 30-minute arguments daily. Compliance is therapeutic (they gain control over arguing). Resistance is therapeutic (they stop arguing to avoid the assignment). Either way, the pattern changes.

Ordeal: Making the symptom more difficult than the alternative. A child who throws tantrums is required to practice tantrums for 20 minutes—making them tiresome and less appealing.

Pretend: Having someone pretend to have the symptom, which gives them control and reveals the symptom is controllable.

Strategic therapy is brief and problem-focused. It's less concerned with insight than with behavior change.

Bowenian family therapy (Murray Bowen) focuses on differentiation—the ability to separate thinking from feeling and maintain a clear sense of self in relationships.

Key concepts:

Differentiation of self: The ability to think independently while maintaining emotional connection to others. Low differentiation means emotions dominate, and the person is fused with others—can't distinguish their feelings from others' feelings. High differentiation means balancing emotion and reason, maintaining clear self while connected to others.

Emotional triangles: When tension exists between two people, they pull in third to reduce anxiety. Understanding triangles helps people address relationships directly rather than through others.

Family projection process: Parents project their anxiety onto a child, who becomes the focus of family worry and develops problems. Multiple generations might participate in focusing on this child.

Multigenerational transmission: Patterns transmit across generations. Understanding family history reveals current patterns' origins.

Interventions:

Genogram: Creating three-generation family diagram showing relationships, patterns, and significant events. This visual map reveals patterns across generations.

Process questions: Asking questions that reduce emotional reactivity and increase thoughtful responding. "What do you think about that?" instead of "How do you feel?"

Detriangulation: Helping family members relate directly instead of through third parties. Teaching parents to address their conflicts directly rather than through children.

Differentiation work: Helping individuals develop clearer sense of self while maintaining connection—thinking independently while staying emotionally engaged.

Bowen therapy moves slowly, emphasizing understanding over rapid change. It's intellectual and less emotionally intense than other approaches.

Emotionally Focused Therapy (Sue Johnson) for families and couples focuses on attachment—the emotional bonds between family members. When attachment is secure, family members function well. When attachment is threatened or insecure, problems emerge.

Key concepts:

Attachment needs: People have innate needs for connection, security, and reassurance. These aren't weaknesses—they're fundamental human needs. Problems arise when attachment needs aren't met.

Negative cycles: Families develop negative interaction patterns that threaten attachment. Common cycle: one person pursues connection desperately, the other distances to protect themselves, pursuing increases, distancing increases. Both feel disconnected.

Primary vs. secondary emotions: Secondary emotions (anger, frustration) are surface reactions. Primary emotions (fear, hurt, loneliness, shame) are underlying vulnerable feelings. Accessing primary emotions creates change.

Interventions:

Identifying cycles: Helping family see the pattern they're stuck in. "Do you see what happens? You reach for him, he steps back, you reach harder, he steps back further. You're both trying to protect yourselves, but you're moving apart."

Accessing primary emotions: Helping family members identify and express vulnerable emotions beneath defensive reactions. Anger often protects against hurt. Withdrawal often protects against fear of rejection.

Restructuring interactions: Creating new emotional experiences where attachment needs are met. A distancing partner expresses need for the pursuing partner instead of withdrawing. The pursuing partner expresses fear of abandonment instead of criticizing.

Consolidating change: Practicing new interactions until they become natural. Creating new positive cycles replacing negative ones.

EFT is structured with specific stages and steps, but emotionally focused on attachment and vulnerability.

Case Example: Structural Family Therapy - Martinez Family

The Martinez family comes to therapy for their 15-year-old daughter Sofia's "oppositional behavior." Parents Maria (42) and Carlos (45) describe Sofia as disrespectful, defiant, and failing school. Older brother Diego (18) is away at college. Younger sister Elena (12) is "perfect"—compliant, high-achieving.

First session assessment:

You observe the family's structure through their seating arrangement, interactions, and communication patterns:

Seating: Sofia sits far from parents. Maria and Elena sit close together. Carlos sits slightly apart from everyone.

Communication: Maria speaks for everyone, answering questions you direct to others. Carlos is silent unless directly addressed, then defers to Maria. Sofia interrupts and argues. Elena is quiet, watching anxiously.

Patterns: When you ask Sofia about her perspective, Maria immediately jumps in to correct or explain. When Carlos tries to discipline Sofia's interruption, Maria undermines him ("Let her express herself"). Sofia escalates when father attempts discipline but negotiates when mother does.

Structural problems identified:

Weak parental subsystem: Parents aren't united. Maria makes decisions alone, Carlos is peripheral. No clear parental hierarchy.

Enmeshment between Maria and Elena: Overly close, with unclear boundaries. Elena looks to Maria constantly for cues.

Maria-Sofia conflict: Constant battling, with no clear resolution process.

Father's peripheral position: Carlos is disengaged from family process. When he tries to engage, Maria blocks him.

Sofia's inappropriate power: She has too much influence, arguing as if she's equal to parents.

Formulation: Sofia's "oppositional behavior" serves multiple functions—she's fighting for normal adolescent autonomy against an enmeshed system, she's the focus keeping parents from addressing their relationship, and she's scapegoated as "the problem" while family structure remains unaddressed. The real problem isn't Sofia—it's the family organization.

Treatment plan: Restructure the family to create clear generational boundaries, strengthen the parental subsystem, appropriate Sofia's power level, and help Maria and Carlos function as united leadership team.

Intervention 1: Strengthening parental subsystem (Session 2)

You meet with Maria and Carlos alone, excluding the children. This immediately restructures—the parents have private space for their relationship.

You: "Sofia's behavior is a problem, but it's also a symptom of the parents not being aligned. Sofia knows she can split you—when Dad disciplines, Mom rescues. When Mom sets limits, Dad is silent. You're not working as a team."

Maria: "Carlos isn't involved enough. I have to make all the decisions."

Carlos: "When I try to be involved, you tell me I'm doing it wrong."

You: "This is the pattern. Carlos, you feel shut out and retreat. Maria, you feel alone and do more yourself, which pushes Carlos further out. Both of you feel resentful. Meanwhile, Sofia operates in the vacuum of parental unity."

You help them develop unified approach to discipline and communication. They agree to discuss parenting decisions privately before presenting to children. You assign homework: daily 20-minute private conversation (without kids) about their day, relationship, and parenting.

Intervention 2: Enactment (Session 3)

Whole family present. You create enactment to reveal and change patterns.

You: "Sofia, I hear you've been staying out past curfew. Let's not talk about it—let's handle it right now. Mom, Dad, discuss with Sofia what the consequence will be."

Maria (immediately): "Sofia, you know the rules. You're grounded for a week."

You (interrupting): "Maria, wait. I asked you and Carlos to discuss it together first, then present a united decision to Sofia."

Maria (frustrated): "Fine. Carlos, what do you think?"

Carlos: "I agree. Grounded."

You: "That didn't look like a discussion—that looked like Carlos agreeing with Maria's decision. Let me see you actually discuss it. Take a minute together, really talk about what makes sense."

They turn to each other and actually discuss—something they don't usually do. They negotiate: one week seems long, maybe three days plus extra chores. They reach agreement.

You: "Now present your decision to Sofia."

Carlos (more engaged): "Sofia, we discussed it, and we agree. You broke curfew, so you're grounded for three days and you'll do extra chores this weekend."

Sofia: "That's not fair! Mom, you said—"

You: "Sofia, your father just spoke to you. Respond to him."

Sofia: "Dad, I had a good reason. I was—"

Maria (starting to intervene): "Sofia, you should have called—"

You (gently): "Maria, let Carlos handle this. Let's see how he and Sofia work this out."

Carlos and Sofia negotiate directly. Maria watches anxiously but stays out of it. Sofia accepts the consequence without the usual explosion. This is new pattern—parents united, father engaged, Sofia responding appropriately.

Intervention 3: Boundary work (Session 5)

You address Maria and Elena's enmeshment.

You: "Elena, you're very tuned in to your mom. You watch her constantly, checking how she's feeling. That's a lot of responsibility for a 12-year-old."

Elena: "I just want to make sure she's okay."

You: "That's kind, but taking care of your mom's emotions is a parent's job, not yours. Maria, I think Elena is parentified—carrying responsibility for your emotional state. That's too much for a child."

You help Maria reassure Elena that she's fine and doesn't need taking care of. You create opportunities for Elena to be appropriately separate—spending time alone, developing her own interests, having privacy.

Sessions 6-10: Consolidating changes. The family practices new structure. Sofia's "oppositional behavior" decreases dramatically as the system reorganizes. Parents are more united, Carlos is more engaged, Maria is less overwhelmed. Elena relaxes as she's freed from caretaking. Sofia still tests limits (she's 15), but parents respond consistently and United.

The problem wasn't Sofia—it was family structure. By reorganizing the system, the symptom resolved.

Couples Therapy Interventions

Couples come to therapy in pain. One or both feel unhappy, disconnected, or attacked. They might present with specific complaints—infidelity, sexual problems, financial disagreements, parenting conflicts—or vague dissatisfaction—"We just don't connect anymore." Your job is understanding what's not working and helping them build something better.

Assessment priorities in couples work:

Presenting problem: What brings them now? Why now? What's the precipitant?

Relationship history: How did they meet? What attracted them? What were early years like? When did problems start?

Current functioning: How much time together? How do they communicate? How do they handle conflict? Sexual relationship? Division of labor? Extended family involvement?

Individual functioning: Mental health history? Substance use? Trauma history? Each partner's issues affect the relationship.

Commitment: Are both partners committed to improving the relationship? Or is one ambivalent? Is there active affair? Commitment affects treatment approach.

Strengths: What's working? What are positive qualities? Past successes? Shared values or goals? Building on strengths is more effective than only addressing problems.

Communication assessment reveals how couples interact:

Gottman's Four Horsemen: Criticism (attacking character), contempt (disrespect and disgust), defensiveness (refusing responsibility), stonewalling (withdrawing). Presence of these—especially contempt—predicts relationship failure.

Positive-to-negative ratio: Gottman found successful couples have 5:1 ratio of positive to negative interactions. Couples heading for divorce have 1:1 or worse. Even during conflict, successful couples maintain positive moments—humor, affection, interest.

Repair attempts: When conflict escalates, successful couples make repair attempts—humor, affection, apology, de-escalation. Unsuccessful couples ignore or reject repair attempts, allowing conflict to escalate unchecked.

Demand-withdraw: One partner demands discussion or change, the other withdraws. This creates escalating cycle—more demand leads to more withdrawal leads to more demand. Often gender-patterned (women demand, men withdraw) but not always.

Pursue-distance: Similar pattern around intimacy. One partner pursues connection, the other distances. Pursuer feels rejected, distancer feels suffocated.

Flooding: Becoming so emotionally overwhelmed that productive conversation is impossible. Heart rate increases, stress hormones surge, the person can't process information well. When flooded, taking breaks helps.

Emotionally Focused Couples Therapy helps partners identify negative cycles, access underlying emotions, and create new positive patterns:

Stage 1: De-escalation

Step 1: Identify negative cycle. "Do you see the pattern? You feel lonely and reach for him. He feels criticized and pulls away. You feel more alone and reach harder. He feels more overwhelmed and pulls further. You're stuck in pursue-distance."

Step 2: Identify underlying emotions. The pursuer isn't just angry—they're terrified of abandonment. The distancer isn't just avoidant—they're terrified of failure and criticism. Accessing these vulnerable emotions creates empathy.

Step 3: Reframe the problem. The problem isn't "he's distant" or "she's clingy"—the problem is "you're both scared and trying to protect yourselves, but your protection strategies push you apart."

Step 4: Each partner shares underlying emotions. "I get angry because underneath I'm terrified you'll leave." "I withdraw because I'm afraid nothing I do will be enough."

Stage 2: Restructuring interactions

Step 5: Identify disowned attachment needs. People often disown needs for connection, viewing them as weakness. "I need you" feels vulnerable. Therapy helps partners reclaim and express attachment needs.

Step 6: Accept partner's experience. Each partner listens to and accepts the other's experience without defending or problem-solving. Just accepting.

Step 7: Express needs and wants. Partners practice expressing needs directly. "I need to know I matter to you." "I need to feel competent as your partner."

Step 8: Establish new patterns. Create new emotional experiences where attachment needs are met. The distancer moves toward the pursuer. The pursuer expresses needs calmly. New cycles replace old ones.

Stage 3: Consolidation

Step 9: Consolidate new positions. Practice new ways of interacting until they feel natural. Identify and disrupt old patterns when they emerge.

EFT creates lasting change by changing the emotional bond between partners.

Gottman Method Couples Therapy based on decades of research on what makes marriages succeed or fail:

Assessment phase: Couples complete questionnaires, participate in structured interview, and engage in conflict discussion you observe. This comprehensive assessment identifies strengths and problems.

Interventions:

Building Love Maps: Knowing detailed information about partner's world—their worries, hopes, dreams, history. You help couples update their knowledge and maintain curiosity.

Sharing Fondness and Admiration: Counteracting negativity by identifying and expressing positive qualities and gratitude. Couples practice appreciation daily.

Turning Toward Instead of Away: Responding to partner's bids for connection. A bid might be small—"Look at that bird"—but response matters. Turning toward builds connection. Turning away creates distance.

Managing Conflict: Teaching conflict management skills:

Softened startup: Beginning difficult conversations gently rather than with criticism. "I feel worried when..." instead of "You never..."

Accepting influence: Being open to partner's perspective and willing to compromise. Not insisting on being right or having your way.

Compromise: Finding middle ground where both partners' needs are somewhat met.

Self-soothing: Taking breaks when flooded to calm physiology before continuing discussion.

Creating Shared Meaning: Building shared rituals, goals, roles, and symbols. Couples who create shared meaning together have stronger relationships.

Trust and Betrayal: After affairs or major betrayals, specific interventions rebuild trust: atoning (betrayer takes full responsibility), attunement (betrayer demonstrates understanding of pain caused), and attachment (rebuilding connection).

Imago Relationship Therapy (Harville Hendrix) proposes that people unconsciously choose partners who resemble early caregivers, then try to heal childhood wounds through the relationship. When this doesn't work, conflict erupts.

Key concepts:

Imago: Unconscious composite image of early caregivers. You're attracted to people who match this image because you unconsciously hope to heal childhood wounds.

Wounded child: Everyone carries childhood pain—unmet needs, hurts, and disappointments. Adult conflicts often activate these old wounds.

Power struggle: After romantic phase, couples enter power struggle where each tries to change the other to meet unmet childhood needs. This is normal but painful.

Interventions:

Imago dialogue: Structured communication process ensuring each partner feels heard:

1. **Mirroring**: Repeat back what partner said. "Let me see if I got that. You're saying..."
2. **Validation**: Acknowledge partner's perspective makes sense. "That makes sense because..."
3. **Empathy**: Imagine how partner feels. "I imagine you might feel..."

This slows conversation down and ensures understanding before responding.

Childhood wounds exploration: Identifying unmet childhood needs and how they show up in current relationship. Understanding that partner's frustrating behavior might be attempt to get childhood needs met.

Reimaging: Intentionally meeting partner's unmet childhood needs. If someone's father was emotionally distant, their partner practices emotional availability. This creates healing experiences.

Behavioral Couples Therapy focuses on increasing positive behaviors and improving communication and problem-solving:

Interventions:

Behavioral exchange: Each partner identifies desired behaviors from the other. "I'd like you to kiss me goodbye in morning." They agree to increase these positive behaviors. This creates immediate positive experiences.

Communication training: Teaching specific skills—active listening, I-statements, avoiding criticism and contempt, expressing feelings and needs clearly.

Problem-solving training: Systematic approach to problems:

1. Define problem specifically
2. Brainstorm possible solutions
3. Evaluate each option
4. Choose solution
5. Implement
6. Evaluate results

Cognitive restructuring: Identifying and challenging negative thoughts about partner. "He doesn't care" becomes "He shows care differently than I do."

Case Example: EFT with Pursue-Distance Couple - James and Maria

James (48) and Maria (46) have been married 20 years. Maria initiated therapy, complaining James is emotionally unavailable. James came reluctantly, saying Maria is never satisfied. They have two teenage children. No affairs or abuse. Both committed to marriage.

Session 1-2: Assessment and identifying the cycle

Maria describes feeling lonely and unimportant. James works long hours, comes home tired, watches TV, and goes to bed. When she tries to talk, he gives short answers or changes the subject. She's tired of "pulling teeth."

James says Maria is always unhappy with him. Nothing he does is enough. He provides well financially, doesn't cheat, doesn't drink. But she constantly wants "deep conversations" and "emotional connection." He feels criticized and inadequate.

You observe their interaction: Maria speaks rapidly, emotionally, with frustration and sadness. James is measured, factual, sitting back with arms crossed. When Maria expresses hurt, James explains or defends. When James withdraws, Maria escalates.

You identify the cycle: "I'm seeing a pattern. Maria, when you feel disconnected, you reach for James—asking questions, wanting to talk, expressing frustration. James, when you feel pressure or criticism, you pull back—giving short answers, changing subjects, withdrawing. Maria, when James pulls back, you feel more alone and reach harder. James, when Maria reaches harder, you feel more criticized and pull back further. You're caught in pursue-distance cycle. You're both hurting and protecting yourselves, but your protections push you apart. Does this sound accurate?"

Both recognize the pattern. Just naming it reduces blame—the problem isn't his coldness or her clinginess; the problem is the cycle they're stuck in.

Session 3-4: Accessing underlying emotions

You: "Maria, when James withdraws, you say you feel frustrated. What's underneath the frustration?"

Maria (crying): "I feel alone. Like I don't matter to him. Like he'd be fine if I disappeared."

You: "You're terrified he doesn't need you. That you're not important."

Maria (nodding): "I'm afraid I've become just the person who manages the kids and house. Not someone he wants."

You: "James, you're hearing that Maria's pursuing isn't criticism—it's fear. She's afraid she's lost you. Does that land differently than when you think she's just demanding?"

James (softening): "I didn't know that. I thought she was just disappointed in me."

You: "James, when Maria reaches for you and you pull back, what's happening for you?"

James: "I feel like I'm failing. Like I'm not doing it right. So I shut down."

You: "You're afraid you won't be enough. That you'll disappoint her."

James: "Yeah. It feels safer to not try than to try and fail."

You: "Maria, James isn't cold. He's scared. He's protecting himself from what feels like inevitable failure. Does that change how you see his withdrawal?"

Maria: "I had no idea. I thought he just didn't care."

You: "So both of you are scared. Maria, you're scared James doesn't want you. James, you're scared you'll fail Maria. And your protection strategies—Maria pursuing, James withdrawing—confirm each other's fears. Your pursuing tells James he's failing. His withdrawing tells you he doesn't care. The cycle maintains itself."

Session 5-7: Restructuring interactions

You: "Maria, what do you need from James?"

Maria: "I need to know I matter to him. That he wants to be close, not that he has to be."

You: "Can you tell him that? Not the anger—the need. 'James, I need...'"

Maria (to James): "I need to know you want me. That connecting with me matters to you."

You: "James, what happens when you hear that?"

James: "It's hard to hear 'I need' without hearing criticism. But this feels different. More... vulnerable."

You: "Exactly. The vulnerable need feels different than the angry pursuit. Can you respond to that need?"

James (to Maria): "I do want you. I always have. I just... I don't know how to give you what you need."

Maria: "What if you didn't have to know how? What if you just stayed instead of leaving when I get emotional?"

James: "I could try that."

You: "Let's practice right now. Maria, tell James about feeling alone—the vulnerable version, not the angry one."

Maria: "James, I miss you. I miss feeling like we're together. I feel like we're just coexisting."

You: "James, instead of withdrawing or defending, can you just stay with that? Just be present with her feeling without fixing it or leaving?"

James (uncomfortable but trying): "I'm here. I hear you."

Maria (tearful): "That's all I needed. Just you here, not running away."

This creates new emotional experience. Maria gets her need met (James stays present with her emotion). James succeeds at being enough (he doesn't have to fix anything, just be present). The new pattern contradicts old fears.

Session 8-12: Consolidating change

Over subsequent sessions, they practice new patterns. Maria expresses needs vulnerably. James stays present instead of withdrawing. When old patterns emerge (Maria escalates, James shuts down), you help them recognize and shift.

They create new rituals—20-minute daily conversation where James practices being emotionally present and Maria practices appreciating his efforts. They schedule weekly date nights rebuilding their connection.

Termination (Session 12)

Maria and James report feeling significantly closer. Conflicts still happen, but they navigate them differently. Maria can express needs without anger. James can stay engaged without withdrawing. They understand their cycle and can interrupt it.

The pursue-distance cycle that once drove them apart now rarely emerges. They've created new patterns where both feel secure in the relationship.

Practice Questions

1. Yalom's therapeutic factor "universality" refers to:

A. Common therapeutic techniques
B. Discovering you're not alone in your struggles
C. Universal truths
D. Group agreement

2. Group cohesiveness is:

A. Unimportant
B. Feeling accepted and valued by the group
C. Always present immediately
D. Only about agreement

3. The "storming" stage of group development involves:

A. No conflict
B. Conflict and challenges emerging
C. Perfect harmony
D. Only positive interactions

4. In group therapy, "here-and-now" focus means:

A. Ignoring outside problems
B. Focusing on current interactions in the room
C. Only discussing the present week
D. Avoiding all past discussion

5. Safety behaviors in groups:

A. Create safety
B. Subtle avoidance preventing full participation
C. Should be encouraged
D. Don't exist

6. Altruism in groups refers to:

A. Being nice
B. Helping others which builds self-esteem
C. Avoiding conflict
D. Financial generosity

7. The "performing" stage is when:

A. Groups just start
B. Groups function effectively with deep work
C. Groups avoid conflict
D. Members act fake

8. Subgrouping outside of group sessions:

A. Should be encouraged
B. Can undermine the group through secrets and alliances
C. Has no impact
D. Always helps

9. Interpersonal learning in groups involves:

A. Only reading about relationships
B. Learning about your patterns through real-time interactions
C. Avoiding all interaction
D. Only listening

10. Family homeostasis refers to:

A. Physical balance
B. Families resisting change to maintain stability
C. Health
D. Agreement

11. Triangulation occurs when:

A. Three people communicate openly
B. Tension between two people leads them to pull in a third
C. Geometry is discussed
D. Families are healthy

12. Enmeshed families have:

A. Healthy boundaries
B. Overly diffuse boundaries with little privacy
C. Rigid boundaries
D. No relationship

13. The "identified patient" often:

A. Is the only problem
B. Manifests symptoms of broader family dysfunction
C. Doesn't exist
D. Is always correct

14. Structural family therapy focuses on:

A. Only individuals
B. Family organization, boundaries, hierarchies
C. Building structure literally
D. Avoiding change

15. An enactment in family therapy involves:

A. Acting classes
B. Having family interact with each other during session
C. Avoiding interaction
D. Only discussion

16. Reframing means:

A. Buying new frames
B. Relabeling behavior to change its meaning
C. Avoiding problems
D. Criticism

17. Strategic family therapy uses:

A. Military tactics
B. Directives and tasks to change patterns
C. No interventions
D. Only medication

18. A paradoxical directive involves:

A. Straightforward instructions
B. Prescribing the symptom to create change
C. Confusion
D. Avoiding problems

19. Bowen's concept of differentiation refers to:

A. Being different
B. Separating thinking from feeling while maintaining relationships
C. Isolation
D. Agreement with everyone

20. A genogram is:

A. Genetic testing
B. Three-generation family diagram showing patterns
C. Unnecessary
D. Only about medical history

21. Emotionally Focused Therapy focuses on:

A. Suppressing emotions
B. Attachment bonds and emotional connection
C. Only cognition
D. Avoiding feelings

22. Primary emotions in EFT are:

A. Surface reactions
B. Underlying vulnerable feelings like fear and hurt
C. Always anger
D. Unimportant

23. Gottman's "Four Horsemen" predict:

A. Success
B. Relationship failure
C. Horse racing
D. Nothing meaningful

24. Contempt in relationships involves:

A. Healthy disagreement
B. Disrespect, disgust, mockery
C. Normal conflict
D. Affection

25. The demand-withdraw pattern involves:

A. Equal communication
B. One demanding discussion while other withdraws
C. Healthy negotiation
D. No specific pattern

26. Flooding occurs when:

A. Houses flood
B. Someone becomes emotionally overwhelmed
C. Communication is perfect
D. Problems are solved

27. Gottman found successful couples have:

A. No conflict
B. 5:1 ratio of positive to negative interactions
C. 1:1 ratio
D. Only negative interactions

28. Repair attempts are:

A. Fixing furniture
B. Efforts to de-escalate conflict
C. Always unsuccessful
D. Unnecessary

29. Imago Relationship Therapy proposes:

A. Random partner selection
B. People choose partners resembling early caregivers
C. Compatibility doesn't matter
D. Relationships are easy

30. Imago dialogue includes:

A. Normal conversation
B. Mirroring, validation, empathy
C. Arguing
D. Ignoring partner

31. The "forming" stage of groups involves:

A. Deep trust immediately
B. Anxiety and politeness with low trust
C. Conflict
D. Perfect cohesion

32. Catharsis in groups means:

A. Medical procedure
B. Expressing intense emotions in supportive environment
C. Avoiding emotions
D. Only positive feelings

33. Linking in group leadership means:

A. Chain reactions
B. Connecting members who share similarities
C. Internet connections
D. Avoiding relationships

34. A psychoeducational group:

A. Avoids teaching
B. Teaches information and skills
C. Only provides support
D. Has no structure

35. Process groups focus on:

A. Manufacturing
B. Interpersonal learning through here-and-now interactions
C. Only education
D. Avoiding emotion

36. Clear boundaries in families mean:

A. No connection
B. Connected while maintaining appropriate separation
C. Enmeshment
D. Conflict

37. Disengaged families:

A. Are very connected
B. Have rigid boundaries with little involvement
C. Are healthy
D. Communicate well

38. The family "scapegoat" role involves:

A. Leading the family
B. Being blamed for family problems
C. Success
D. Invisibility

39. Circular causality means:

A. Going in circles
B. Family interactions are mutually influencing, not linear
C. One person causes everything
D. Nothing is connected

40. Joining in structural therapy means:

A. Becoming family member
B. Connecting with family while positioning to influence
C. Avoiding family
D. Criticism

41. Unbalancing in structural therapy involves:

A. Physical balance
B. Temporarily siding with one person to destabilize homeostasis
C. Avoiding sides
D. Equal time always

42. The multigenerational transmission process involves:

A. Genetics only
B. Patterns transmitting across generations
C. Random change
D. No family influence

43. Detriangulation helps people:

A. Learn geometry
B. Relate directly instead of through third parties
C. Avoid all triangles
D. Increase distance

44. Softened startup means:

A. Slow beginnings
B. Beginning difficult conversations gently not critically
C. Avoiding conversations
D. Aggressive approach

45. Accepting influence means:

A. Being controlled
B. Being open to partner's perspective and willing to compromise
C. Never having your way
D. Always agreeing

46. Installation of hope in groups occurs when:

A. Everyone is hopeless
B. Seeing others improve creates hope for own improvement
C. The leader lectures
D. Nothing happens

47. The "norming" stage involves:

A. Continued conflict
B. Conflict resolving into cooperation with developing cohesion
C. No interaction
D. Only rules

48. The "adjourning" stage focuses on:

A. Starting group
B. Processing termination and saying goodbye
C. Avoiding endings
D. Adding members

49. Corrective recapitulation of family means:

A. Repeating family patterns
B. Reworking family issues in safer group context
C. Avoiding all family topics
D. Only positive family talk

50. Love maps in Gottman method refer to:

A. Geographic maps
B. Knowing detailed information about partner's world
C. Romance only
D. Physical intimacy

Answer Key with Detailed Explanations

1. B. Discovering you're not alone in your struggles
Universality is the therapeutic factor where group members discover others share similar struggles, feelings, and experiences. This normalizes problems and reduces shame. The isolated person realizes "I'm not the only one" and feels immediate relief. Universality is particularly powerful early in groups when members first share their stories and recognize commonalities.

2. B. Feeling accepted and valued by the group
Group cohesiveness is feeling accepted, valued, and connected to the group—the sense of "we're in this together." Cohesive groups feel like safe families where you can be yourself, take risks, and know you'll be supported. Cohesion is the group equivalent of therapeutic alliance in individual therapy. It develops over time, not immediately, and is necessary for deep therapeutic work.

3. B. Conflict and challenges emerging
The storming stage involves conflict emerging as members challenge the leader and each other, form subgroups, and compete for attention. This stage is uncomfortable but necessary—working through conflict builds trust and cohesion. The leader facilitates conflict constructively rather than shutting it down. Storming follows the initial polite forming stage.

4. B. Focusing on current interactions in the room
Here-and-now focus means attending to what's happening in the room right now between group members, not just discussing outside problems. "Tom, you just criticized yourself. That's the third time this session. Has anyone else noticed?" This reveals interpersonal patterns and creates opportunities for immediate learning and change. Balance between discussing outside problems and focusing on current group processes is needed.

5. B. Subtle avoidance preventing full participation
Safety behaviors in groups are subtle forms of avoidance that prevent full participation and authentic interaction—sitting in specific seats, avoiding eye contact, staying silent during difficult topics, leaving early. These behaviors protect against anxiety but prevent the full engagement necessary for change. Leaders gently explore and challenge safety behaviors.

6. B. Helping others which builds self-esteem
Altruism is the therapeutic factor where helping others feels good and builds self-esteem. Members who feel worthless discover they have something valuable to offer. The depressed person who provides support to another member experiences purpose and competence. Giving help is as therapeutic as receiving it, demonstrating that the person has value and can contribute.

7. B. Groups function effectively with deep work
The performing stage is when the group functions effectively with members working deeply on problems, giving direct but caring feedback, and largely self-managing. Therapeutic factors are

maximized. This is the most productive phase. The group has moved through forming, storming, and norming to reach optimal functioning.

8. B. Can undermine the group through secrets and alliances
Subgrouping outside group sessions—private friendships, conversations, or alliances between members—can undermine the group by creating secrets and preventing full disclosure in group. Relationships between members bypass group process. Many leaders discourage outside socializing or, if it occurs, require that it be brought into group discussion to prevent undermining group cohesion and safety.

9. B. Learning about your patterns through real-time interactions
Interpersonal learning is learning about your relational patterns through actual interactions with group members. The way you act in group reflects how you act in life. The leader helps members recognize patterns ("You're doing with Sarah what you described doing with your sister"), understand impact on others, and try new behaviors. This real-time interpersonal work is uniquely powerful in groups.

10. B. Families resisting change to maintain stability
Family homeostasis is the tendency of family systems to resist change to maintain stability and equilibrium. Even dysfunctional patterns are familiar and predictable—the system pushes back against change to restore what's known. When one person improves, another might develop symptoms. Understanding homeostasis helps anticipate and address resistance to change in family therapy.

11. B. Tension between two people leads them to pull in a third
Triangulation occurs when tension exists between two people and they pull a third person in to stabilize the relationship. Parents in marital conflict focus on child's problems instead of their relationship. Two siblings pull in parent to mediate. The triangle reduces immediate tension but prevents resolution between the original two people and burdens the third person.

12. B. Overly diffuse boundaries with little privacy
Enmeshed families have overly diffuse, permeable boundaries where members are overly involved in each other's lives with little privacy, individuality, or autonomy. Everyone knows everything about everyone. Members are overly reactive to each other's moods and problems. This prevents healthy individuation and independence. It's different from healthy closeness by interfering with development of separate identity.

13. B. Manifests symptoms of broader family dysfunction
The "identified patient" is the family member who manifests symptoms, but their problems often reflect broader family dysfunction rather than being solely individual pathology. A child's acting out might maintain parental homeostasis by giving them something to unite against. An adult's depression might allow them to avoid difficult life transitions. Understanding the symptom's function in the family system guides intervention.

14. B. Family organization, boundaries, hierarchies
Structural family therapy (Minuchin) focuses on family structure—organization, boundaries between subsystems, and power hierarchies. The therapist assesses and restructures family organization. Key

questions: Are boundaries clear, enmeshed, or disengaged? Do parents lead? Are generational boundaries appropriate? Interventions restructure the family to create healthier organization.

15. B. Having family interact with each other during session
Enactment involves having family members interact with each other during session rather than talking to the therapist about problems. "Don't tell me about the argument—have the argument here." This reveals actual patterns and allows the therapist to intervene in real-time. Enactment is more powerful than discussion because it shows rather than tells what happens.

16. B. Relabeling behavior to change its meaning
Reframing is relabeling behavior to change its meaning and reduce defensiveness. An "oppositional" teenager is reframed as "fiercely independent." An "overinvolved" mother is "deeply caring." Reframing doesn't change the behavior initially but changes how it's perceived, opening possibilities for change by reducing blame and increasing understanding of positive intentions.

17. B. Directives and tasks to change patterns
Strategic family therapy (Haley, Madanes) uses directives—tasks assigned to families to change patterns maintaining problems. These can be direct (straightforward assignments) or paradoxical (prescribing the symptom). Strategic therapy is brief and problem-focused, less concerned with insight than with behavior change. Directives are designed strategically to interrupt problematic patterns.

18. B. Prescribing the symptom to create change
Paradoxical directives involve prescribing the symptom—telling someone to do the very thing they're trying to stop. Tell a couple who argues constantly to schedule two 30-minute arguments daily. Compliance is therapeutic (gaining control over arguing). Resistance is therapeutic (stopping arguing to avoid the assignment). Either way, the spontaneous, uncontrolled pattern is disrupted.

19. B. Separating thinking from feeling while maintaining relationships
Differentiation (Bowen's concept) is the ability to separate thinking from feeling and maintain a clear sense of self while in relationships. Low differentiation means emotions dominate, and the person is fused with others—can't distinguish their feelings from others' feelings. High differentiation means balancing emotion and reason, maintaining clear self while connected to others. It's not isolation but thoughtful independence within relationships.

20. B. Three-generation family diagram showing patterns
A genogram is a three-generation family diagram showing relationships, patterns, significant events, and sometimes medical/psychiatric history. This visual map reveals patterns across generations—divorce, addiction, triangulation, enmeshment. Creating a genogram helps families see multigenerational patterns and understand how current problems have historical roots. It's used particularly in Bowen family therapy.

21. B. Attachment bonds and emotional connection
Emotionally Focused Therapy (Sue Johnson) focuses on attachment bonds—the emotional connections between family members or partners. When attachment is secure, people function well. When attachment is threatened or insecure, problems emerge. EFT helps partners identify negative

cycles threatening attachment, access vulnerable emotions beneath defensive reactions, and create new positive patterns that strengthen attachment security.

22. B. Underlying vulnerable feelings like fear and hurt
Primary emotions in EFT are underlying vulnerable feelings like fear, hurt, loneliness, and shame. Secondary emotions (anger, frustration, criticism) are surface reactions protecting against primary emotions. Accessing primary emotions creates change because they reveal underlying attachment needs. When partners express and respond to primary emotions, attachment security increases and problems decrease.

23. B. Relationship failure
Gottman's Four Horsemen—criticism, contempt, defensiveness, and stonewalling—predict relationship failure with high accuracy based on decades of research. Presence of these communication patterns, especially contempt, indicates relationships heading toward divorce. Identifying these patterns helps couples recognize destructive communication and learn alternatives that support relationship health.

24. B. Disrespect, disgust, mockery
Contempt involves treating partner with disrespect, disgust, mockery, sarcasm, or superiority—eye-rolling, name-calling, hostile humor, treating partner as inferior. Contempt is the most toxic of the Four Horsemen and the strongest predictor of divorce. It communicates "I'm better than you" and destroys the respect and admiration necessary for relationship health. Contempt must be eliminated for relationships to survive.

25. B. One demanding discussion while other withdraws
The demand-withdraw pattern involves one partner demanding discussion, change, or connection while the other withdraws and avoids. This creates escalating cycle—more demand triggers more withdrawal triggers more demand. Often (but not always) women demand and men withdraw. Both partners feel misunderstood—the demander feels unheard, the withdrawer feels attacked. Breaking this cycle requires new responses from both.

26. B. Someone becomes emotionally overwhelmed
Flooding occurs when someone becomes so emotionally overwhelmed during conflict that productive conversation becomes impossible. Heart rate increases significantly, stress hormones surge, and the person can't process information well or think clearly. When flooded, taking breaks to calm physiology before continuing discussion is helpful. Recognizing flooding and taking appropriate breaks prevents destructive escalation.

27. B. 5:1 ratio of positive to negative interactions
Gottman found that successful couples maintain approximately 5:1 ratio of positive to negative interactions—five positive moments for every negative one. Even during conflict, successful couples maintain positive moments through humor, affection, and interest. Couples heading for divorce have 1:1 or worse ratios. This research finding emphasizes the importance of maintaining positivity, not just reducing negativity.

28. B. Efforts to de-escalate conflict
Repair attempts are efforts to de-escalate conflict and restore connection—humor, affection, apology, acknowledgment, change of topic. Successful couples make repair attempts during conflict and accept their partner's repair attempts. Unsuccessful couples ignore or reject repair attempts, allowing conflict to escalate unchecked. The presence and acceptance of repair attempts predict relationship success.

29. B. People choose partners resembling early caregivers
Imago Relationship Therapy (Hendrix) proposes that people unconsciously choose partners who resemble early caregivers (the "imago"—composite image of caregivers) because they unconsciously hope to heal childhood wounds through the relationship. When partners can't meet these unconscious needs, conflict erupts. Understanding this dynamic helps couples work consciously to heal each other's wounds.

30. B. Mirroring, validation, empathy
Imago dialogue is a structured communication process ensuring partners feel heard: (1) Mirroring—repeat back what partner said ("Let me see if I got that..."), (2) Validation—acknowledge their perspective makes sense ("That makes sense because..."), (3) Empathy—imagine their feelings ("I imagine you might feel..."). This slows conversation and ensures understanding before responding, reducing reactivity.

31. B. Anxiety and politeness with low trust
The forming stage (first stage of group development) involves members being anxious and polite. They seek acceptance, test boundaries, figure out group norms. Trust is low. Cohesion hasn't developed. Members look to leader for guidance and structure. Conflict is avoided. Discussion stays surface-level. This initial uncertainty is normal and precedes deeper work.

32. B. Expressing intense emotions in supportive environment
Catharsis is the therapeutic factor involving expression of intense emotions in a supportive environment, providing relief and helping process feelings. The group provides safe container for emotional expression. However, catharsis alone isn't sufficient—it must be combined with interpersonal learning, cognitive understanding, and support to be therapeutic. Expression plus processing creates change.

33. B. Connecting members who share similarities
Linking is a leader intervention connecting members who share similarities or whose issues relate. "Mary, what Tom described sounds similar to what you said last week." Linking builds universality, encourages member-to-member interaction rather than all communication going through the leader, and helps members support each other. It creates the interconnections that make group cohesive.

34. B. Teaches information and skills
Psychoeducational groups teach information and skills systematically. Examples: anger management, social skills training, parenting skills, illness education. These are structured with curriculum, homework, and specific skill practice. The leader actively teaches content. While support occurs, the primary purpose is education. These differ from support groups (mutual aid) and therapy groups (interpersonal learning).

35. B. Interpersonal learning through here-and-now interactions
Process groups focus on interpersonal learning through examining here-and-now interactions between members. The way members interact in group reveals their interpersonal patterns. The leader helps members recognize patterns, understand their impact on others, and try new behaviors. Process groups are less structured than psychoeducational groups, with focus on group dynamics and relationships rather than curriculum.

36. B. Connected while maintaining appropriate separation
Clear boundaries in families mean being connected and involved while maintaining appropriate separation, privacy, and autonomy. Clear boundaries allow both connection and independence. This is healthier than either enmeshed boundaries (no separation, no privacy) or disengaged boundaries (no connection, excessive separation). Clear boundaries support both relationship and individuation.

37. B. Have rigid boundaries with little involvement
Disengaged families have rigid, impermeable boundaries where members are disconnected with little involvement, emotional connection, or mutual support. When someone has a problem, others don't notice or help. Members function independently but lack the connection and support families should provide. This represents one extreme of boundary problems, with enmeshment at the other extreme.

38. B. Being blamed for family problems
The scapegoat role involves being blamed for family problems and acting out to manifest family dysfunction. This child's problems allow the family to avoid addressing deeper issues—particularly parental conflicts or family dysfunction. The scapegoat serves a function in the system, and their improvement might destabilize the family temporarily. Treatment addresses the family system, not just the scapegoated individual.

39. B. Family interactions are mutually influencing, not linear
Circular causality describes how family interactions are circular and mutually influencing rather than linear (A causes B). Dad criticizes, son withdraws, mom rescues son, dad feels undermined and criticizes more—who started it? There's no beginning or end to the cycle. Each person's behavior influences and is influenced by others. Understanding circular causality prevents blame and opens multiple intervention points—you can enter the cycle anywhere to create change.

40. B. Connecting with family while positioning to influence
Joining in structural family therapy means the therapist connects with and accommodates to the family's style and organization while positioning to influence change. You respect their structure initially to gain credibility and alliance, then use that connection to guide restructuring. Joining isn't becoming a family member or avoiding necessary confrontation—it's strategic connection that allows you to work effectively with the system.

41. B. Temporarily siding with one person to destabilize homeostasis
Unbalancing is a structural therapy technique where the therapist temporarily sides with one family member to destabilize existing homeostasis and create change. You might support a disempowered parent against an overly powerful child, challenging the family's usual pattern. This strategic imbalance creates disequilibrium that opens possibilities for reorganization. It's temporary and purposeful, not permanent alliance.

42. B. Patterns transmitting across generations
The multigenerational transmission process (Bowen concept) describes how patterns, beliefs, and relationship styles transmit across generations. Divorce patterns, triangulation, enmeshment, communication styles, and coping strategies are passed down through modeling and family culture. Understanding family history reveals how current patterns have multigenerational roots. The genogram makes these transmissions visible, helping families recognize and potentially change inherited patterns.

43. B. Relate directly instead of through third parties
Detriangulation helps people relate directly with each other rather than communicating through third parties. Instead of parents discussing their conflict with a child who carries messages between them, they address each other directly. Detriangulation reduces the burden on the third person and allows the two people with the issue to resolve it. This is particularly important for freeing children from adult conflicts.

44. B. Beginning difficult conversations gently not critically
Softened startup (Gottman concept) means beginning difficult conversations gently rather than with criticism, blame, or harsh approach. "I feel worried when bills aren't paid on time—can we talk about our budget?" instead of "You never pay the bills on time! What's wrong with you?" How you start a conversation largely predicts how it ends. Soft startups increase likelihood of productive resolution.

45. B. Being open to partner's perspective and willing to compromise
Accepting influence means being open to your partner's perspective, considering their input seriously, and being willing to compromise rather than insisting on being right or having your way. Gottman found that men who accept influence from their wives have more successful marriages. Accepting influence doesn't mean having no opinions—it means valuing partnership over being right.

46. B. Seeing others improve creates hope for own improvement
Installation of hope occurs when group members see others improve, which creates hope for their own improvement. When someone who was severely depressed six months ago now functions well, newer members think "If she can recover, maybe I can too." Hope is particularly powerful when members are at different stages—those further along model possibility for those beginning the journey.

47. B. Conflict resolving into cooperation with developing cohesion
The norming stage (third stage of group development) occurs when conflict from the storming stage resolves into cooperation. Cohesion develops, trust increases, members feel accepted and valued. The group develops its own identity and culture. Members interact more with each other and less exclusively through the leader. This sets the stage for the performing stage where deep therapeutic work occurs.

48. B. Processing termination and saying goodbye
The adjourning stage (final stage of group development) focuses on processing termination feelings, reviewing progress and learning, and saying goodbye. Grief and loss are expected and normal. This stage is therapeutically powerful—members practice healthy endings and separations. The leader helps members articulate what they've gained, process feelings about ending, and plan for maintaining gains after group ends.

49. B. Reworking family issues in safer group context
Corrective recapitulation of the primary family is a therapeutic factor where the group recreates family dynamics, allowing members to work through unresolved family issues in the safer group context. Someone who couldn't express anger to a parent might learn to express it appropriately with a group member who reminds them of that parent. The group becomes a corrective family experience where old wounds can be healed.

50. B. Knowing detailed information about partner's world
Love maps (Gottman concept) refers to knowing detailed information about your partner's world—their current worries, hopes, dreams, stresses, friends, preferences, and life experiences. Partners with strong love maps know what matters to their partner and maintain curiosity about their inner world. Building and updating love maps through asking questions and listening attentively strengthens relationship connection.

Reflecting on Relational Work

Group and family therapy tap into something powerful—the healing that happens through connection with others. We're social creatures. We develop in relationships, we're wounded in relationships, and we heal in relationships. Individual therapy provides focused attention and safety, but groups and families offer unique opportunities for change through multiple relationships simultaneously.

Working with systems requires different thinking. You're not just tracking one person's thoughts, feelings, and behaviors. You're tracking patterns across people, understanding how everyone affects everyone else, seeing the larger picture. A symptom in one person often reflects system-level problems. Real change requires system-level intervention.

Groups teach us we're not alone. Families show us how we learned to be who we are. Couples reveal how our attachment needs and fears play out in intimate relationships. These modalities are complex, challenging, and powerful. They require you to think systemically, manage multiple relationships, facilitate difficult interactions, and tolerate the intensity that emerges when people work on problems together.

The skills you develop leading groups and working with families will make you a better therapist in all settings. You'll see patterns more clearly. You'll understand how problems develop and maintain themselves in relational contexts. You'll intervene more effectively because you understand that problems rarely exist in isolation—they're embedded in relationships and systems.

Essential Understanding for Systemic Work

- Yalom's therapeutic factors explain how groups create change through universality, altruism, hope, interpersonal learning, and cohesion
- Groups progress through predictable stages: forming (polite, anxious), storming (conflict), norming (cooperation), performing (deep work), adjourning (termination)
- Here-and-now focus in groups addresses current interactions revealing interpersonal patterns and creating immediate learning opportunities

- Family homeostasis is the system's resistance to change to maintain stability, even when patterns are dysfunctional
- Triangulation occurs when two people pull a third into their relationship to manage tension between them
- Enmeshed families have diffuse boundaries with little privacy; disengaged families have rigid boundaries with little connection
- The identified patient often manifests symptoms of broader family dysfunction rather than having purely individual pathology
- Structural family therapy restructures organization, boundaries, and hierarchies to create healthier family functioning
- Enactment has families interact during sessions, revealing actual patterns rather than just discussing problems
- Strategic family therapy uses directives including paradoxical interventions to interrupt patterns maintaining problems
- Bowen's differentiation describes separating thinking from feeling while maintaining clear self in relationships
- Emotionally Focused Therapy addresses attachment bonds, accessing primary emotions beneath secondary defensive reactions
- Gottman's Four Horsemen (criticism, contempt, defensiveness, stonewalling) predict relationship failure, with contempt most toxic
- Successful couples maintain 5:1 positive-to-negative ratio even during conflicts through repair attempts and positive interactions
- The demand-withdraw pattern creates escalating cycles where one partner's pursuit triggers the other's withdrawal in vicious cycle
- Effective systemic therapy requires understanding circular causality, intervening at system level, and facilitating new patterns replacing dysfunctional ones

Chapter 12: Case Management and Coordination of Care

Here's what nobody tells you when you start doing this work: being a good therapist isn't enough. You can be brilliant at CBT, masterful at reading family dynamics, exceptional at building therapeutic alliance—but if you can't coordinate care, connect clients to resources, and work with other providers, your impact is limited.

Real people have complex needs that exceed what any single provider can offer. Your depressed client also needs housing assistance. Your anxious client needs disability benefits. Your trauma survivor needs medical care for chronic pain. The teenager you're seeing needs school accommodations. The older adult needs home health services. You're not just a therapist—you're a coordinator, advocate, navigator, and bridge between your client and the multiple systems they interact with.

Case management isn't separate from clinical work—it's integrated with it. You can't treat someone's depression effectively if they're homeless. You can't address anxiety if they can't afford their medications. You can't process trauma if they're in active crisis without support. Maslow was right—basic needs come first. Your clinical skills matter most when clients have stability to engage in treatment.

Service Coordination

Service coordination means ensuring clients receive all needed services in organized, integrated manner. You don't provide everything yourself—that's impossible and inappropriate. Instead, you assess what's needed, connect clients to appropriate services, ensure they can access those services, and monitor whether services are effective.

Assessment of needs goes beyond diagnosis and symptoms. You assess the whole person in their whole life:

Basic needs: Housing, food, income, safety, transportation, utilities. Without these, treatment can't progress. A person focused on where they'll sleep tonight can't engage in cognitive restructuring.

Medical needs: Physical health problems, medications, coordination with medical providers. Physical and mental health are intertwined—untreated medical conditions worsen mental health and vice versa.

Mental health and substance use needs: What level of care is appropriate? Outpatient therapy? Intensive outpatient? Partial hospitalization? Inpatient? Residential treatment? Medication management?

Social and support needs: Family support, social connections, peer support, community involvement. Isolation worsens mental health. Connection supports recovery.

Educational and vocational needs: School accommodations, special education services, vocational rehabilitation, job training, supported employment. Purpose and productivity matter.

Legal needs: Criminal justice involvement, child welfare involvement, guardianship, protective orders, disability hearings. Legal problems create enormous stress and require specialized assistance.

Financial needs: Benefits (SSI, SSDI, TANF, SNAP), medical insurance, debt management, money management. Financial stress worsens mental health. Financial stability supports recovery.

The resource assessment identifies what's available in your community:

Mental health services: Outpatient clinics, private practitioners, intensive services, crisis services, peer support, support groups. Know what exists, admission criteria, costs, waitlists.

Medical services: Primary care, specialty care, emergency services, community health centers, free clinics. Where can clients access affordable medical care?

Substance use services: Detox, residential treatment, intensive outpatient, outpatient counseling, medication-assisted treatment, recovery support. What levels of care exist locally?

Housing services: Emergency shelter, transitional housing, permanent supportive housing, affordable housing, housing subsidies. How do clients access each?

Income support: SSI/SSDI, TANF, General Assistance, unemployment. What are eligibility criteria and application processes?

Food assistance: SNAP, food banks, meal programs, WIC. Where can clients get food if they're hungry?

Transportation: Public transit, paratransit, transportation vouchers, volunteer services. How do clients get to appointments?

Legal services: Legal aid, public defenders, victim advocates, disability law centers. Where can clients get free or low-cost legal help?

Educational and vocational services: Vocational rehabilitation, job training, supported employment, adult education, GED programs. What exists for skill building and employment?

You can't know every resource, but you need to know how to find information. Maintain resource lists, connect with 211 information lines, network with other providers, and know key resources your population frequently needs.

Making effective referrals requires more than handing someone a phone number:

Assess readiness: Is the client ready for this service? Do they understand why you're suggesting it? If they're not ready, what would help them become ready?

Provide warm handoff when possible: Call the agency while the client is with you. Introduce the client. Schedule the first appointment. This dramatically increases follow-through compared to "Here's a number—call them."

Explain clearly: What is this service? What will happen? What should the client expect? Unknown situations create anxiety, especially for clients with limited experience navigating systems.

Address barriers: Transportation? Cost? Childcare? Anxiety about new situations? Problem-solve barriers before they prevent access.

Ensure appropriateness: Does the client meet eligibility criteria? Is this the right level of service? Inappropriate referrals waste everyone's time and frustrate clients.

Obtain consent: Get written consent to communicate with other providers. You need permission to coordinate care.

Follow up: Did the client make the appointment? Did they go? Did they engage? If not, what got in the way? Follow-up shows you care and allows troubleshooting.

Documentation of referrals protects everyone:

Who: What service/provider you referred to
Why: Reason for referral
When: Date referral was made
What information was provided: Did you explain the service? Give written information? Make appointment?
Consent: Did you obtain consent for communication?
Follow-up: What happened with the referral?

Advocacy means using your position to help clients access services they're entitled to but struggling to obtain:

System navigation: Helping clients understand complex systems—how to apply for benefits, how to appeal denials, how to access services. Many systems are deliberately confusing. Your knowledge helps.

Documentation: Writing letters supporting applications—disability applications, housing applications, school accommodations. Your professional documentation carries weight.

Direct advocacy: Sometimes you need to call directly—advocating with insurance companies for coverage, with schools for appropriate services, with hospitals for appropriate discharge planning. Be professional but persistent.

Teaching self-advocacy: Don't do for clients what they can do themselves. Teach them to advocate. Practice with them. But when they can't effectively advocate (due to symptoms, cognitive limitations, or power imbalances), you step in.

Barriers to service access are common and need addressing:

Financial barriers: Can't afford copays, deductibles, or services not covered by insurance. Connect to financial assistance programs, sliding scale services, or free services.

Transportation barriers: No car, can't use public transit, too anxious to drive. Arrange medical transportation, schedule telehealth when appropriate, or connect to volunteer transportation.

Knowledge barriers: Don't know services exist, don't understand how to access them, don't know they're eligible. Education and navigation help.

Stigma barriers: Afraid of being judged, worried about records, fear of being "weak." Normalize service use, explain confidentiality, validate concerns while encouraging care.

Language barriers: Limited English proficiency. Connect to services with interpreters, use telephonic interpretation, provide materials in preferred language.

Cultural barriers: Services don't match cultural values or practices. Connect to culturally specific services when available, work with providers to increase cultural responsiveness.

Systemic barriers: Long waitlists, restrictive eligibility, limited hours, inconvenient locations. Advocate for system changes while helping clients navigate current reality.

Case Example: Comprehensive Case Management - Michael

Michael, 38, presents with depression and panic disorder. Initial assessment reveals complexity beyond mental health symptoms:

Mental health: Major Depression, Panic Disorder, suicidal ideation (no current intent)
Medical: Type 2 diabetes (poorly controlled), hypertension, chronic back pain
Substance use: Previously used alcohol heavily, currently sober 4 months
Housing: Living in friend's basement, unstable, friend wants him out
Income: Unemployed 8 months, lost job due to panic attacks, no income
Insurance: Lost employer insurance, uninsured
Support: Divorced, limited contact with two adult children, few friends
Legal: $40,000 medical debt, creditors calling

Your assessment: Michael needs multiple services coordinated simultaneously. Mental health treatment alone won't succeed without addressing basic needs.

Service coordination plan:

Immediate needs (week 1-2):

Health insurance: You help Michael apply for Medicaid—completing application, gathering documents, submitting. Medicaid will cover mental health treatment and medical care. This is first priority because it enables access to other services.

Mental health treatment: Begin weekly therapy sessions. Given suicide risk and severity, discuss whether outpatient is sufficient or if higher level needed. Michael is appropriate for outpatient with close monitoring.

Medical care: Help Michael establish with primary care physician for diabetes and hypertension management. His uncontrolled diabetes affects mood and energy. You call community health center, make appointment, ensure they accept Medicaid.

Food: Michael has $30 to last two weeks. You help him apply for SNAP (food stamps) online. While application processes, you connect him to food bank. He can eat while waiting for benefits.

Crisis plan: Develop safety plan given suicidal ideation. Identify warning signs, coping strategies, supports, professional contacts, and means restriction.

Short-term needs (week 3-8):

Housing: Michael's current housing ends in one month. You help him apply for housing assistance and emergency shelter if needed. You also discuss whether staying sober in friend's basement (where friend drinks) is sustainable. You connect Michael to transitional housing program for people in recovery.

Income: You help Michael apply for General Assistance (minimal cash aid while waiting for other benefits). You also help him file for unemployment—he may be eligible despite panic attacks causing job loss. You refer to vocational rehabilitation for assessment—might he be eligible for disability benefits?

Substance use support: You connect Michael to AA meetings and recovery support services. Maintaining sobriety is crucial. He's doing well but needs support as stress increases.

Debt: You refer Michael to legal aid for assistance with overwhelming medical debt. They may negotiate settlements or help with bankruptcy if appropriate.

Medium-term needs (month 2-6):

Disability application: Given severity of panic disorder and history of job loss, you help Michael apply for Social Security Disability Insurance (SSDI). This requires extensive documentation. You provide detailed letter documenting functional limitations from panic disorder and depression. You connect him to disability attorney who works on contingency.

Medication management: Once Medicaid approves, you refer Michael to psychiatrist for medication evaluation. Medication could significantly improve panic and depression symptoms.

Medical stability: Monitor whether Michael is attending medical appointments and whether diabetes and blood pressure are controlled. Poor physical health worsens mental health.

Vocational rehabilitation: If Michael's panic improves, vocational rehabilitation can help with job retraining, accommodations, or supported employment. But first, he needs stability.

Coordination challenges and solutions:

Challenge 1: Michael misses psychiatry appointment.

Your response: You call Michael. He was overwhelmed by paperwork and anxiety about new doctor. You problem-solve: offer to attend first appointment with him for support. You call psychiatry office, explain situation, reschedule. You prepare Michael for what to expect.

Challenge 2: Medicaid application denied due to missing documentation.

Your response: You call Medicaid office, identify what's missing. You help Michael obtain documents (birth certificate, tax return). You resubmit. This time, approved.

Challenge 3: Food bank requires ID, Michael has no current ID.

Your response: You help Michael order birth certificate and apply for ID. Meanwhile, you advocate with food bank supervisor—given emergency situation, can they make exception? They agree to provide food with social security card while ID processes.

Challenge 4: Michael stops coming to therapy after four sessions.

Your response: You call and leave message. No response. You send letter saying you're concerned and offering to reschedule. Finally, Michael calls—he's overwhelmed with appointments (medical, vocational rehabilitation, housing interviews). You validate how overwhelming this is and help him prioritize and schedule more sustainably.

Outcomes after 6 months:

- **Mental health**: Depression improved significantly (PHQ-9 from 20 to 9). Panic attacks decreased from daily to 2-3 times weekly. No longer suicidal.
- **Medical**: Diabetes under better control, blood pressure normalized, managing chronic pain better.
- **Substance use**: Maintaining sobriety, active in AA.
- **Housing**: Moved to transitional housing program with stable rent and recovery support.
- **Income**: Receiving SNAP and General Assistance while SSDI application processes. Not yet working but making progress.
- **Insurance**: Medicaid approved, accessing all needed medical and mental health services.
- **Legal**: Legal aid negotiated medical debt settlements, substantial reduction in what he owes.

Michael's depression and panic didn't improve from therapy alone. They improved because basic needs were met, medical conditions were treated, housing was stabilized, and he wasn't in constant crisis. Case management and therapy together created change that neither would alone.

Interdisciplinary Collaboration

You don't work alone. Effective treatment involves multiple providers—physicians, psychiatrists, nurses, case managers, peer specialists, vocational counselors, teachers, probation officers. Collaboration isn't optional—it's necessary for comprehensive care.

The treatment team includes everyone contributing to client's care. For a child, this might include: therapist, psychiatrist, pediatrician, school counselor, special education teacher, family therapist. For an adult with serious mental illness: therapist, psychiatrist, case manager, nurse, peer specialist, vocational rehabilitation counselor, primary care physician.

Roles and responsibilities need clarity. Who does what? What's each person's scope? Who coordinates? Confusion about roles creates gaps (important tasks undone) or duplication (multiple people doing the same thing).

Common provider roles:

Therapist: Provides psychotherapy, assessment, treatment planning, sometimes case management. You're reading this, so this is probably you.

Psychiatrist: Evaluates for medication, prescribes and monitors medication, provides medical perspective on symptoms. They don't typically provide therapy (though some do). Coordination with psychiatrists ensures integrated medication and therapy.

Primary care physician: Addresses physical health, prescribes medication for some mental health conditions, provides medical clearance, identifies medical causes of psychiatric symptoms.

Nurse: In mental health settings, provides medication administration, health education, medical monitoring. Psychiatric nurse practitioners prescribe and monitor medication.

Case manager: Coordinates services, helps with benefits applications, provides practical assistance with housing/employment/daily living. Often works with people with serious mental illness.

Peer specialist: Person with lived experience of mental health challenges who provides support, hope, practical guidance. Peers offer unique perspective—they've been there.

Vocational rehabilitation counselor: Assists with employment—job training, job placement, supported employment, workplace accommodations.

School personnel: Teachers, school counselors, school psychologists, special education staff. Critical for children and adolescents.

Probation/parole officers: Monitor compliance with court orders, provide structure, connect to services. Important partners for justice-involved clients.

Effective communication between providers requires structure:

Get consent: You need written consent to communicate about the client with other providers. HIPAA allows sharing information necessary for treatment, but explicit consent is best practice. Explain to clients why communication matters.

Use secure methods: Email without encryption isn't HIPAA-compliant. Use secure messaging systems, encrypted email, or phone. Fax is still common (archaic but considered secure). Never discuss identifiable patient information on unsecured platforms.

Be concise and relevant: Busy providers don't have time for lengthy narratives. Communicate relevant information clearly: diagnosis, current treatment, medications, important symptoms or concerns, and what you need from them.

Document communication: Every contact with another provider should be documented—date, who you spoke with, what was discussed, any decisions or actions. This protects everyone and ensures continuity.

Respond promptly: When another provider contacts you, respond within 24-48 hours when possible. Timely communication prevents crises and shows respect.

Treatment team meetings occur regularly for complex cases. Everyone involved meets to discuss progress, coordinate interventions, and problem-solve. These can be formal (scheduled, structured) or informal (calling to discuss).

Effective meetings include:

Clear purpose: Why are we meeting? What do we need to accomplish?

Relevant participants: Only people directly involved in the client's care. Too many people creates inefficiency.

Client participation: Include the client when appropriate. They're the expert on their own life. Their input is crucial.

Structured agenda: What will we discuss? In what order? How much time for each topic?

Clear documentation: Who will document? What was decided? Who will do what by when?

Follow-up plan: When will we meet again? What needs to happen before then?

Disagreements between providers happen and need addressing professionally:

Different perspectives are normal: A psychiatrist focused on medication might see things differently than a therapist focused on trauma. Both perspectives have value. Look for synthesis, not victory.

Focus on client welfare: What's best for the client? Keep that central. Personal preferences and professional turf battles harm clients.

Communicate directly: Don't talk about another provider to the client or to other providers. Address concerns directly with the person involved.

Respect expertise: Recognize that others have specialized knowledge. The psychiatrist knows medication better than you. You know psychotherapy better than them. Value what each brings.

Seek consultation: If you and another provider fundamentally disagree, consult with a supervisor or colleague. Fresh perspective helps.

Common collaboration challenges:

Challenge: Provider doesn't respond to your calls or messages.

Solution: Try different communication methods. Document attempts. If truly urgent and no response, escalate to their supervisor. Most providers are busy, not deliberately ignoring you.

Challenge: Provider gives client contradictory advice.

Solution: Call provider, discuss discrepancy professionally. Often it's miscommunication or the client hearing things differently. Clarify together, then provide client with consistent message.

Challenge: Client lies to different providers, creating inconsistent information.

Solution: Team meeting where everyone shares information (with client's consent). Address directly with client about honesty and why accurate information matters.

Challenge: You believe client needs service another provider controls access to (higher level of care, specific service) but provider disagrees.

Solution: Present your reasoning clearly with documentation. Ask for their perspective. Try to understand their decision. If you still disagree and client is at risk, you may need to escalate or document your concern.

Case Example: Interdisciplinary Collaboration - Sarah's Treatment Team

Sarah, 16, has anorexia nervosa, Major Depression, and self-harm through cutting. Her treatment team includes:

- **You (therapist)**: Provide individual therapy, family therapy
- **Dr. Martinez (psychiatrist)**: Prescribe/monitor antidepressant, assess need for higher level of care
- **Dr. Chen (pediatrician)**: Monitor medical stability (heart rate, blood pressure, labs)
- **Ms. Johnson (school counselor)**: Monitor school functioning, provide accommodations
- **Emily (dietitian)**: Provide nutrition counseling, meal planning
- **Parents (Maria and David)**: Implement meal support at home

Weekly team meeting (phone conference):

You: "Sarah's weight is stable at 88 pounds but hasn't increased. She's more resistant in therapy lately, minimizing concerns. Self-harm decreased—one cutting episode this week vs. three last week. Depression seems improved but eating disorder behaviors are entrenched."

Dr. Martinez: "I agree she's not progressing on eating. Medication helping depression but doesn't address anorexia directly. I'm concerned we're not intensive enough. Has anyone discussed partial hospitalization?"

Dr. Chen: "Medically, she's currently stable enough for outpatient. Heart rate is 54—low but not dangerous yet. If weight drops below 85 pounds or heart rate goes below 50, we need higher level of care immediately."

Emily (dietitian): "Sarah's following meal plan minimally—maybe 60%. She's not lying but she's not progressing either. Parents report battles at every meal. Family is exhausted."

You: "I've noticed same resistance. Parents are burned out from food battles. Sarah's not motivated to change—she sees being thin as success, not problem. I think we need more structure than outpatient provides."

Ms. Johnson (school counselor): "Academically, Sarah's maintaining good grades but teachers report she seems increasingly isolated. She eats lunch in counseling office now, not cafeteria."

Dr. Martinez: "I recommend we present partial hospitalization option to Sarah and parents. Sounds like we need more intensive structure—meal support multiple times daily, therapy, group. Sarah's not making progress at this level."

Team agrees: You will present partial hospitalization recommendation to family next session. If family agrees, Dr. Martinez will provide referral to program. Dr. Chen will provide medical records. Emily will provide nutrition assessment. Ms. Johnson will coordinate school absences/make-up work.

Follow-up: Team meets again in one week to confirm whether family accepted recommendation and Sarah enrolled in partial program.

This coordination ensures everyone is aligned, no one's working at cross-purposes, and the team responds decisively when treatment isn't working. Without this collaboration, Sarah might have continued in outpatient too long, risking medical crisis.

Referral Processes

Making appropriate referrals is a core clinical skill. You can't treat every problem or provide every service. Knowing when to refer, where to refer, and how to refer effectively ensures clients get what they need.

When to refer:

Outside your scope of practice: You're not trained in or don't have expertise in what's needed. Examples: complex medical conditions, formal psychological testing, specialized trauma treatment you're not trained in.

Outside your competence: You have basic training but not sufficient experience or expertise for this particular case. Ethics require practicing within competence boundaries.

Conflict of interest: Relationship with client makes you unable to provide objective service. Example: you can't treat your neighbor's child.

Client needs different service: The service needed isn't therapy. Examples: medication evaluation, vocational rehabilitation, housing assistance, legal services.

Treatment isn't working: Despite your best efforts and reasonable time, the client isn't improving or is getting worse. Fresh perspective needed.

You can't maintain objectivity: Personal reactions prevent you from being helpful. Example: client reminds you too much of someone from your own life and you can't manage countertransference.

Types of referrals:

Medication evaluation: Refer to psychiatrist or psychiatric nurse practitioner when medication might help. You provide context—diagnosis, symptoms, treatment response, relevant history. Don't just say "maybe medication would help"—give clinical rationale.

Psychological testing: Refer to psychologist for formal assessment when diagnosis is unclear, learning disabilities or cognitive impairment suspected, or documentation needed for accommodations.

Medical evaluation: Refer to physician when physical symptoms might explain psychiatric symptoms (thyroid problems, neurological conditions), medical clearance needed, or you're concerned about medical causes.

Higher level of mental health care: Refer to intensive outpatient, partial hospitalization, residential, or inpatient when outpatient isn't sufficient. Criteria vary by level but generally based on severity, safety, and failure of less intensive treatment.

Specialized treatment: Refer to provider with specific expertise—trauma specialist for complex PTSD, eating disorder program for anorexia, substance use treatment for addiction.

Concrete services: Case management, benefits assistance, housing services, vocational rehabilitation, legal aid, financial counseling, transportation assistance.

The referral conversation with the client matters:

Explain why: "I'm suggesting you see a psychiatrist because medication might help your depression alongside our therapy. Medication can make it easier to use the skills we're learning."

Address concerns: "What concerns do you have about seeing a psychiatrist?" Common concerns: cost, stigma, side effects, not wanting medication. Address each directly.

Clarify the process: "Here's what will happen: you'll meet with the psychiatrist for evaluation—about an hour. They'll ask about symptoms, history, and what you've tried. Then they'll discuss options and, if you both agree, start medication. You'll see them monthly to monitor."

Provide warm handoff: "I'm going to call Dr. Johnson now while you're here and introduce you. Let's schedule your first appointment together."

Ensure understanding: "Do you have questions? What will you tell the receptionist when you call?"

Follow up: "Let's check in next session about how the appointment went."

Information to provide when making referral:

To the client:

- Why you're making this referral
- What service/provider you're referring to
- What will happen (process)
- Practical information (location, phone, cost, insurance)
- What to bring (insurance card, ID, medication list)
- How to prepare (write questions, bring support person)

To the receiving provider:

- Reason for referral
- Diagnosis
- Current symptoms and functioning
- Current treatment and response
- Medications
- Relevant history
- Safety concerns
- Specific questions or needs

Tracking referrals:

Who: Client name
What: What you referred them for
Where: Specific provider or agency
When: Date referral made
Status: Appointment scheduled? Kept appointment? Engaged?
Outcome: Did client access service? Is it helping?

Without tracking, referrals fall through cracks. Clients say they'll call and don't. Appointments are missed. Services aren't accessed. Your follow-up increases success.

When referrals fail:

Client doesn't follow through: Call to explore what happened. Anxiety about new provider? Transportation problem? Forgot? Not ready? Problem-solve barriers or process ambivalence.

Provider can't see client: Waitlist full, client doesn't meet criteria, insurance not accepted. Find alternatives, help client appeal decisions, or connect to different service.

Client goes but doesn't engage: Attend first appointment but don't return, or participate minimally. Explore what happened—poor fit? Bad experience? Unmet expectations? Help decide whether to try again or find different provider.

Service doesn't help: Client engages but doesn't improve. Reassess—was this the right referral? Did something important get missed? Does client need different approach or level of care?

Case Example: Referral Process - Marcus's Medication Evaluation

Marcus, 35, has been in therapy with you for eight weeks for Major Depression. Despite good engagement and compliance with behavioral activation and cognitive restructuring, improvement is minimal. PHQ-9 remains at 19 (severe). Marcus is functioning but suffering significantly.

Your assessment: Marcus would likely benefit from antidepressant medication in addition to therapy. You've discussed this possibility before; Marcus was hesitant.

Session 8 conversation:

You: "Marcus, we've been working together for two months now. You've been doing everything right—coming to sessions, completing homework, practicing skills. I see some small improvements, but you're still suffering a lot. Your PHQ-9 score is still 19—same as when we started. I'm wondering if we should add medication to our work together."

Marcus: "I really don't want to take medication. I don't like the idea of being dependent on pills."

You: "I hear that concern. A lot of people worry about dependence. Here's the thing—antidepressants aren't addictive. You won't become dependent on them. They correct chemical imbalances that make depression harder to overcome. Think of it like diabetes—people with diabetes need insulin not because they're weak but because their body needs help. Depression is similar."

Marcus: "I've heard antidepressants change your personality."

You: "That's a common worry but not accurate. Antidepressants don't change who you are—they help you be more yourself by reducing the depression that's covering up who you are. You'll still be Marcus, just not weighed down by this suffering."

Marcus: "What about side effects?"

You: "All medications have potential side effects, but most people tolerate antidepressants well. Common initial side effects—nausea, headache—usually resolve in a week or two. The psychiatrist will discuss specific options and their side effects. You'll also monitor closely and can stop if side effects outweigh benefits."

Marcus (pause): "If I meet with a psychiatrist, does that mean I have to take medication?"

You: "No. The evaluation is just gathering information and discussing options. You make the final decision about whether to start medication. The psychiatrist will recommend what they think would help, but you're in control."

Marcus: "Okay. I'll at least talk to them."

You: "Great. I'm going to call Dr. Patel now while you're here. She's excellent—really listens and explains things well. Let's schedule your appointment."

You call Dr. Patel's office, introduce Marcus (he says hello), schedule appointment for next week. You give Marcus written appointment information (date, time, location, phone number, what to bring).

You: "Before next week, write down any questions you have for Dr. Patel. Bring your insurance card and photo ID. The appointment takes about an hour. Dr. Patel will ask about your symptoms, history, and what we've been working on in therapy. Then she'll discuss medication options. Come back next week prepared to tell me how it went."

Following up: You send Dr. Patel written referral:

To: Dr. Patel
Re: Marcus Johnson, DOB 5/12/1990
Referral for: Medication evaluation and management

Marcus is a 35-year-old male I've been treating for Major Depression for 8 weeks. Despite good engagement in therapy (behavioral activation, cognitive restructuring), improvement has been minimal. Current PHQ-9: 19 (severe). Symptoms include depressed mood, anhedonia, fatigue, sleep disturbance (early morning awakening), poor concentration, guilt, hopelessness. No suicidal ideation currently. No prior medication trials. No substance use. No medical problems. He's ambivalent about medication but agreed to evaluation. Would appreciate your assessment regarding whether medication might augment psychotherapy.

Thank you,
[Your name]

Next session: Marcus reports he met with Dr. Patel, liked her, and agreed to start escitalopram 10mg. He has questions about how long until it works and whether he should tell his employer. You answer questions, encourage patience (medication takes 4-6 weeks for full effect), and continue therapy while medication takes effect.

One month later: Marcus reports significant improvement. PHQ-9 dropped to 10 (mild). He feels "like a fog lifted." Energy is better. Anhedonia reduced. He's grateful he agreed to medication evaluation.

This referral succeeded because you: (1) explained rationale clearly, (2) addressed concerns directly, (3) provided warm handoff, (4) gave detailed information to receiving provider, (5) followed up, and (6) continued supporting client through process.

Crisis Intervention

Crises happen. Clients become suicidal, decompensate psychotically, experience traumatic events, or face overwhelming stressors. Your response in crisis moments can save lives and prevent deterioration.

Crisis defined: A crisis is a time-limited, intense emotional response to a hazardous event that exceeds the person's usual coping resources. The person is in disequilibrium—normal functioning is disrupted. Crisis intervention stabilizes and returns the person to baseline, not comprehensive treatment.

Types of crises:

Suicidal crisis: Active suicidal ideation with plan and intent. Imminent risk of suicide attempt.

Psychiatric emergency: Psychotic break, severe manic episode, dissociative episode, severe self-harm. The person can't care for themselves safely.

Traumatic event: Sexual assault, violent crime, sudden death, accident, natural disaster. Acute trauma response.

Situational crisis: Overwhelming life stress—eviction, job loss, relationship ending, medical diagnosis. The person's coping is overwhelmed.

Substance-related crisis: Overdose, severe intoxication, withdrawal, drug-induced psychosis.

Violence risk: Risk of harm to others. Homicidal ideation with plan and intent.

Immediate crisis assessment determines severity and needed response:

Safety: Is the person danger to self or others right now? Do they need emergency intervention?

Current functioning: Can they care for themselves? Make decisions? Execute basic tasks?

Support: Are there people who can help? Or are they completely alone?

Resources: What coping strategies have they used before? What's worked?

Mental status: Are they thinking clearly? Reality testing intact? Following conversation?

Substance use: Are they intoxicated? Withdrawing? Has substance use contributed to crisis?

Medical issues: Could medical problems be contributing? Do they need medical evaluation?

Crisis intervention principles:

Be present: The most powerful intervention is being fully present—calm, attentive, focused. Your presence provides stability when the client's world is chaos.

Ensure safety: Physical safety is first priority. If imminent danger exists, call 911 or initiate involuntary hold. Safety allows other intervention.

Provide hope: Crises feel permanent but are temporary. "This is terrible right now, but you won't always feel this way. We'll get through this together."

Reduce arousal: High emotional intensity impairs thinking. Help the person calm somewhat—slow breathing, grounding, validating emotions while preventing escalation.

Focus on current crisis: Don't explore childhood, process trauma, or address longstanding problems during crisis. Focus on what's happening now and how to stabilize.

Be directive: Crises aren't times for open-ended exploration. Give clear direction—"Here's what we need to do," "I need you to..." Decisiveness is reassuring.

Mobilize supports: Who can help? Family? Friends? Other providers? Community resources? Activate support systems.

Make concrete plan: What happens next? Who will do what? When will you have contact again? Concrete plans reduce anxiety.

Follow up: Call next day. Schedule appointment soon. Don't leave people alone after crisis without follow-up plan.

Suicide risk assessment is crucial crisis skill:

Ask directly: "Are you thinking about killing yourself?" Direct questions don't cause suicidal thoughts—they show you take concerns seriously and create opening for honest conversation.

Assess components:

Ideation: Thoughts about death or suicide. How frequent? How intense? How long-lasting?

Intent: Do they want to die, or just want pain to stop? Intent indicates higher risk.

Plan: Do they have specific plan? More specific and detailed plans indicate higher risk.

Means: Do they have access to means? Firearms are most lethal. Access to means dramatically increases risk.

Prior attempts: History of attempts, especially recent or multiple attempts, increases risk.

Rehearsal: Have they taken steps toward plan (buying pills, writing note, giving away possessions)? Rehearsal indicates high risk.

Timing: When are they planning to act? "Tonight" is higher risk than vague "someday."

Risk factors: Depression, substance use, recent loss, isolation, hopelessness, chronic pain, previous attempts, family history of suicide, access to firearms.

Protective factors: Reasons for living, social support, religious beliefs, responsibility to children, engagement in treatment, future plans.

Intervention based on assessment:

Low risk (thoughts but no plan, strong protective factors): Safety plan, frequent contact, remove means if possible, activate supports, close monitoring.

Moderate risk (thoughts with vague plan, mixed protective factors): Consider intensive outpatient or partial hospitalization, daily contact, safety plan, involve family/supports, possibly start/adjust medication.

High risk (plan with intent and means, few protective factors): Voluntary or involuntary hospitalization. Outpatient treatment insufficient.

Safety planning structure for ongoing risk:

1. **Warning signs**: What tells you crisis is building? (thoughts, feelings, behaviors, situations)
2. **Internal coping**: What can you do yourself to feel better or distract? (exercise, relaxation, hobbies)

3. **Social contacts**: People/places that provide distraction (friends, family, activities—not discussing suicide)
4. **People to ask for help**: Who can you tell when in crisis? (family, friends, sponsors)
5. **Professionals to contact**: Therapist number, crisis line, mobile crisis team, emergency services
6. **Making environment safe**: Removing means—firearms, pills, other lethal methods

Client keeps written copy accessible. Review and update regularly. Research shows safety planning reduces suicide attempts.

Involuntary hospitalization is sometimes necessary but always difficult:

Criteria (vary by state but generally):

- Imminent danger to self (active suicide plan with intent, severe self-harm)
- Imminent danger to others (credible homicidal threat)
- Gravely disabled (can't meet basic needs due to mental illness)

Process:

- Complete evaluation documenting criteria are met
- Contact mobile crisis team or call 911
- Stay with person until they're safely in care
- Complete required forms for involuntary hold
- Contact family/emergency contact if possible
- Document thoroughly

After:

- Maintain contact with hospital for discharge planning
- Attend discharge meeting if possible
- Schedule follow-up appointment soon after discharge
- Ensure client has medications, prescriptions, and clear plan

Involuntary hospitalization isn't punishment—it's protection. Most people are grateful afterward, even if angry initially. When someone is at imminent risk, hospitalization can save their life.

Working with mobile crisis teams: Many areas have mobile crisis teams who come to wherever the person is (home, your office, community) to assess and provide immediate intervention. They can assess whether hospitalization is needed or crisis can be managed with intensive community support.

When available, use them—they prevent unnecessary emergency room visits and provide expert crisis assessment.

Case Example: Crisis Intervention - Lisa's Suicide Crisis

Lisa, 29, calls you at 8 PM (your office hours are 9-5, but you gave her your cell for emergencies). She's crying, barely coherent. "I can't do this anymore. I'm going to end it."

Immediate response:

You: "Lisa, I'm glad you called. I'm here with you. First, I need to know—are you safe right now? Are you somewhere safe?"

Lisa: "I'm in my apartment. I have pills. I was just going to take them all."

You: "Do you have the pills right there with you now?"

Lisa: "Yes. In my hand."

You: "Okay. I need you to put the pills down and step away from them. Can you do that for me right now?"

Lisa (crying): "I don't know. I just want the pain to stop."

You: "I know you're in terrible pain right now. I hear that. And there are ways to stop the pain that don't involve ending your life. But first, I need you to be safe. Put the pills down and step into another room. Can you do that?"

Lisa: "Okay." (sounds of movement) "I put them down. I'm in my living room."

You: "Good. Thank you. That took courage. Now, is anyone there with you?"

Lisa: "No, I'm alone."

You: "Is there anyone you can call to come be with you? Family? Friends?"

Lisa: "My sister. But I don't want to bother her."

You: "This is exactly when you need to call her. This is an emergency. I need you to call your sister right now and ask her to come over. Will you do that?"

Lisa: "Okay."

You: "While we're on the phone, I want you to tell me what happened. What made tonight so unbearable?"

Lisa explains: her boyfriend broke up with her this morning, she got written up at work, she feels like a complete failure, she's been having suicidal thoughts for weeks but tonight they became overwhelming. She's been drinking. She feels hopeless that anything will get better.

You: "Lisa, I hear how much you're hurting. This has been building, and tonight pushed you to the edge. But you did the right thing calling me. That tells me part of you wants to live. Part of you knows this pain is temporary even though it feels permanent."

Lisa (crying): "I just can't keep going like this."

You: "You can't keep going like THIS—I agree. We need to make changes. But ending your life isn't the change we need. We need to get you more support and address this suffering. Here's what's going to happen: you're going to call your sister to come stay with you tonight. Tomorrow morning, I'm going to see you first thing. We're going to figure out whether you need a higher level of care—maybe intensive outpatient or partial hospitalization. But tonight, you need to be safe and not alone."

Lisa: "I don't want to go to the hospital."

You: "I'm not saying hospital yet. Let's get through tonight safely, then tomorrow we'll figure out next steps. Can you commit to staying safe tonight? No taking those pills? Your sister will be there with you?"

Lisa: "Yes. I promise."

You: "Good. Call your sister right now. Then call me back and let me know she's coming. I'll stay on the phone until I know you're not alone."

Lisa calls her sister, who lives nearby and can be there in 20 minutes. Lisa calls you back. Her sister is coming. You talk with Lisa until sister arrives. You speak briefly with sister, explaining Lisa's in crisis and shouldn't be alone. Sister will stay the night.

You: "Lisa, I'm going to call you tomorrow at 9 AM, and you'll come to my office at 10 AM. We're going to make a clear plan for keeping you safe and getting you the help you need. Between now and then, if the thoughts get overwhelming again, you call me or you go to the emergency room. Your sister has my number too. I'm glad you reached out. See you tomorrow."

Next morning:

Lisa comes in, exhausted but alive. You complete thorough suicide risk assessment. She still has thoughts but less intense. She's embarrassed about last night. You normalize—crises happen, reaching out was brave.

Assessment: Moderate to high risk. Contributing factors: recent loss (breakup), work stress, alcohol use, social isolation, history of depression. But protective factors exist: sister support, willingness to engage in treatment, no prior attempts.

Plan: Refer to intensive outpatient program starting Monday (provides daily structure and support). See Lisa daily until IOP starts. Refer for medication evaluation (her depression needs more than weekly therapy). Sister agrees to stay with Lisa through the weekend. Lisa gives sister the pills to hold. You create written safety plan with warning signs, coping strategies, supports, and crisis numbers.

Outcome: Lisa enters IOP, starts medication, begins addressing underlying depression and relationship patterns. The crisis was turning point—she couldn't continue as she had been. With intensified treatment, she makes progress. Three months later, she's functioning better than before the crisis.

This crisis intervention worked because you: (1) prioritized immediate safety, (2) removed means, (3) reduced isolation, (4) provided concrete next steps, (5) followed up, and (6) arranged appropriate level of care.

Termination and Aftercare Planning

All therapeutic relationships end. Sometimes it's planned—client achieves goals, you're leaving the agency, insurance coverage ends. Sometimes it's unexpected—client moves, client stops coming, you're terminated due to budget cuts. How you handle endings affects whether clients maintain gains and can engage in future treatment.

Planned termination is the goal. You and client together decide treatment goals have been met and it's time to end:

When to terminate:

Goals achieved: The problems that brought the client to treatment have been resolved or significantly improved. They have skills and support to maintain gains.

Plateau reached: Progress has stalled at "good enough" level. Continued treatment isn't producing additional gains. Client is functioning adequately.

Client ready: Even if you see room for more work, the client feels ready. Respecting client autonomy means honoring their readiness to end.

Treatment isn't helping: Despite adequate time and effort, treatment isn't working. Continuing wastes resources and may harm therapeutic relationship.

Transition to different service: Client needs different level or type of service. You terminate from your service while ensuring smooth transition to new one.

Preparing for termination:

Discuss several sessions in advance: Don't surprise clients with sudden ending. Give time to process.

Review progress: What did you work on? What changed? What did client learn? Articulating progress helps consolidate gains and build self-efficacy.

Discuss feelings: Ending evokes feelings—sadness, anxiety, pride, abandonment. Make space for these. Normalizing feelings about endings is therapeutic.

Relapse prevention: What are warning signs client is struggling? What coping strategies will they use? When should they seek help again?

Address dependency concerns: Some clients worry they can't function without therapy. Review evidence of their competence. Emphasize that ending therapy doesn't mean ending progress.

Create continuity plan: What will client do for ongoing support? Support groups? Continued skills practice? Periodic booster sessions?

Final session: The last session focuses on closure:

Summarize journey: Where did you start? Where are you now? What obstacles did you overcome?

Highlight client's strengths and efforts: "You did this work. You showed up, you practiced skills, you faced difficult feelings. I'm proud of you, but you should be proud of yourself."

Discuss possibility of return: "Ending therapy doesn't mean you can never come back. If you struggle in the future, you can return. That wouldn't be failure—it would be good self-care."

Express your experience: "It's been meaningful for me to work with you. I've seen your courage and growth. Thank you for trusting me." Be genuine but maintain boundaries.

Say goodbye: Simple, direct goodbye. Don't minimize—"This is hard for me too. Goodbye, and I wish you well."

Unplanned termination happens frequently:

Client stops attending: They cancel, no-show, don't reschedule. You don't know why.

Your response:

- Call and leave message expressing concern, inviting contact
- Send letter if no response: "I noticed you haven't been coming to sessions. I'm concerned and want to make sure you're okay. If you'd like to resume therapy, please call. If you've decided to stop, that's your right, but I'd appreciate the chance to say goodbye and ensure you have resources for the future."
- Document your attempts to contact
- Close case if no response after reasonable attempts (typically 2-3 contacts over 2-4 weeks)

You're leaving agency: Job change, relocation, career transition.

Your response:

- Notify clients as soon as you know, giving maximum advance notice
- Help clients transfer to another therapist at agency if available
- Provide referrals if clients need to find new therapist elsewhere
- Offer to have one session with new therapist for warm handoff
- Be available for questions during transition

- Process feelings about the change

Client moves or circumstances change: Life happens—new job, relocation, lost insurance coverage, changed life circumstances.

Your response:

- Honor whatever time remains for proper termination
- Provide referrals for new location if applicable
- Summarize progress and provide written treatment summary they can share with new provider
- Discuss how they'll maintain gains with new circumstances
- Offer to consult with new provider if client wishes

Premature termination is when client leaves before goals are achieved:

Common reasons:

- Couldn't afford continued treatment
- Practical barriers (transportation, childcare, time)
- Didn't feel treatment was helping
- Conflict with therapist or treatment approach
- Feeling better, doesn't think they need more help
- Too uncomfortable with therapy process
- External pressure to stop (partner, family)

Your response:

- Explore why client wants to stop
- Validate their reasons while sharing your perspective
- If leaving due to barriers, problem-solve (sliding scale, telehealth, different appointment times)
- If leaving due to feeling better, discuss relapse prevention
- If leaving due to not helping, discuss whether different approach might help or whether referral to different provider makes sense
- Don't pressure client to stay, but ensure they know door is open for return
- Offer at least one termination session to close properly

Aftercare planning helps clients maintain gains:

Support groups: Al-Anon for family members of alcoholics, NAMI support groups for families affected by mental illness, DBSA for mood disorders, grief support groups. Ongoing peer support maintains progress.

Booster sessions: Schedule one appointment 1-3 months after termination to check in, troubleshoot, reinforce skills. Prevents small setbacks from becoming relapses.

Continued skill practice: Clients should keep practicing skills learned in therapy—thought records, mindfulness, communication skills. Skills maintained through practice.

Regular self-monitoring: Encourage clients to monitor their own symptoms—continuing to complete PHQ-9 monthly, noticing warning signs early. Early detection prevents crises.

Clear plan for return: If symptoms worsen significantly or new problems emerge, client should return to treatment. Normalize that returning isn't failure—it's good self-care.

Connection to recovery resources: Recovery isn't just absence of symptoms—it's presence of meaningful life. Connect clients to activities, relationships, work, volunteering, hobbies that provide purpose.

Documentation of termination:

Termination note includes:

- Date of last session
- Reason for termination
- Summary of treatment provided (duration, frequency, modalities)
- Summary of progress (goals achieved, improvements, ongoing concerns)
- Client's current functioning
- Discharge diagnosis
- Aftercare plan (recommendations, referrals provided, follow-up scheduled)
- Client's understanding of aftercare plan

Thorough termination documentation protects you legally and provides clear record if client returns or needs information for future treatment.

Case Example: Planned Termination - Jennifer

Jennifer, 42, began therapy 14 months ago for Generalized Anxiety Disorder and social anxiety. At intake, her GAD-7 was 18 (severe). She avoided social situations, worried constantly, had panic attacks, and struggled at work due to anxiety about presentations.

Session 60 (month 14):

You: "Jennifer, I've been thinking about where you are now compared to when we started. Your GAD-7 last week was 4—minimal anxiety range. You're attending social events regularly, you gave two presentations at work without panic attacks, and you're using your skills consistently. How do you feel about your progress?"

Jennifer: "I feel so much better. I still get anxious sometimes, but I can manage it. It doesn't control my life anymore."

You: "That's significant change. I'm wondering if we should start thinking about termination—ending our regular therapy because you've achieved your goals."

Jennifer (anxious): "Really? I'm not sure I'm ready. What if the anxiety comes back?"

You: "That's a normal worry. Here's what I notice: you have strong skills now—you challenge anxious thoughts, you use relaxation techniques, you face feared situations instead of avoiding. You don't need me to tell you what to do anymore—you're doing it yourself. That's the goal of therapy—helping you become your own therapist."

Jennifer: "I guess you're right. I have been handling things on my own more."

You: "What if we plan for four more sessions over the next two months? That gives us time to review everything you've learned, create a relapse prevention plan, and say goodbye properly. And termination doesn't mean never coming back—if you struggle in the future, you can always return for tune-up sessions."

Jennifer: "Okay. That sounds manageable."

Sessions 61-63: You review Jennifer's progress, identify warning signs of relapse (sleep disruption, avoiding social situations, increased worry), create written relapse prevention plan with specific coping strategies, discuss continuing to practice skills even without weekly therapy. Jennifer expresses pride in her progress and sadness about ending. You validate both feelings.

Session 64 (final session):

You: "This is our last session. I want to start by reviewing how far you've come."

Jennifer: "When I started, I was barely functioning. I couldn't go to social events without panic attacks. I avoided presentations at work. I worried about everything constantly. Now I'm doing all those things. I'm not perfect, but I'm living my life instead of being controlled by anxiety."

You: "You achieved every goal we set. More than that, you learned skills you'll have forever. You know how to challenge catastrophic thinking. You know how to use exposure instead of avoidance. You know how to relax your body when it's tense. These skills don't disappear when therapy ends."

Jennifer: "I'm going to miss coming here. This has been such a safe place."

You: "I'm going to miss our sessions too. Working with you has been meaningful to me—I've watched you go from someone paralyzed by anxiety to someone facing fears and building the life you want. That takes real courage. You should be incredibly proud."

Jennifer (crying): "Thank you. You've helped me so much."

You: "You did the work. I guided, but you took the risks, faced the fears, practiced the skills. Remember that—this progress is yours. And remember, ending therapy doesn't mean you can never come back. If you struggle in the future, call me. That's not failure—that's good self-care."

Jennifer: "I will. Thank you for everything."

You: "You're welcome. Goodbye, Jennifer. I wish you well."

Follow-up: You send Jennifer brief note two weeks later congratulating her on completing therapy and reminding her you're available if needed. Six months later, Jennifer calls to schedule a booster session—she's doing well overall but wants to troubleshoot new work stress. You schedule one session, review skills, and she's back on track.

This termination was successful because: (1) it was planned and gradual, (2) client's readiness was assessed, (3) progress was reviewed thoroughly, (4) relapse prevention plan was created, (5) feelings about ending were processed, (6) possibility of return was normalized, and (7) follow-up contact occurred.

Practice Questions

1. Service coordination involves:

A. Doing everything yourself
B. Ensuring clients receive all needed services in organized manner
C. Avoiding other providers
D. Only therapy

2. A "warm handoff" means:

A. Shaking hands
B. Calling agency while client is present and scheduling appointment
C. Just giving phone numbers
D. Avoiding referrals

3. When advocating for clients, you:

A. Do everything for them
B. Use your position to help them access entitled services
C. Never get involved
D. Only write letters

4. Assessment of needs includes:

A. Only mental health
B. Basic needs, medical, mental health, social, vocational, legal, financial
C. Just diagnosis
D. Only what insurance covers

5. Effective interdisciplinary collaboration requires:

A. Working alone
B. Clear roles, communication, and coordination
C. Avoiding other providers
D. Only calling in emergencies

6. Treatment team meetings should include:

A. Everyone in the agency
B. Relevant participants directly involved in client's care
C. Only administrators
D. Never the client

7. When making referrals, you should:

A. Just give phone numbers
B. Explain rationale, address concerns, provide information, follow up
C. Force clients to go
D. Assume they'll follow through

8. Consent for communication with other providers:

A. Isn't needed
B. Requires written permission from client
C. Is automatic
D. Doesn't matter

9. A crisis is:

A. Any problem
B. Time-limited intense response exceeding usual coping
C. Always requires hospitalization
D. Chronic difficulty

10. When assessing suicide risk, you should:

A. Avoid asking
B. Ask directly about thoughts, intent, plan, means
C. Assume client will tell you
D. Only ask once

11. Safety planning includes:

A. Only phone numbers
B. Warning signs, coping strategies, supports, professional contacts, means restriction
C. Just hospitalization
D. Avoiding discussion

12. Involuntary hospitalization is appropriate when:

A. Client refuses outpatient treatment
B. Person is imminent danger to self or others
C. Family requests it
D. Therapist is frustrated

13. Mobile crisis teams:

A. Only work in hospitals
B. Come to where person is to assess and provide immediate intervention
C. Only transport to hospitals
D. Aren't helpful

14. Crisis intervention should:

A. Process childhood trauma
B. Focus on stabilization and current crisis
C. Be long-term
D. Avoid directiveness

15. Primary emotions in crisis often are:

A. Just anger
B. Fear, hurt, helplessness beneath defensive reactions
C. Unimportant
D. Should be ignored

16. When clients stop attending without explanation, you should:

A. Do nothing
B. Call, leave message, send letter offering to resume or say goodbye
C. Just close the case
D. Be angry

17. Planned termination should:

A. Be sudden
B. Be discussed in advance with review of progress
C. Avoid feelings
D. Happen after one session

18. Relapse prevention planning includes:

A. Nothing specific
B. Warning signs, coping strategies, plan for return if needed
C. Just hoping for the best
D. Only medication

19. When you leave an agency, you should:

A. Just disappear
B. Notify clients early, help transfer to new therapist, process feelings
C. Not tell anyone
D. Only tell supervisor

20. Premature termination means:

A. Client achieved goals quickly
B. Client leaves before goals achieved
C. Only after one session
D. Therapist decides

21. Aftercare planning might include:

A. Nothing
B. Support groups, booster sessions, continued practice, clear return plan
C. Only medication
D. Avoiding all contact

22. Case management includes:

A. Only therapy
B. Coordinating services, connecting to resources, advocacy
C. Avoiding practical issues
D. Only crisis work

23. When referrals fail, you should:

A. Give up
B. Explore what happened and problem-solve barriers
C. Blame the client
D. Never refer again

24. Documentation of termination should include:

A. Nothing specific
B. Reason, treatment summary, progress, discharge diagnosis, aftercare plan
C. Just the date
D. Only billing information

25. Booster sessions after termination:

A. Show failure
B. Help maintain gains and prevent small setbacks from becoming relapses
C. Aren't helpful
D. Should be avoided

Answer Key with Detailed Explanations

1. B. Ensuring clients receive all needed services in organized manner
Service coordination means ensuring clients receive all needed services in organized, integrated manner. You assess needs, connect clients to appropriate services, ensure access, and monitor effectiveness. You don't provide everything yourself (impossible and inappropriate), but you orchestrate multiple services to work together addressing the client's complex needs comprehensively.

2. B. Calling agency while client is present and scheduling appointment
A warm handoff is calling the receiving agency or provider while the client is with you, introducing the client, and scheduling the first appointment. This dramatically increases follow-through compared to just giving phone numbers and telling clients to call themselves. It reduces barriers (anxiety, procrastination, confusion) and ensures the connection actually happens.

3. B. Use your position to help them access entitled services
Advocacy means using your professional position to help clients access services they're entitled to but struggling to obtain. This includes system navigation (explaining processes), documentation (writing supporting letters), and direct advocacy (calling on their behalf when needed). You don't do everything for them (teach self-advocacy when possible), but when they can't effectively advocate due to symptoms or power imbalances, you intervene.

4. B. Basic needs, medical, mental health, social, vocational, legal, financial
Comprehensive needs assessment goes beyond mental health diagnosis and symptoms to include: basic needs (housing, food, income), medical needs, mental health and substance use needs, social support, educational and vocational needs, legal needs, and financial needs. You assess the whole person in their whole life because problems in any area affect mental health and recovery.

5. B. Clear roles, communication, and coordination
Effective interdisciplinary collaboration requires clarity about who does what (roles and responsibilities), regular communication (meetings, calls, messages) using secure methods, and intentional coordination ensuring everyone works toward shared goals without duplication or gaps. You don't work in isolation or avoid other providers—effective treatment involves multiple professionals working as team.

6. B. Relevant participants directly involved in client's care
Treatment team meetings should include relevant participants directly involved in the client's care—not everyone in the agency or only administrators. Include the client when appropriate since they're expert on their own life. Too many participants creates inefficiency. Too few means important perspectives are missing. Focus on those actively providing services or making decisions about the client's care.

7. B. Explain rationale, address concerns, provide information, follow up
Effective referrals require explaining why you're suggesting the service, addressing client's concerns, providing practical information (location, cost, what to expect), making warm handoffs when possible, and following up to ensure connection happened. Just giving phone numbers results in low follow-through. Forcing clients is unethical. Assuming they'll follow through without support means many fall through cracks. Comprehensive referral process increases success.

8. B. Requires written permission from client
Communication with other providers about the client requires written permission from the client. While HIPAA allows some sharing for treatment purposes, explicit written consent is best practice. You explain to clients why communication matters (coordinated care is better care), obtain signature on release of information form, and only share information relevant to coordination. This protects confidentiality while allowing necessary collaboration.

9. B. Time-limited intense response exceeding usual coping
A crisis is a time-limited (not chronic), intense emotional response to a hazardous event that exceeds the person's usual coping resources. The person is in disequilibrium—normal functioning disrupted. Not every problem is a crisis. Not all crises require hospitalization. Crises are acute situations where usual coping isn't working and immediate intervention is needed to stabilize.

10. B. Ask directly about thoughts, intent, plan, means
When assessing suicide risk, ask directly and specifically: "Are you thinking about killing yourself?" "Do you have a plan?" "What is the plan?" "Do you have access to means?" Direct questions don't cause suicidal thoughts—they show you take concerns seriously and create space for honest conversation. Never avoid asking or assume clients will volunteer information. One assessment isn't sufficient—reassess regularly.

11. B. Warning signs, coping strategies, supports, professional contacts, means restriction
Safety planning includes: (1) warning signs indicating crisis is building, (2) internal coping strategies the person can use themselves, (3) social contacts for distraction, (4) people to ask for help, (5) professional contacts including therapist and crisis lines, and (6) making environment safe by removing means. This structured plan provides concrete steps for managing suicidal crises and reduces suicide attempts according to research.

12. B. Person is imminent danger to self or others
Involuntary hospitalization is appropriate when the person is imminent danger to self (active suicide plan with intent), imminent danger to others (credible homicidal threat), or gravely disabled (can't meet basic needs due to mental illness). It's not appropriate just because client refuses outpatient treatment, family requests it, or therapist is frustrated. Specific dangerousness criteria must be met. It's protection, not punishment.

13. B. Come to where person is to assess and provide immediate intervention
Mobile crisis teams come to wherever the person is—home, your office, community location—to assess crisis and provide immediate intervention. They can determine whether hospitalization is needed or whether crisis can be managed with intensive community support. When available, mobile crisis teams prevent unnecessary emergency room visits, provide expert crisis assessment, and offer alternatives to hospitalization when safe.

14. B. Focus on stabilization and current crisis
Crisis intervention focuses on stabilization and current crisis, not processing childhood trauma, exploring longstanding problems, or providing long-term therapy. The goal is returning the person to baseline functioning quickly. You can be appropriately directive during crises—giving clear guidance

rather than open-ended exploration. Once stabilized, comprehensive treatment can address underlying issues.

15. B. Fear, hurt, helplessness beneath defensive reactions
Primary emotions during crises are often vulnerable feelings—fear, hurt, helplessness, shame—beneath defensive secondary emotions like anger or numbness. Accessing primary emotions creates connection and understanding. The angry person is often terrified. The withdrawn person is often deeply hurt. Understanding and validating primary emotions helps de-escalate crises and builds therapeutic alliance.

16. B. Call, leave message, send letter offering to resume or say goodbye
When clients stop attending without explanation, make reasonable efforts to contact them: call and leave message expressing concern, send letter inviting them to resume or say goodbye properly. Document contact attempts. If no response after 2-3 contacts over 2-4 weeks, close case. Don't do nothing (shows you don't care), but don't pursue indefinitely. Respect client autonomy while offering chance for closure.

17. B. Be discussed in advance with review of progress
Planned termination should be discussed several sessions in advance (not suddenly), include review of progress (what changed, what was learned), process feelings about ending (sadness, anxiety, pride), and prepare for maintaining gains. Adequate time for termination work helps consolidate learning, process the relationship ending, and prevent feelings of abandonment. One-session terminations after extended therapy feel abrupt.

18. B. Warning signs, coping strategies, plan for return if needed
Relapse prevention planning identifies warning signs of relapse (symptom increases, behavior changes, stressors), reviews coping strategies learned in treatment, and creates clear plan for returning if needed. This normalizes that setbacks can occur but provides tools for managing them. It's not just hoping for best or only medication—it's concrete preparation including when to seek help again.

19. B. Notify clients early, help transfer to new therapist, process feelings
When you leave an agency, notify clients as soon as you know (giving maximum advance notice), help them transfer to another therapist at the agency or provide referrals elsewhere, and process their feelings about the change. Don't just disappear or only tell your supervisor. Clients have feelings about endings—abandonment, anger, sadness. Processing this is therapeutic and shows respect for the relationship.

20. B. Client leaves before goals achieved
Premature termination is when the client leaves before treatment goals are achieved. This differs from quick achievement of goals or therapist-initiated termination. Common reasons include financial barriers, practical obstacles, feeling better (though not fully improved), or dissatisfaction with treatment. Your response is exploring why, validating concerns, problem-solving barriers when possible, and ensuring door remains open for return.

21. B. Support groups, booster sessions, continued practice, clear return plan
Aftercare planning might include: connection to support groups for ongoing peer support, scheduled

booster sessions (1-3 months after termination) to check in, continued practice of skills learned in therapy, regular self-monitoring of symptoms, and clear plan for returning if symptoms worsen significantly. Aftercare helps clients maintain gains and prevents small setbacks from becoming full relapses.

22. B. Coordinating services, connecting to resources, advocacy
Case management includes coordinating multiple services, connecting clients to needed resources (housing, income, medical care, vocational services), advocating for access to services, ensuring services work together effectively, and monitoring whether services are helping. It's not only therapy or only crisis work—it's comprehensive attention to all factors affecting the person's functioning and recovery.

23. B. Explore what happened and problem-solve barriers
When referrals fail (client doesn't follow through, provider can't accept, service doesn't help), explore what happened and problem-solve barriers. Was it anxiety about new provider? Transportation problem? Poor fit? Insurance issue? Unmet expectations? Understanding why allows you to address obstacles and try again differently. Don't give up, blame client, or never refer again—learn and adjust approach.

24. B. Reason, treatment summary, progress, discharge diagnosis, aftercare plan
Termination documentation should include: reason for termination, treatment summary (duration, frequency, modalities used), summary of progress (goals achieved, improvements, ongoing concerns), client's current functioning, discharge diagnosis, aftercare plan (recommendations, referrals, follow-up), and client's understanding of plan. Thorough documentation protects legally and provides clear record if client returns or needs information shared with future providers.

25. B. Help maintain gains and prevent small setbacks from becoming relapses
Booster sessions after termination (scheduled 1-3 months later to check in, troubleshoot, reinforce skills) help maintain treatment gains and prevent small setbacks from escalating into full relapses. They're not signs of failure—they're proactive maintenance supporting long-term success. Research shows booster sessions improve sustained outcomes. Normalizing their use encourages clients to return before problems become severe.

Bringing It All Together

Case management and care coordination separate adequate therapists from excellent ones. You can be brilliant at CBT, but if your depressed client is homeless and you don't help them find housing, your therapy won't work. You can masterfully process trauma, but if your client can't afford their blood pressure medication and has a stroke, the trauma work becomes irrelevant.

Real people exist in complex systems—medical, social, economic, legal. Their problems don't exist in isolation. Depression doesn't float in space—it exists in a person who needs housing, income, medical care, social connection, and purpose. Your job includes addressing or connecting them to services addressing all these needs.

This work is messy. Clients miss appointments. Referrals fail. Other providers don't return calls. Systems are confusing and often deliberately so. Resources are inadequate. You'll feel frustrated trying to get someone disability benefits when you know they deserve them but bureaucracy says no. You'll be angry that someone can't access mental health care because they don't have insurance. You'll be exhausted coordinating seven different services for one person.

But this work matters. When you help someone get housing after years of homelessness, you've changed their life. When you coordinate medical and mental health care so both are addressed, you've improved their health on multiple levels. When you advocate successfully for school accommodations, you've given a child a chance at education. When you manage a crisis well, you may have saved a life.

Case management isn't glamorous. It's phone calls and paperwork and problem-solving logistics. But it's as essential as therapy itself—maybe more so. Maslow was right. Basic needs first. Stability before growth. You provide both, and that makes you invaluable.

Core Principles for Effective Care Coordination

- Service coordination ensures clients receive all needed services addressing basic needs, medical care, mental health, social support, vocational, legal, and financial needs comprehensively
- Effective referrals require explaining rationale, addressing concerns, providing warm handoffs when possible, giving detailed information, and following up consistently
- Advocacy involves using your professional position to help clients navigate systems, document needs, and access services they're entitled to but struggle to obtain
- Interdisciplinary collaboration requires clear roles, regular communication, coordination around shared goals, and mutual respect for each provider's expertise
- Written consent is required before communicating about clients with other providers, protecting confidentiality while allowing necessary coordination
- Crisis intervention focuses on immediate safety, stabilization, and concrete planning rather than exploring underlying long-term issues
- Suicide risk assessment requires direct questioning about ideation, intent, plan, means, prior attempts, and protective factors with regular reassessment
- Safety planning includes warning signs, coping strategies, social supports, professional contacts, and means restriction, reducing suicide attempts when implemented
- Involuntary hospitalization is appropriate when person is imminent danger to self or others or gravely disabled, not simply for refusing treatment or family request
- Mobile crisis teams provide expert assessment and intervention in community settings, often preventing unnecessary hospitalizations when available
- Planned termination discussed in advance includes reviewing progress, processing feelings, creating relapse prevention plans, and normalizing possibility of return

- Premature termination requires exploration of reasons, validation of concerns, problem-solving barriers, and ensuring door remains open for future care
- Aftercare planning with support groups, booster sessions, continued skills practice, and clear return plans helps maintain treatment gains long-term
- When referrals fail, exploring what happened and problem-solving barriers allows adjustment of approach rather than giving up on needed services
- Thorough documentation of service coordination, referrals, crises, and termination protects legally and ensures continuity of care across providers and time

Chapter 13: NASW Code of Ethics

Something interesting happens when you start practicing. Everything you learned in school—theories, techniques, interventions—suddenly meets reality. And reality is messy. A client asks you to lie to their insurance company. Your supervisor tells you to do something you believe is harmful. You discover your colleague is impaired and treating clients. A client wants to be friends on Facebook. Your agency pressures you to see more clients than you can handle safely.

The Code of Ethics doesn't make these decisions for you. It won't tell you exactly what to do in every situation. What it does is provide a framework—values, principles, and standards guiding your decision-making when the right answer isn't obvious. And trust me, the right answer is rarely obvious.

Ethics isn't about memorizing rules. It's about developing ethical sensitivity—recognizing when situations have ethical dimensions. It's about ethical reasoning—thinking through dilemmas systematically. It's about ethical courage—doing the right thing even when it's uncomfortable, costly, or unpopular.

You'll face ethical dilemmas throughout your career. Some will be dramatic—a client threatening violence, a colleague engaged in exploitation. Most will be everyday challenges—managing boundaries, balancing competing obligations, practicing within competence, being honest when it's easier to avoid. Your ethical compass matters more than you realize. It protects clients, protects you, and protects the profession.

Ethical Principles and Core Values

The NASW Code of Ethics rests on six core values that define what social work is about. These aren't just nice ideas—they're foundational commitments shaping everything we do.

Service: Social workers' primary goal is helping people in need and addressing social problems. Service comes before self-interest. You chose this profession to help others—that commitment remains central even when you're exhausted, frustrated, or dealing with difficult clients. Your convenience, comfort, or personal preferences take a backseat to client welfare.

This doesn't mean you sacrifice yourself completely. You can't help anyone if you're burned out or impaired. But it means that in the moment-to-moment decisions of practice, you ask: "What serves the client best?" not "What's easiest for me?"

Social justice: Social workers challenge social injustice and pursue change on behalf of vulnerable and oppressed individuals and groups. You're not politically neutral—you're explicitly committed to social justice. This means understanding how poverty, discrimination, and oppression create the problems clients face. It means advocating for policy changes, not just helping individuals cope with unjust systems.

Social justice work happens at multiple levels. You challenge discrimination in your agency. You advocate for policy changes. You help clients access resources they're entitled to. You recognize that a client's depression might be reasonable response to poverty and discrimination, not just individual pathology.

Dignity and worth of the person: Social workers treat each person with care and respect, mindful of individual differences and cultural and ethnic diversity. Every person has inherent worth regardless of their actions, beliefs, or circumstances. You respect the dignity of the person who committed horrific crimes. You respect the worth of the person whose values oppose yours. You respect the humanity of the person who's difficult, angry, or rejecting your help.

This gets tested. The client who's racist, who abuses their children, who relapses repeatedly—they still deserve respect. Not for their actions but for their humanity. Dignity isn't earned through good behavior. It's inherent.

Importance of human relationships: Social workers recognize that relationships between and among people are important vehicles for change. The therapeutic relationship isn't just pleasant—it's central to change. Your connection with clients, their connections with others, community connections—relationships are where healing and growth happen.

This is why we emphasize therapeutic alliance. Research shows relationship quality predicts outcomes as strongly as specific techniques. You're not just a technician applying interventions. You're a person in relationship with another person, and that relationship itself is therapeutic.

Integrity: Social workers behave in a trustworthy manner. You're honest. You follow through on commitments. You practice congruently with the profession's mission, values, and ethical standards. Clients trust you with their most vulnerable selves—you honor that trust by being consistently trustworthy.

Integrity means doing the right thing when no one's watching. It means acknowledging mistakes. It means being honest even when dishonesty would be easier. It means your actions match your words and the profession's values.

Competence: Social workers practice within their areas of competence and develop and enhance their professional expertise. You don't pretend to know what you don't know. You don't practice beyond your training. You continually learn and improve. Competence isn't a static achievement—it's ongoing commitment to growth.

This creates tension. How do you develop new competencies without initially being competent? The answer: training, supervision, and gradual expansion of skills. You don't treat complex trauma without training. You don't work with populations you don't understand. You build competence deliberately and ethically.

Ethical principles expand on core values:

Principle 1: Service: Social workers' primary goal is to help people in need and to address social problems. You elevate service above self-interest, but you can also engage in scholarly research and teaching. Your primary responsibility remains helping people and addressing social problems.

Principle 2: Social Justice: Social workers challenge social injustice by pursuing social change particularly with and on behalf of vulnerable and oppressed individuals and groups. Focus areas include poverty, unemployment, discrimination, and other forms of social injustice. These activities promote sensitivity to and knowledge about oppression and cultural and ethnic diversity.

Principle 3: Dignity and Worth of the Person: Social workers respect the inherent dignity and worth of every person. You treat people in a caring and respectful manner, mindful of individual differences and cultural and ethnic diversity. You promote clients' socially responsible self-determination, seek to enhance clients' capacity and opportunity to change and to address their own needs, and are cognizant of dual responsibility to clients and to broader society.

Principle 4: Importance of Human Relationships: Social workers understand that relationships between and among people are important vehicles for change. You engage people as partners in the helping process and seek to strengthen relationships among people to restore, promote, and enhance their well-being.

Principle 5: Integrity: Social workers behave in a trustworthy manner. You are continually aware of the profession's mission, values, ethical principles, and ethical standards and practice in manner consistent with them. You act honestly and responsibly and promote ethical practices on the part of organizations you're affiliated with.

Principle 6: Competence: Social workers practice within their areas of competence and develop and enhance professional expertise. You continually strive to increase your professional knowledge and skills and to apply them in practice. You aspire to contribute to the knowledge base of the profession.

Using values and principles in practice: When facing ethical dilemmas, return to these core values and principles. They provide foundation for decision-making. Ask yourself:

- How does each option align with social work values?
- Which option best serves the client?
- Which option promotes social justice?
- Which option respects human dignity?
- Which option preserves relationship and trust?
- Which option demonstrates integrity?
- Which option reflects my competence limits?

The values don't always point to the same action. Service to client might conflict with broader social responsibility. Respecting self-determination might conflict with protecting someone from harm. When values conflict, you engage in ethical reasoning—weighing competing considerations thoughtfully.

Ethical Responsibilities to Clients

Your primary responsibility is to clients. The Code provides specific standards governing this central relationship.

Commitment to clients: Clients' interests are primary. You have dual responsibility to clients and to broader society, but when responsibilities conflict, clients' interests generally prevail. Exception: when client interests would result in serious, foreseeable, imminent harm to themselves or others.

Example: Client tells you they're undocumented and working under false social security number. Your commitment to client means you don't report this—no serious imminent harm exists. But if client threatens to harm someone, commitment to client yields to protection of potential victims.

Self-determination: You respect and promote clients' right to self-determination and assist them in identifying and clarifying their goals. You may limit clients' self-determination only when their actions pose serious, foreseeable, imminent risk to themselves or others.

This gets complex. A depressed client refuses medication that would likely help. You can't force it—respect for self-determination means allowing people to make decisions you disagree with. But if client is so impaired they can't make informed decisions, you may need to act protectively.

Self-determination doesn't mean abandonment. A client choosing to continue drinking doesn't mean you say "Okay, good luck." You continue providing services, expressing concern, offering alternatives—while respecting their ultimate choice.

Informed consent: You provide services to clients only in context of professional relationship based on valid informed consent. You use clear and understandable language to inform clients of:

- Purpose of services
- Risks related to services
- Limits to services because of requirements of third-party payer
- Relevant costs
- Reasonable alternatives
- Clients' right to refuse or withdraw consent
- Time frame covered by consent

Informed consent isn't just signing a form. It's ongoing conversation ensuring clients understand what's happening, why, and what their options are. You check understanding, not just whether they signed something.

Competence: You provide services only within boundaries of your education, training, license, certification, consultation received, supervised experience, or other relevant professional experience. When new knowledge and skills are needed, you obtain appropriate education and consultation. In emergencies, you may provide services for which you lack full competence, but only to extent necessary and only with appropriate consultation and supervision.

This means saying "I'm not qualified to treat that" even when client needs help and you want to help. It means seeking consultation when you're unsure. It means recognizing your limits protects clients.

Cultural competence and social diversity: You understand culture and its function in human behavior and society, recognizing strengths in all cultures. You have and continue to develop specialized knowledge about cultures of clients you serve. You seek education about nature of social diversity and oppression regarding race, ethnicity, national origin, color, sex, sexual orientation, gender identity or expression, age, marital status, political belief, religion, immigration status, and mental or physical ability.

Cultural competence isn't achieved through one workshop. It's career-long commitment to learning, humility, and self-examination. You recognize your own biases, learn about cultures different from yours, and adapt practice to be culturally responsive.

Conflicts of interest: You avoid conflicts of interest that interfere with exercise of professional discretion and impartial judgment. When unavoidable dual or multiple relationships exist, you take steps to protect clients and are responsible for setting clear, appropriate, and culturally sensitive boundaries.

Example: You work in small town and your hairdresser becomes client. You can't avoid seeing each other in community. You acknowledge the dual relationship, discuss how to manage it (professional boundaries in therapy, normal interaction in community), and monitor for problems.

Privacy and confidentiality: You respect clients' right to privacy and don't solicit private information unless essential to providing services or conducting social work evaluation or research. Once obtained, you protect confidentiality except for compelling professional reasons. General expectation that you'll keep information confidential doesn't apply when disclosure is necessary to prevent serious, foreseeable, imminent harm to client or others or when laws or regulations require disclosure without client consent.

You inform clients to extent possible about disclosure of confidential information and potential consequences before disclosure. You discuss with clients and other interested parties conditions under which information may be disclosed. You don't disclose confidential information in any setting unless privacy can be ensured—you don't discuss clients in hallways, elevators, public places.

Access to records: You provide clients with reasonable access to records concerning them. You limit access to portions of records that could cause serious harm to client, making every effort to discuss rationale for withholding and assist client in dealing with harmful effects. You develop policies consistent with applicable laws and regulations regarding storage, retrieval, and disposal of records.

Sexual relationships: You don't engage in sexual activities or sexual contact with current clients, whether such contact is consensual or forced. You don't engage in sexual activities with clients' relatives or other individuals whom clients maintain close personal relationship when there's risk of exploitation or potential harm. You don't provide clinical services to individuals with whom they've had prior sexual relationship.

This is absolute. No exceptions. No matter how attracted you are. No matter if they initiate. No matter if "it's true love." Sexual relationships with current clients are prohibited. Period.

Sexual relationships with former clients are prohibited for at least two years after termination and even then are strongly discouraged unless social worker can demonstrate extraordinary circumstances showing relationship hasn't been exploitative.

Physical contact: You don't engage in physical contact with clients when there's possibility of psychological harm. You're responsible for setting clear, appropriate, culturally sensitive boundaries.

Appropriate physical contact (handshake, pat on shoulder, hug when culturally appropriate and client-initiated) is acceptable. Sexual or potentially harmful contact is not. When uncertain, err on side of less contact.

Sexual harassment: You don't sexually harass clients. Sexual harassment includes sexual advances, sexual solicitation, requests for sexual favors, and other verbal or physical conduct of sexual nature.

Derogatory language: You don't use derogatory language in communication with or about clients. You use accurate and respectful language.

This includes private conversations with colleagues. Referring to clients with derogatory terms—even when client isn't present—violates respect for dignity and worth. It changes how you see them and how colleagues see them.

Payment for services: You establish and maintain billing practices that accurately reflect nature and extent of services and identify who provided service. You don't accept goods or services from clients as payment for professional services. Bartering may be considered only in limited circumstances when it's essential to provision of services, client requests it, relationship isn't exploitative, and arrangement is in client's best interest.

Accepting gifts requires judgment. Small gifts of nominal value as expression of gratitude may be acceptable. Expensive gifts or gifts creating obligation aren't. Consider cultural context—in some cultures, refusing gifts is deeply offensive.

Interruption of services: You make reasonable efforts to ensure continuity of services in event services are interrupted by factors such as unavailability, relocation, illness, disability, or death. You notify clients promptly and seek transfer, referral, or continuation of services.

Termination of services: You terminate services to clients when services are no longer required or no longer serve clients' needs or interests. You take reasonable steps to avoid abandonment—withdrawing services precipitously except under unusual circumstances, giving due consideration to all factors and making reasonable efforts to arrange continuation of services.

You may terminate services when client no longer needs services, client isn't benefiting from services, client or third-party payer is not paying, you're at risk of harm, or continued services would result in violation of ethical or legal standards. You provide pretermination counseling and suggest appropriate alternatives.

Case Example: Ethical Responsibilities to Clients - Maria's Dilemma

Maria, a social worker at community mental health center, sees David, 28, for depression. After three months of good progress, David reveals he's been having sexual fantasies about Maria. He says he's "falling in love" with her and wants to pursue relationship after therapy ends.

Maria's ethical considerations:

Commitment to clients: Maria's primary responsibility is David's welfare, not her own comfort or convenience. She must address this therapeutically, not just shut it down because it's uncomfortable.

Self-determination: David has right to his feelings, but not right to relationship with Maria. This isn't area for self-determination—ethical standards clearly prohibit sexual relationships with clients.

Informed consent: Maria should have discussed boundaries at treatment outset, but she'll address them now clearly.

Cultural competence: Maria considers whether cultural factors affect David's expression or her interpretation. In some cultures, direct expression of feelings like this is very unusual; in others it's more normative.

Boundaries: Maria must set and maintain clear boundaries. The prohibition on sexual relationships with current clients is absolute.

Maria's response (session):

Maria: "David, I appreciate your honesty in sharing your feelings. That took courage. I want to address this directly. First, I can't have romantic or sexual relationship with you—not now, not after therapy ends. The ethics of my profession prohibit relationships with current clients and strongly discourage them with former clients. More importantly, pursuing relationship would harm you. These feelings are important material for our therapy work, but they can't become actual relationship."

David (hurt, embarrassed): "I shouldn't have said anything."

Maria: "I'm glad you did. Keeping these feelings secret would have interfered with our work. Now we can explore them. Often, strong feelings toward a therapist—what we call transference—reflect patterns from other relationships. Let's explore what these feelings might tell us about your relationship patterns, your needs, your fears."

David: "You're saying my feelings aren't real?"

Maria: "Your feelings are absolutely real. I'm suggesting they might have meanings beyond just 'I'm attracted to my therapist.' They might connect to your longing for connection, your pattern of idealizing people, your desire to be understood and accepted. This is valuable therapeutic material. But understanding them in therapy is very different from acting on them outside therapy."

Maria documents the conversation thoroughly. She consults with her supervisor about managing the situation. She continues working with David therapeutically, addressing the feelings within therapeutic frame, but maintaining clear boundaries. She monitors carefully whether she can continue to help David effectively or whether his feelings make that impossible.

If David can't accept boundaries and continues pursuing relationship, Maria may need to terminate and refer—not as punishment but because effective therapy requires appropriate boundaries. But her first effort is addressing this therapeutically while maintaining ethical standards.

This example demonstrates multiple ethical responsibilities: prioritizing client welfare, maintaining boundaries, using situations therapeutically when possible, seeking consultation, and being willing to terminate if necessary to protect client.

Ethical Responsibilities to Colleagues

You work with other social workers and professionals from other disciplines. These relationships have ethical dimensions requiring attention.

Respect: You treat colleagues with respect and represent accurately their qualifications, views, and obligations. You avoid unwarranted negative criticism, particularly regarding colleagues' competence or attributes such as level of education, experience, or licensure.

Disagreeing with colleague's approach is fine. Respectfully discussing different perspectives is professional. Gossip, personal attacks, and undermining colleagues violates this standard.

Confidentiality: You respect confidential information shared by colleagues in course of professional relationships and transactions. You ensure such information is shared only for professional purposes and only with people clearly concerned with the matter.

Your colleague mentions in case consultation that she's worried about her client's suicidal ideation. You don't share this information socially ("You won't believe what Sarah's dealing with..."). You maintain confidentiality of colleague communications just as you maintain client confidentiality.

Interdisciplinary collaboration: You who are members of interdisciplinary team should participate in and contribute to decisions affecting well-being of clients by drawing on perspectives, values, and experiences of social work profession. Professional and ethical obligations of interdisciplinary team as whole and of individual members should be clearly established.

You represent social work perspective on teams. When team decisions conflict with social work values, you advocate for change while respecting team process. You don't simply defer to other disciplines—you bring social work expertise and values.

Disputes involving colleagues: You don't exploit disputes between colleagues or engage in partisan behavior that undermines colleagues. When you believe colleague has acted unethically, you attempt to resolve issue through discussion with colleague when feasible. If not resolved, you take action through appropriate channels—agency procedures, NASW committees, licensing boards.

Finding out a colleague violated ethics is hard. Your first step is usually direct conversation if safe and appropriate—"I'm concerned about..." Sometimes that's not feasible (colleague has power over you, safety concerns exist). Then you report through proper channels. You don't ignore unethical behavior to avoid conflict.

Consultation: You keep current with emerging knowledge and consult with other professionals when this best serves clients' interests. You seek advice and counsel of colleagues when such consultation is in best interests of clients.

Consultation isn't sign of weakness—it's professional responsibility. The complex case you can't figure out needs fresh perspective. The intervention you're unfamiliar with needs expert input. You seek consultation regularly.

Referral for services: You refer clients to other professionals when others' specialized knowledge or expertise is needed or when you believe they're not being effective. You're knowledgeable about colleagues' qualifications and competencies, making appropriate referrals. If case is transferred, you appropriately share information and follow up to ensure transfer has been properly accomplished.

Sexual relationships with supervisees and students: You don't engage in sexual activities or contact with supervisees, students, trainees, or other colleagues over whom they exercise professional authority.

This is like sexual relationships with clients—absolutely prohibited. The power differential makes consent questionable and exploitation likely.

Sexual harassment: You don't sexually harass supervisees, students, trainees, or colleagues. Sexual harassment includes sexual advances, sexual solicitation, requests for sexual favors, and other verbal or physical conduct of sexual nature.

Impairment of colleagues: When you have direct knowledge of colleague's impairment interfering with practice effectiveness, you consult with that colleague when feasible and assist colleague in taking remedial action. If colleague hasn't taken adequate steps, you take action through appropriate channels.

This is difficult. Your colleague and friend shows up to work smelling like alcohol. Your supervisor seems increasingly erratic and you suspect substance use. A colleague mentions their depression is so severe they can barely function. You don't ignore these situations because they're uncomfortable. You address them—first with colleague if possible, then through supervisory or licensing channels if necessary—because impaired practitioners harm clients.

Incompetence of colleagues: When you have direct knowledge of colleague's incompetence, you consult with that colleague when feasible and assist in taking remedial action. If colleague hasn't taken adequate steps, you take action through appropriate channels.

Incompetence differs from impairment. Colleague lacks necessary skills, practices outside competence, uses discredited or harmful techniques. Again, you address directly when possible, then through appropriate channels.

Unethical conduct of colleagues: You take adequate measures to discourage, prevent, expose, and correct unethical conduct of colleagues. You're knowledgeable about established policies and procedures for handling concerns about colleagues' ethical behavior and are familiar with national, state, and local procedures for handling ethics complaints.

When you know colleague is acting unethically—violating boundaries, exploiting clients, misrepresenting credentials, billing fraudulently—you have responsibility to act. Report through appropriate channels. Ignoring unethical behavior makes you complicit.

Case Example: Ethical Responsibilities to Colleagues - Reporting Impairment

James, a social worker at hospital, increasingly notices that his colleague Linda seems impaired. She arrives late, seems disorganized, and twice he's smelled alcohol on her breath in the afternoon. Yesterday, a nurse mentioned concern that Linda seemed "out of it" when meeting with a patient's family.

James's ethical considerations:

Impairment of colleagues: James has direct knowledge suggesting impairment interfering with practice. He has ethical obligation to address this.

Respect: He should treat Linda with respect while addressing concerns.

Client welfare: Linda's impairment may be harming clients—this is primary concern.

Due process: Linda deserves opportunity to address concerns before formal reporting.

James's actions:

Step 1: Direct conversation (when feasible and safe):

James asks Linda to coffee. "Linda, I'm concerned about you. I've noticed you seem stressed lately—arriving late, seeming overwhelmed. Yesterday the nurse mentioned you seemed unwell when meeting with the Johnson family. I'm worried about you and I'm worried about client care. What's going on?"

Linda could respond several ways:

Scenario A: Linda acknowledges problem:
"You're right. I've been drinking too much. My marriage is falling apart and I'm not coping well. I know I need help."

James's response: "I appreciate your honesty. Let's figure out next steps. Have you considered EAP? Taking medical leave while you get treatment? I'll support you, but we need to ensure clients are safe and you're getting help. What do you think makes sense?"

They develop plan together: Linda contacts EAP, takes leave for treatment, James helps cover her cases temporarily.

Scenario B: Linda denies problem:
"I'm fine. I've been stressed but I'm managing. There's no problem."

James's response: "I hear you, but I remain concerned. I've smelled alcohol on your breath twice at work. The nurse observed you seeming impaired with clients. These aren't minor concerns. I'd like you to address this—talk to our supervisor, access EAP, something. If you don't, I'll need to take it further myself because client safety is at stake."

Linda refuses to acknowledge problem or take action.

Step 2: Report to supervisor:
James documents his observations and conversation with Linda. He meets with their supervisor: "I need to report concerns about Linda's potential impairment affecting client care." He provides specific observations, documentation, and notes about his conversation with Linda.

The supervisor investigates, following agency protocol. This might involve requiring Linda to undergo evaluation, requiring treatment, placing her on leave, or other administrative actions.

Step 3: Report to licensing board if necessary:
If agency doesn't address the issue adequately and Linda continues practicing while impaired, James reports to state licensing board. He doesn't want to harm Linda's career, but client safety comes first.

This situation demonstrates the difficulty of ethical responsibilities to colleagues. James doesn't want to betray Linda or damage their relationship. But his responsibility to clients and profession requires addressing impairment. He follows appropriate steps—direct conversation when possible, then escalating through proper channels—balancing respect for colleague with protection of clients.

Ethical Responsibilities to Practice Settings

You work in organizational contexts—agencies, hospitals, schools, private practices. Your ethical responsibilities extend to these settings.

Supervision and consultation: You provide supervision and consultation only within areas of knowledge and competence. You provide appropriate direction and feedback to supervisees on regular basis. You don't engage in sexual activities with supervisees or students or colleagues over whom you exercise professional authority.

As supervisor, you're responsible for supervisees' work with clients. You ensure they practice competently, ethically, and effectively. You provide regular supervision—not just crisis management. You teach, support, monitor, and evaluate.

Education and training: You function as educators, field instructors, or trainers provide instruction only within areas of knowledge and competence and provide instruction based on most current information and knowledge.

Don't teach what you don't know. If you're training students in MI and you've only read about it but never practiced it, that's inadequate. Your teaching should reflect current best practices, not outdated or discredited approaches.

Performance evaluation: You who have responsibility for evaluating performance of others do so in fair and respectful manner and on basis of clearly stated criteria. You take reasonable steps to ensure evaluations based on assessments made at appropriate intervals that use established measures when available.

Evaluations shouldn't be subjective or personal. They should be based on clear criteria applied fairly. You document performance concerns, provide feedback and opportunity to improve, and use evaluation processes ethically.

Client records: You accurately record information and ensure access to records is limited to people authorized to have access. You take precautions to ensure records are stored appropriately and disposed of properly. Records should include sufficient and timely documentation to facilitate service delivery and ensure continuity.

Sloppy documentation harms clients (information is lost, services aren't coordinated) and exposes you to liability. You document promptly, accurately, and comprehensively. You protect records from unauthorized access.

Billing: You establish and maintain billing practices that accurately reflect nature and extent of services provided. You don't misrepresent services for purpose of obtaining financial gain.

Billing fraud—claiming services you didn't provide, upcoding to higher reimbursement levels, billing for time you didn't work—is unethical and illegal. You bill honestly for services actually provided.

Client transfer: When individual receiving services is transferred to another professional or agency, you carefully consider needs and preferences. You notify clients of options, potential consequences, benefits, and risks of alternative services.

You don't transfer clients for your convenience without considering their needs. When transfer is necessary, you ensure smooth transition with appropriate information sharing (with consent).

Administration: Administrative obligations don't supersede obligations to clients. Administrators allocate resources and make decisions using sound management principles and professional judgment.

When administrators pressure you to see more clients than safe, document inadequate time for supervision, or impose policies harmful to clients, you advocate for change. You don't simply comply with harmful administrative demands because "boss said so."

Continuing education and staff development: Administrators and supervisors provide ongoing educational opportunities for staff. You who work in agencies evaluate performance of staff with respect to degree to which staff maintain and improve practice skills.

Professional development isn't luxury—it's ethical obligation. Agencies should provide supervision, training, and education supporting competent practice. Staff should actively pursue learning.

Commitments to employers: You adhere to commitments made to employers and employing organizations. You don't engage in activities that conflict with employers' interests unless conflict concerns ethical issues and organization's policies violate social work ethics.

You owe loyalty to employers, but not blind loyalty. When employer policies or actions violate ethics—discrimination, exploitation, substandard care—your commitment to social work ethics trumps commitment to employer. You advocate for change through appropriate channels.

Labor-management disputes: During labor-management disputes, you're concerned first and foremost with welfare of clients and should work to ensure clients have access to services. You may engage in organized action, including formation of and participation in labor unions, to improve services to clients and working conditions.

Strike or work action that harms clients is problematic. You balance rights to fair working conditions with responsibilities to clients. When action is necessary, you ensure client care continues.

Case Example: Ethical Responsibilities to Practice Settings - Unsafe Caseloads

Sarah works at community mental health center. Administration announces that due to budget cuts, all clinicians will increase caseloads from 30 to 45 clients. Sarah knows this is unsafe—she can't provide adequate care to 45 clients.

Sarah's ethical considerations:

Competence: Increased caseload will compromise her ability to provide competent care.

Commitment to clients: Primary responsibility is client welfare. This policy harms clients.

Administration: She has obligations to employer, but not when policies violate ethics.

Advocacy: She should advocate for change through appropriate channels.

Sarah's actions:

Step 1: Document concerns:
Sarah writes memo to supervisor detailing how 45-client caseload compromises care:

- Inadequate time per client (20 minutes weekly vs. needed 50 minutes)
- Inability to respond to crises
- Missed warning signs due to limited contact
- Compromised treatment planning and documentation

She includes research on recommended caseload sizes and potential risks to clients.

Step 2: Discuss with supervisor and administration:
Sarah meets with supervisor: "I understand budget pressures, but this caseload size compromises client safety. I've documented specific concerns. Can we explore alternatives—hiring per diem staff, reducing services, prioritizing highest-risk clients?"

If supervisor is receptive, they work on solutions. If not, Sarah escalates to administration.

Step 3: Collective action:
Sarah talks with colleagues. All share concerns. Together, they meet with administration presenting united front with data, specific concerns, and proposed alternatives.

Administration may reconsider, negotiate, or stand firm.

Step 4: External advocacy if necessary:
If internal advocacy fails, Sarah considers:

- Consulting with licensing board about regulatory standards for caseloads
- Contacting NASW chapter for guidance
- Documenting that she informed administration of unsafe conditions
- If truly untenable, seeking other employment

Meanwhile, Sarah manages her caseload ethically:

- She's transparent with clients about limited time
- She prioritizes highest-risk clients
- She refers clients needing more intensive care to other resources
- She documents inadequate time and resources
- She doesn't compromise care quality to see more clients—she acknowledges realistic limits

This example shows ethical responsibilities to employers don't supersede responsibilities to clients. Sarah works within system to advocate for change, but she doesn't silently comply with policies that harm clients. She documents, advocates, and if necessary, takes external action or leaves—but she doesn't compromise ethics just because administration pressures her.

Ethical Responsibilities to the Profession

You represent social work profession to clients, the public, and other professionals. Your behavior reflects on the entire profession.

Integrity of the profession: You work toward maintenance and promotion of high standards of practice. You uphold and advance values, ethics, knowledge, and mission of profession. You protect, enhance, and improve integrity of profession through appropriate study and research, active discussion, and responsible criticism of profession.

When you see profession falling short, you work to improve it. You contribute to knowledge base, participate in professional organizations, mentor students, and advocate for professional standards.

Evaluation and research: You monitor and evaluate policies, implementation of programs, and practice interventions. You promote and facilitate evaluation and research, discuss collected information only for professional purposes and only with people professionally concerned, and ensure anonymous or confidential responses are protected.

You contribute to evidence base. You evaluate whether your interventions work. You participate in research ethically, protecting participants and using findings to improve practice.

Case Example: Ethical Responsibilities to Colleagues - Impaired Colleague

Tom works at a private practice. His colleague Amanda has been acting strangely—arriving late, missing appointments, seeming confused. A client complained that Amanda seemed "not herself" and fell asleep briefly during session. Tom suspects substance use.

Tom's ethical response:

Tom invites Amanda for coffee. "Amanda, I'm concerned. Clients have mentioned you seem tired, you've missed appointments, and yesterday a client said you fell asleep during session. What's going on?"

Amanda breaks down. She's been taking prescription painkillers since back surgery three months ago. What started as legitimate pain management has become addiction. She's taking more than prescribed and it's affecting her work.

Tom responds with compassion but clarity: "I'm glad you told me. You need help, and your clients need protection. Here's what needs to happen: You need to stop seeing clients immediately until you get treatment. Let's contact the EAP today and figure out treatment options. I'll help cover your clients temporarily. But this can't continue—you're impaired and that's harming people."

Amanda agrees. She enters treatment, takes medical leave, and works with licensing board (she reports herself) to ensure appropriate monitoring when she returns to practice. Tom supports her recovery while protecting clients.

If Amanda had refused help, Tom would have reported to licensing board himself. Colleague loyalty doesn't supersede client safety.

Ethical Responsibilities to the Broader Society

Social work's commitment to social justice extends beyond individual clients to society.

Social welfare: You promote general welfare of society, from local to global levels, and development of people, their communities, and environments. You advocate for living conditions conducive to fulfillment of basic human needs and promote social, economic, political, and cultural values and institutions compatible with realization of social justice.

This means policy advocacy, community organizing, political action—not just clinical work. You're advocates for systemic change.

Public participation: You facilitate informed participation by public in shaping social policies and institutions. You engage in social and political action to ensure all people have equal access to resources, employment, services, and opportunities and to ensure meaningful participation in decision-making for all.

Democracy requires informed citizens. You help people participate effectively—registering to vote, understanding issues, accessing decision-makers, organizing for change.

Public emergencies: During emergencies, you provide appropriate professional services to greatest extent possible. Services should be provided without regard to race, ethnicity, nationality, color, sex, sexual orientation, gender identity or expression, age, marital status, political belief, religion, immigration status, or mental or physical ability.

During disasters, pandemics, or crises, you help. You don't discriminate based on who deserves help—you provide services based on need.

Case Example: Broader Social Responsibility - Advocacy

Individual level: Your client Juan, an undocumented immigrant, can't access mental health services due to insurance limitations. You help him find free clinic providing services regardless of immigration status.

Agency level: You notice your agency routinely denies services to undocumented immigrants. You research relevant laws (emergency services must be provided regardless of status), document discriminatory practices, and advocate internally for policy change.

Policy level: You join coalition advocating for state-level policy expanding mental health access regardless of immigration status. You provide testimony about how current policies harm vulnerable populations.

Professional level: You publish article about mental health needs of undocumented immigrants and ethical imperatives to provide care, contributing to profession's knowledge and advocacy.

Each level addresses injustice at different scale. Effective social workers operate at all levels—helping individual clients, changing organizational policies, advocating for legislative change, and contributing to professional knowledge.

Practice Questions

1. The core value "service" means:

A. Social workers charge appropriate fees
B. Primary goal is helping people, service before self-interest
C. Only providing services you enjoy
D. Limiting services to those who can pay

2. Social justice commitment requires:

A. Political neutrality
B. Challenging social injustice on behalf of vulnerable populations
C. Avoiding political topics
D. Only individual treatment

3. Dignity and worth of the person applies:

A. Only to clients you like
B. Only to those who behave well
C. To every person regardless of actions or circumstances
D. Only to those with similar values

4. When values conflict, you:

A. Always prioritize client wishes
B. Engage in ethical reasoning weighing competing considerations
C. Follow agency policy
D. Do what's easiest

5. Clients' interests are primary except when:

A. You disagree with their choices
B. Actions would cause serious, foreseeable, imminent harm
C. It's inconvenient
D. Insurance won't pay

6. Self-determination means:

A. Clients can do whatever they want
B. Respect clients' right to make their own decisions
C. You make decisions for clients
D. Avoiding all influence

7. Informed consent requires:

A. Just getting a signature
B. Clear communication about purpose, risks, costs, alternatives, rights
C. Only explaining at intake
D. Assuming clients understand

8. You should practice only within:

A. What interests you
B. Boundaries of your competence
C. What insurance covers
D. Your comfort zone

9. Cultural competence involves:

A. One training course
B. Career-long learning, humility, and adaptation to diverse clients
C. Treating everyone the same
D. Avoiding cultural topics

10. Conflicts of interest:

A. Should be exploited for maximum benefit
B. Should be avoided; when unavoidable, manage carefully with clear boundaries
C. Don't matter
D. Are always unethical

11. Confidentiality must be broken when:

A. You're curious
B. Necessary to prevent serious, foreseeable, imminent harm
C. Convenient
D. Anyone asks

12. Sexual relationships with current clients are:

A. Acceptable if consensual
B. Absolutely prohibited
C. Okay after termination
D. Fine if you love each other

13. Sexual relationships with former clients:

A. Are prohibited for at least two years and discouraged after
B. Are fine immediately after termination
C. Are encouraged
D. Don't matter

14. When client can't pay, you should:

A. Immediately terminate
B. Consider sliding scale, refer to free services, don't abandon
C. Demand payment
D. Report to collections

15. Bartering for services:

A. Is always acceptable
B. May be considered only when essential, requested by client, not exploitative
C. Should be encouraged
D. Is always prohibited

16. When terminating services, you:

A. Can stop anytime
B. Make reasonable efforts to avoid abandonment and ensure continuity
C. Don't need to explain
D. Just stop showing up

17. You should represent colleagues:

A. Inaccurately to make yourself look better
B. Accurately and avoid unwarranted criticism
C. However benefits you
D. With exaggeration

18. When colleague acts unethically, you:

A. Ignore it
B. Attempt to resolve through discussion, then through appropriate channels
C. Gossip about it
D. Do nothing

19. Consultation with colleagues:

A. Shows weakness
B. Is professional responsibility serving clients' best interests
C. Should be avoided
D. Is only for new practitioners

20. Sexual relationships with supervisees:

A. Are fine if consensual
B. Are absolutely prohibited
C. Are encouraged
D. Don't matter

21. When colleague is impaired, you:

A. Ignore it to preserve friendship
B. Consult with colleague if feasible, then take action through channels
C. Just gossip about it
D. Cover for them

22. Supervisors should provide:

A. Only crisis management
B. Regular supervision within areas of competence
C. No feedback
D. Supervision they're not qualified to provide

23. Performance evaluations should be:

A. Subjective and personal
B. Fair, respectful, based on clearly stated criteria
C. Punitive
D. Based on personal feelings

24. Client records should:

A. Be accessible to everyone
B. Be accurate, timely, protected, with limited access
C. Be vague
D. Include personal opinions

25. Billing practices must:

A. Maximize revenue regardless of accuracy
B. Accurately reflect services provided
C. Include services not rendered
D. Upcode for higher payment

26. When administrative demands conflict with ethics:

A. Always comply
B. Advocate for change, don't compromise client care
C. Quit immediately
D. Ignore both

27. During labor disputes, primary concern is:

A. Your paycheck
B. Client welfare and ensuring access to services
C. Administration's interests
D. Union politics

28. You should contribute to the profession through:

A. Just doing your job
B. Research, discussion, evaluation, responsible criticism
C. Avoiding all involvement
D. Only if paid extra

29. In emergencies, services are provided:

A. Only to those who can pay
B. Without regard to race, religion, status, ability to pay
C. Based on who deserves help
D. Only to certain groups

30. Ethical principles:

A. Always point to one clear answer
B. Sometimes conflict, requiring ethical reasoning
C. Are simple and obvious
D. Don't apply in real situations

31. When client requests you lie to insurance:

A. Comply to maintain relationship
B. Refuse, explain ethical obligation to honesty
C. Do it if client insists
D. Avoid the topic

32. Gifts from clients:

A. Should always be accepted
B. Require judgment considering value, meaning, cultural context
C. Should always be refused
D. Don't matter

33. Physical contact with clients:

A. Is always prohibited
B. Requires careful judgment about appropriateness and potential harm
C. Is always appropriate
D. Doesn't need consideration

34. Derogatory language about clients:

A. Is fine in private
B. Is prohibited in all communication
C. Is acceptable with colleagues
D. Doesn't matter if client doesn't hear

35. Access to records:

A. Can be completely denied
B. Should be provided with reasonable limits if serious harm likely
C. Is never appropriate
D. Requires court order

36. Multiple relationships:

A. Should be pursued
B. When unavoidable, require clear boundaries and protection
C. Are always prohibited
D. Don't need management

37. Competence:

A. Is achieved once in school
B. Requires ongoing development and staying current
C. Isn't necessary
D. Means knowing everything

38. When you lack competence for client's needs:

A. Fake it
B. Refer or obtain training/consultation
C. Hope for the best
D. Try anyway

39. Privacy means:

A. Never asking personal questions
B. Not soliciting information unless essential for services
C. Knowing everything
D. Avoiding all personal topics

40. Cultural adaptation of practice:

A. Treats everyone identically
B. Adapts approaches to be culturally responsive
C. Isn't necessary
D. Is discriminatory

41. Self-determination limits exist when:

A. You disagree
B. Actions pose serious, foreseeable, imminent risk
C. It's inconvenient
D. Family objects

42. Informed consent is:

A. One-time signature
B. Ongoing process ensuring understanding
C. Not necessary
D. Just a formality

43. When colleague lacks competence:

A. Ignore it
B. Consult with colleague, assist remedial action, report if needed
C. Gossip about it
D. Let clients suffer

44. Interdisciplinary collaboration requires:

A. Deferring to other disciplines
B. Contributing social work perspective while respecting team
C. Dominance
D. Avoiding other professionals

45. Sexual harassment includes:

A. Only physical contact
B. Advances, solicitation, favors, verbal or physical conduct
C. Only serious behaviors
D. Nothing specific

46. Professional boundaries:

A. Aren't necessary
B. Protect clients and maintain appropriate professional relationship
C. Only matter in some settings
D. Can be ignored

47. Integrity means:

A. Only being honest when convenient
B. Consistent trustworthy behavior aligned with values
C. Flexibility with truth
D. Self-interest

48. Social welfare promotion involves:

A. Only individual treatment
B. Advocacy from local to global level for basic needs and justice
C. Avoiding politics
D. Clinical work only

49. When services are interrupted:

A. Just stop without explanation
B. Ensure continuity through transfer, referral, or arrangement
C. Don't worry about it
D. Let client figure it out

50. Commitment to clients means:

A. Doing whatever they want
B. Their interests are primary within ethical bounds
C. Your interests first
D. Equal weight to all concerns

51. Dual responsibility exists to:

A. Clients only
B. Clients and broader society
C. Agency and self
D. Profession only

52. Accurate representation of qualifications:

A. Can be exaggerated
B. Must be honest about education, experience, credentials
C. Doesn't matter
D. Should inflate achievements

53. When client relatives request information:

A. Always provide it
B. Only with client consent unless specific exceptions
C. Share freely
D. Avoid all communication

54. Education you provide should be:

A. Based on outdated material
B. Within competence and based on current information
C. About anything
D. Without preparation

55. Conflicts between values:

A. Mean you've failed
B. Require thoughtful weighing of competing ethical considerations
C. Should be avoided
D. Have obvious answers

56. Client transfer should consider:

A. Only your convenience
B. Client needs, preferences, and ensuring smooth transition
C. Only agency needs
D. Financial factors only

57. Professional development:

A. Ends after school
B. Is career-long ethical obligation
C. Is optional
D. Isn't necessary

58. Evaluating research participants:

A. Harm is acceptable
B. Must protect anonymity and confidentiality
C. Doesn't require consent
D. Ignores safety

59. Discrimination in service provision:

A. Is sometimes acceptable
B. Is prohibited based on race, religion, status, orientation, etc.
C. Is fine if you have reasons
D. Doesn't matter

60. When agency policies violate ethics:

A. Always comply
B. Advocate for change through appropriate channels
C. Quit without trying to fix it
D. Ignore ethics

61. Misrepresenting services for financial gain:

A. Is smart business
B. Is unethical and illegal
C. Is acceptable if you need money
D. Doesn't matter

62. Client wishes for unethical action:

A. Must be followed
B. Should be refused with explanation
C. Are binding
D. Override ethics

63. Colleague sexual harassment should be:

A. Ignored
B. Addressed directly or through proper channels
C. Encouraged
D. Kept secret

64. Public participation means:

A. Avoiding politics
B. Facilitating informed participation in policy shaping
C. Making decisions for people
D. Limiting involvement

65. Values of the profession:

A. Are suggestions
B. Guide all professional conduct and decisions
C. Can be ignored
D. Apply only sometimes

66. Emergency services:

A. Can be denied based on ability to pay
B. Should be provided to greatest extent possible without discrimination
C. Are only for some people
D. Require insurance

67. When colleague competence is questioned:

A. Gossip about them
B. Follow due process - discuss, assist, report if needed
C. Do nothing
D. Publicly criticize

68. Importance of relationships means:

A. Being friends with clients
B. Recognizing relationships as vehicles for change
C. Avoiding all boundaries
D. Only techniques matter

69. Responsible criticism of profession:

A. Should be avoided
B. Is part of advancing and improving profession
C. Is always negative
D. Isn't allowed

70. Documentation of services:

A. Can be vague or false
B. Must be accurate, timely, and comprehensive
C. Isn't important
D. Is optional

71. Labor organizing:

A. Is prohibited
B. Is permitted to improve services and conditions
C. Harms clients always
D. Isn't professional

72. Colleague confidences:

A. Can be shared socially
B. Must be maintained for professional purposes only
C. Are gossip material
D. Don't matter

73. Evaluation of programs:

A. Isn't necessary
B. Is ethical responsibility to ensure effectiveness
C. Wastes time
D. Harms clients

74. Former clients:

A. Can immediately become friends
B. Require continued boundaries and careful consideration
C. Don't need boundaries
D. Are fair game

75. Core values:

A. Change with situations
B. Are foundational commitments defining social work
C. Are optional
D. Apply only in clinical work

Answer Key with Detailed Explanations

1. B. Primary goal is helping people, service before self-interest
The core value "service" means social workers' primary goal is helping people in need and addressing social problems, elevating service above self-interest. This doesn't mean working for free or ignoring your own needs, but it means that in moment-to-moment practice, you ask "What serves the client best?" not "What's easiest or most convenient for me?" Service is the foundational commitment of the profession.

2. B. Challenging social injustice on behalf of vulnerable populations
Social justice commitment requires actively challenging social injustice, pursuing change particularly with and on behalf of vulnerable and oppressed individuals and groups. Social workers are not politically neutral—the profession explicitly commits to social justice. This includes addressing poverty, discrimination, and oppression at multiple levels from individual advocacy to policy change.

3. C. To every person regardless of actions or circumstances
Dignity and worth of the person applies to every person regardless of their actions, beliefs, or circumstances. Even people who've committed terrible acts, who hold values you oppose, or who are difficult and rejecting help deserve respect for their inherent humanity. Dignity isn't earned through good behavior—it's inherent to being human.

4. B. Engage in ethical reasoning weighing competing considerations
When values conflict (which they often do), you engage in ethical reasoning—thoughtfully weighing competing ethical considerations. There isn't always one obviously right answer. Service to client might conflict with broader social responsibility. Self-determination might conflict with protection from harm. You think through the dilemma systematically, considering which values are most salient and what action best aligns with professional ethics.

5. B. Actions would cause serious, foreseeable, imminent harm
Clients' interests are primary except when those interests would result in serious, foreseeable, imminent harm to themselves or others. For example, client confidentiality generally prevails, but you breach confidentiality to prevent imminent harm. Client self-determination generally prevails, but you may limit it when they pose serious danger. The key is "serious, foreseeable, imminent"—not just any potential harm.

6. B. Respect clients' right to make their own decisions
Self-determination means respecting and promoting clients' right to make their own decisions, even when you disagree with those decisions. It's not abandonment (you continue providing services and expressing concern), but it's recognizing client autonomy. Limits exist only when actions pose serious, foreseeable, imminent risk to self or others, or when client is so impaired they can't make informed decisions.

7. B. Clear communication about purpose, risks, costs, alternatives, rights
Informed consent requires clear, understandable communication about: purpose of services, risks, limitations due to third-party payers, costs, reasonable alternatives, right to refuse or withdraw consent, and timeframe. It's not just getting a signature—it's ongoing conversation ensuring clients understand what's happening and what their options are. You check understanding, not just whether they signed something.

8. B. Boundaries of your competence
You should practice only within boundaries of your education, training, licensure, certification, consultation, supervised experience, or other relevant professional experience. This means saying "I'm not qualified" even when client needs help and you want to help. It means seeking consultation when unsure. Practicing beyond competence harms clients and violates ethics.

9. B. Career-long learning, humility, and adaptation to diverse clients
Cultural competence isn't achieved through one training—it's career-long commitment to learning, humility, self-examination, and adapting practice to be culturally responsive. You recognize your own biases, learn about cultures different from yours, understand how culture affects behavior and well-being, and adapt interventions to be culturally appropriate. It's ongoing process, not destination.

10. B. Should be avoided; when unavoidable, manage carefully with clear boundaries
Conflicts of interest should be avoided when possible. When unavoidable (small communities, complex systems), you take steps to protect clients and are responsible for setting clear, appropriate, culturally sensitive boundaries. You acknowledge the conflict, discuss how to manage it, monitor for problems, and always prioritize client welfare over your own interests.

11. B. Necessary to prevent serious, foreseeable, imminent harm
Confidentiality must be broken when disclosure is necessary to prevent serious, foreseeable, imminent harm to client or others, or when laws require disclosure. The general expectation of confidentiality doesn't apply in these circumstances. You inform clients to the extent possible about disclosure and potential consequences before disclosing. The key criteria are "serious, foreseeable, imminent"—not minor concerns or vague possibilities.

12. B. Absolutely prohibited
Sexual relationships with current clients are absolutely prohibited regardless of consent, mutual attraction, or belief that "it's true love." The prohibition is unequivocal with no exceptions. The power differential makes genuine consent questionable, and such relationships cause profound harm. This is one of the clearest, most absolute ethical prohibitions.

13. A. Are prohibited for at least two years and discouraged after
Sexual relationships with former clients are prohibited for at least two years following termination and even then are strongly discouraged. After two years, such relationships are only acceptable if social worker can demonstrate extraordinary circumstances showing relationship hasn't been and won't be exploitative. The burden of proof is entirely on the social worker.

14. B. Consider sliding scale, refer to free services, don't abandon
When clients can't pay, you don't immediately terminate. You consider sliding scale fees, payment plans, referral to free or low-cost services, or pro bono work if feasible. You make reasonable efforts to ensure continuity of care and don't abandon clients due to inability to pay. Financial hardship shouldn't result in loss of services when alternatives exist.

15. B. May be considered only when essential, requested by client, not exploitative
Bartering may be considered only in limited circumstances when: it's essential to provision of services, client requests it, relationship isn't exploitative, and arrangement is in client's best interest. It's not encouraged due to potential boundary problems and exploitation risks. Cultural context matters—in some communities bartering is normative and refusing may be offensive.

16. B. Make reasonable efforts to avoid abandonment and ensure continuity
When terminating services, you make reasonable efforts to avoid abandonment—withdrawing services precipitously without consideration of client needs. You provide pretermination counseling, suggest alternatives, arrange transfer or referral when appropriate, and ensure continuity of care. Termination should be planned and consider client welfare, not just your convenience.

17. B. Accurately and avoid unwarranted criticism
You should represent colleagues accurately regarding their qualifications, views, and obligations, and avoid unwarranted negative criticism, particularly regarding competence or attributes like education or experience. Disagreeing professionally is acceptable. Spreading false information, gossip, or personal attacks violates this standard. Respect for colleagues maintains professional integrity.

18. B. Attempt to resolve through discussion, then through appropriate channels
When you believe a colleague has acted unethically, you attempt to resolve through discussion with the colleague when feasible. If not resolved, you take action through appropriate channels—agency procedures, NASW committees, licensing boards. You don't ignore unethical behavior to avoid conflict, and you don't gossip. You address it professionally through proper mechanisms.

19. B. Is professional responsibility serving clients' best interests
Consultation with colleagues is professional responsibility, not sign of weakness. You seek consultation when it best serves clients' interests—complex cases, unfamiliar interventions, ethical

dilemmas, when you're stuck. Fresh perspective, expert input, and collaborative problem-solving improve client care. Consultation is expected throughout your career, not just for new practitioners.

20. B. Are absolutely prohibited
Sexual relationships with supervisees, students, trainees, or other colleagues over whom you exercise professional authority are absolutely prohibited. The power differential makes consent questionable and exploitation likely. This is similar to prohibition on sexual relationships with clients—the power imbalance makes ethical relationships impossible.

21. B. Consult with colleague if feasible, then take action through channels
When you have direct knowledge of colleague impairment interfering with practice, you consult with that colleague when feasible and assist them in taking remedial action. If colleague hasn't taken adequate steps, you take action through appropriate channels established by employers, agencies, NASW, licensing boards, or other professional organizations. Impaired practitioners harm clients—protection of clients supersedes loyalty to colleagues.

22. B. Regular supervision within areas of competence
Supervisors should provide supervision and consultation only within areas of their knowledge and competence, and provide appropriate direction and feedback regularly, not just during crises. Supervision is ongoing teaching, support, monitoring, and evaluation. Supervisors are responsible for supervisees' work with clients and must ensure competent, ethical practice.

23. B. Fair, respectful, based on clearly stated criteria
Performance evaluations should be fair and respectful, based on clearly stated criteria, not subjective or personal. Use established measures when available, make assessments at appropriate intervals, document concerns, provide feedback and opportunity to improve. Evaluations shouldn't be punitive or based on personal feelings—they should be objective and professional.

24. B. Be accurate, timely, protected, with limited access
Client records should be accurate, include sufficient and timely documentation, be protected from unauthorized access, and be accessible only to those authorized. You document promptly, comprehensively, and factually. You store records appropriately and dispose of them properly. Sloppy documentation harms clients and creates liability.

25. B. Accurately reflect services provided
Billing practices must accurately reflect the nature and extent of services provided and identify who provided services. You don't misrepresent services, claim services not rendered, upcode to higher reimbursement, or engage in any form of billing fraud. Honest billing is both ethical obligation and legal requirement.

26. B. Advocate for change, don't compromise client care
When administrative demands conflict with ethical obligations, administrative obligations don't supersede obligations to clients. You advocate for change through appropriate channels, but you don't compromise client care simply because administration pressures you. If truly untenable, you may need to seek other employment, but you don't silently comply with harmful policies.

27. B. Client welfare and ensuring access to services
During labor-management disputes, social workers are concerned first and foremost with welfare of clients and work to ensure clients have access to services. You may engage in organized action including union participation to improve services and working conditions, but client welfare remains primary concern. Strike or work action shouldn't harm clients.

28. B. Research, discussion, evaluation, responsible criticism
You should contribute to the profession through study and research, active discussion, responsible criticism, and efforts to maintain and promote high standards. Contributing to knowledge base, participating in professional organizations, mentoring students, evaluating interventions, and advocating for professional standards all fulfill this responsibility.

29. B. Without regard to race, religion, status, ability to pay
In emergencies, social workers provide appropriate professional services to greatest extent possible without regard to race, ethnicity, nationality, color, sex, sexual orientation, gender identity, age, marital status, political belief, religion, immigration status, mental or physical ability, or ability to pay. Emergency services are based on need, not on who deserves help or can pay.

30. B. Sometimes conflict, requiring ethical reasoning
Ethical principles sometimes conflict with each other, requiring thoughtful ethical reasoning. Service to client might conflict with broader social responsibility. Self-determination might conflict with protection from harm. When principles conflict, there isn't always one obviously correct answer—you must weigh competing considerations thoughtfully using ethical decision-making frameworks.

31. B. Refuse, explain ethical obligation to honesty
When a client requests you lie to insurance or engage in billing fraud, you refuse and explain your ethical obligation to honesty and integrity. You explore why client is making this request (financial hardship?) and problem-solve legitimate alternatives (sliding scale, payment plans, appeal for coverage). You maintain professional integrity while being compassionate about client's circumstances.

32. B. Require judgment considering value, meaning, cultural context
Gifts from clients require professional judgment considering value, meaning, and cultural context. Small gifts of nominal value as expression of gratitude may be acceptable. Expensive gifts or gifts creating obligation aren't. Cultural context matters—in some cultures refusing gifts is deeply offensive. You consider whether accepting creates boundary problems or exploitation risk.

33. B. Requires careful judgment about appropriateness and potential harm
Physical contact with clients requires careful judgment about appropriateness and potential for psychological harm. You're responsible for setting clear, culturally sensitive boundaries. Appropriate contact (handshake, brief hug when client-initiated and culturally appropriate) may be acceptable. Sexual or potentially harmful contact is prohibited. When uncertain, err on side of less contact.

34. B. Is prohibited in all communication
Derogatory language about clients is prohibited in all communication—with or about clients, even in private conversations with colleagues. Using derogatory terms violates respect for dignity and worth,

changes how you and others see clients, and degrades professional culture. Accurate, respectful language is required in all contexts.

35. B. Should be provided with reasonable limits if serious harm likely
You provide clients reasonable access to records concerning them. You may limit access to portions that could cause serious harm, making every effort to discuss rationale and assist client with harmful effects. Complete denial is generally not appropriate—reasonable access with protective limitations when necessary is the standard.

36. B. When unavoidable, require clear boundaries and protection
Multiple relationships should be avoided when possible. When unavoidable (small communities, complex systems), you take steps to protect clients and are responsible for setting clear, appropriate, culturally sensitive boundaries. You acknowledge the situation, discuss management strategies, monitor carefully, and always prioritize client welfare.

37. B. Requires ongoing development and staying current
Competence is not achieved once in school—it requires ongoing development and staying current with emerging knowledge and research. You continually strive to increase professional knowledge and skills and apply them in practice. You participate in continuing education, seek supervision and consultation, and maintain awareness of new developments in your practice areas.

38. B. Refer or obtain training/consultation
When you lack competence for a client's needs, you refer to someone qualified or obtain appropriate training, supervision, or consultation before proceeding. You don't fake competence, hope for the best, or try anyway. In emergencies, you may provide services for which you lack full competence but only to extent necessary and with appropriate consultation.

39. B. Not soliciting information unless essential for services
Privacy means respecting clients' right to privacy and not soliciting private information unless essential to providing services or conducting social work evaluation or research. You don't probe out of curiosity. Once obtained, you protect confidential information. You only gather information that serves legitimate professional purposes.

40. B. Adapts approaches to be culturally responsive
Cultural adaptation means adapting approaches to be culturally responsive, not treating everyone identically regardless of culture. You recognize cultural strengths, understand how culture affects presentation and treatment, and modify interventions to fit cultural context. Treating everyone the same ignores meaningful cultural differences and reduces effectiveness.

41. B. Actions pose serious, foreseeable, imminent risk
Self-determination may be limited only when client's actions pose serious, foreseeable, imminent risk to themselves or others. You don't limit self-determination because you disagree with choices, because it's inconvenient, or because family objects. The threshold is high—serious, foreseeable, imminent risk, not just potential concerns or different values.

42. B. Ongoing process ensuring understanding
Informed consent is an ongoing process of ensuring client understanding, not a one-time signature.

You use clear language, check comprehension, update information as circumstances change, and ensure clients understand purpose, risks, alternatives, and rights throughout treatment. It's active communication, not just a formality.

43. B. Consult with colleague, assist remedial action, report if needed
When you have direct knowledge of colleague incompetence, you consult with colleague when feasible and assist in taking remedial action—additional training, supervision, limiting practice scope. If colleague hasn't taken adequate steps, you take action through appropriate channels. You don't ignore incompetence or just gossip—you address it professionally to protect clients.

44. B. Contributing social work perspective while respecting team
Interdisciplinary collaboration requires participating and contributing to decisions by drawing on social work perspectives, values, and experiences. You don't simply defer to other disciplines or dominate. You bring social work expertise, represent social work values, advocate when team decisions conflict with those values, while respecting team process and other disciplines' expertise.

45. B. Advances, solicitation, favors, verbal or physical conduct
Sexual harassment includes sexual advances, sexual solicitation, requests for sexual favors, and other verbal or physical conduct of sexual nature. It's not limited to physical contact or only the most serious behaviors. Unwelcome sexual comments, jokes, looks, or suggestions all constitute harassment. Both supervisors and colleagues can commit and experience sexual harassment.

46. B. Protect clients and maintain appropriate professional relationship
Professional boundaries protect clients and maintain appropriate professional relationship. They distinguish professional relationships from social or romantic ones, preventing exploitation and maintaining the therapeutic frame. Boundaries aren't arbitrary rules—they serve essential protective function ensuring professional relationships serve clients' needs, not workers' needs.

47. B. Consistent trustworthy behavior aligned with values
Integrity means behaving in trustworthy manner consistently aligned with profession's mission, values, and ethical standards. You're honest, follow through on commitments, acknowledge mistakes, and do the right thing even when no one's watching or when dishonesty would be easier. Your actions match your words and professional values.

48. B. Advocacy from local to global level for basic needs and justice
Social welfare promotion involves advocating from local to global levels for development of people, communities, and environments. You advocate for living conditions conducive to fulfillment of basic human needs and for social, economic, political, and cultural values compatible with social justice. This includes but extends far beyond individual treatment.

49. B. Ensure continuity through transfer, referral, or arrangement
When services are interrupted by unavailability, relocation, illness, disability, or death, you make reasonable efforts to ensure continuity of services. You notify clients promptly, discuss options, and seek transfer, referral, or continuation arrangements. You don't just stop without explanation or leave clients without resources or alternative services.

50. B. Their interests are primary within ethical bounds
Commitment to clients means their interests are primary, but not absolute. You have dual responsibility to clients and broader society. When these conflict, clients' interests generally prevail except when this would result in serious, foreseeable, imminent harm or violate laws or ethical standards. Client welfare is central concern guiding practice.

51. B. Clients and broader society
Social workers have dual responsibility to clients and to broader society. You serve individual clients while also promoting general welfare and social justice. When these responsibilities conflict, clients' interests generally prevail unless conflict would result in serious harm or legal/ethical violations. You balance individual and collective responsibilities.

52. B. Must be honest about education, experience, credentials
You must accurately represent your qualifications, including education, experience, credentials, and competencies. You don't exaggerate, claim credentials you don't have, or misrepresent your expertise. Accurate representation allows clients, employers, and colleagues to make informed decisions about your capabilities and appropriate role.

53. B. Only with client consent unless specific exceptions

When client relatives request information, you provide it only with client consent unless specific legal or ethical exceptions apply (danger to self or others, mandated reporting, court order). Family relationships don't automatically grant access to confidential information. The client controls their information unless circumstances require disclosure without consent.

54. B. Within competence and based on current information
Education and training you provide should be within your areas of knowledge and competence and based on most current information and knowledge available. Don't teach what you don't know or use outdated material. Your instruction should reflect current best practices, recent research, and evidence-based approaches. Teaching requires same competence standards as practice.

55. B. Require thoughtful weighing of competing ethical considerations
Conflicts between values don't mean you've failed or that ethics are useless—they require thoughtful weighing of competing ethical considerations through systematic ethical decision-making. You identify which values are at stake, consider which are most salient to the situation, examine possible actions and their consequences, and make reasoned decisions. Ethical dilemmas are inherent to the work.

56. B. Client needs, preferences, and ensuring smooth transition
Client transfer should carefully consider client needs and preferences, not just your convenience or agency needs. You notify clients of options, explain potential consequences and benefits of alternatives, obtain consent for information sharing, and ensure smooth transition with appropriate documentation. Transfer serves client welfare, not administrative ease.

57. B. Is career-long ethical obligation
Professional development doesn't end after school—it's a career-long ethical obligation. You

continually strive to increase professional knowledge and skills through continuing education, supervision, consultation, reading professional literature, attending trainings, and applying new learning to practice. Maintaining competence requires ongoing active learning.

58. B. Must protect anonymity and confidentiality
When evaluating or conducting research with participants, you must protect their anonymity or confidentiality. You obtain informed consent, ensure responses are protected, discuss collected information only for professional purposes and only with people professionally concerned. Research ethics require the same protections as clinical practice plus additional safeguards specific to research.

59. B. Is prohibited based on race, religion, status, orientation, etc.
Discrimination in service provision is prohibited based on race, ethnicity, national origin, color, sex, sexual orientation, gender identity or expression, age, marital status, political belief, religion, immigration status, or mental or physical ability. Services are provided based on need and professional assessment, not on personal biases or prejudices about who deserves help.

60. B. Advocate for change through appropriate channels
When agency policies violate ethical standards, you don't just comply or quit without trying to fix the problem. You advocate for change through appropriate channels—documenting concerns, discussing with supervisors and administration, using agency grievance procedures, consulting with licensing boards or professional organizations. You work within systems to change harmful policies.

61. B. Is unethical and illegal
Misrepresenting services for financial gain—billing fraud, claiming services not provided, upcoding—is both unethical and illegal. It violates integrity, harms clients, defrauds payers, and can result in criminal prosecution. Honest billing reflecting services actually provided is fundamental professional responsibility regardless of financial pressures.

62. B. Should be refused with explanation
When clients wish you to take unethical action (lying to insurance, violating confidentiality inappropriately, providing services outside your competence), you refuse and explain your ethical obligations. You're compassionate about why they're asking (often financial hardship or desperation) and problem-solve legitimate alternatives, but you don't compromise professional ethics to satisfy client wishes.

63. B. Addressed directly or through proper channels
Colleague sexual harassment should be addressed directly when safe and appropriate, or through proper channels—supervisors, HR, NASW ethics committees, licensing boards. You don't ignore, encourage, or keep secret. Sexual harassment creates hostile work environment, harms those experiencing it, and violates professional standards. It must be addressed.

64. B. Facilitating informed participation in policy shaping
Public participation means facilitating informed participation by the public in shaping social policies and institutions. You help people understand issues, access decision-makers, register to vote, organize for change, and participate meaningfully in democratic processes. You don't make decisions for people or limit their involvement—you support and enhance their participation.

65. B. Guide all professional conduct and decisions
Values of the profession—service, social justice, dignity and worth, importance of relationships, integrity, competence—guide all professional conduct and decisions. They're not suggestions or optional—they're foundational commitments defining what social work is. Your practice should consistently align with these values.

66. B. Should be provided to greatest extent possible without discrimination
Emergency services should be provided to greatest extent possible without discrimination based on race, ethnicity, nationality, color, sex, sexual orientation, gender identity, age, marital status, political belief, religion, immigration status, mental or physical ability, or ability to pay. During emergencies, you help based on need, not on who you think deserves help or who can pay.

67. B. Follow due process - discuss, assist, report if needed
When colleague competence is questioned, you follow due process: discuss concerns with colleague when feasible, assist them in taking remedial action (additional training, supervision, limiting scope), and if they don't take adequate steps, report through appropriate channels. You don't gossip, publicly criticize, or ignore—you address professionally through proper mechanisms.

68. B. Recognizing relationships as vehicles for change
Importance of human relationships means recognizing that relationships between and among people are important vehicles for change. The therapeutic relationship, family relationships, community connections—relationships are where healing and growth happen. This value emphasizes that you're not just a technician applying techniques but a person in relationship facilitating change through connection.

69. B. Is part of advancing and improving profession
Responsible criticism of the profession is part of advancing and improving it, not disloyalty. When you see the profession falling short, you engage in thoughtful critique through professional channels—journals, conferences, committees. Responsible criticism is constructive, evidence-based, and aimed at improvement. Protecting the profession means making it better, not defending its flaws.

70. B. Must be accurate, timely, and comprehensive
Documentation of services must be accurate (factual, truthful), timely (recorded promptly while information is fresh), and comprehensive (sufficient detail for continuity and quality care). You don't falsify records, document late with unreliable recall, or provide vague inadequate documentation. Proper documentation protects clients, supports quality care, and meets legal and ethical standards.

71. B. Is permitted to improve services and conditions
Labor organizing including formation of and participation in labor unions is permitted to improve services to clients and working conditions. Workers' rights and client welfare aren't opposed—adequate working conditions support quality client care. You can engage in collective action while maintaining primary concern for client welfare.

72. B. Must be maintained for professional purposes only
Information shared by colleagues in professional relationships and transactions should be respected as confidential and shared only for professional purposes and only with people clearly concerned with

the matter. Your colleague's case consultation about a difficult client isn't social gossip material. You maintain confidentiality of professional communications as you maintain client confidentiality.

73. B. Is ethical responsibility to ensure effectiveness
Evaluation of programs, interventions, and policies is ethical responsibility to ensure effectiveness and accountability. You monitor whether your interventions work, contribute to program evaluation, and use findings to improve practice. Evaluation isn't optional extra—it's how you know whether you're actually helping people and how you improve services.

74. B. Require continued boundaries and careful consideration
Former clients still require continued boundaries and careful consideration of any relationship changes. You can't immediately become friends or social contacts after termination. The professional relationship creates lasting power differential and vulnerability. Any relationship changes require careful consideration of exploitation risk and whether it serves former client's interests.

75. B. Are foundational commitments defining social work
Core values—service, social justice, dignity and worth, importance of relationships, integrity, competence—are foundational commitments that define what social work is. They're not changeable with situations or optional based on setting. They apply across all contexts—clinical, macro, research, administration. These values distinguish social work from other professions and guide all professional activities.

Understanding Ethics in Action

Ethics isn't abstract philosophy—it's daily practice. Every decision about boundaries, every choice about how much to disclose, every moment of advocating or staying silent has ethical dimensions. The Code provides framework, but you provide judgment.

Some situations are clear. Sexual relationships with current clients? Prohibited. Billing fraud? Prohibited. Discrimination? Prohibited. But many situations fall in gray areas. A client who's a casual acquaintance before becoming a client. A gift that's culturally expected but feels excessive. Continuing to work with someone when you're not helping but termination feels like abandonment.

In these gray areas, the Code doesn't provide simple answers. It provides values to consider, principles to apply, and standards to meet. You engage in ethical decision-making: identify the ethical issues, determine which values and principles apply, examine possible courses of action, consult with colleagues or supervisors, make a decision, and reflect on the outcome.

You'll make mistakes. Everyone does. Ethical practice isn't perfection—it's commitment to doing right, recognizing when you fall short, correcting course, and learning. When you make ethical errors, you acknowledge them, repair harm when possible, and use the experience to improve.

The Code protects clients. It protects you by providing clear guidelines. It protects the profession by maintaining standards. But ultimately, ethics is about integrity—being the professional you'd want for yourself or your loved ones. That's the standard worth pursuing.

Essential Ethical Understanding

- Core values (service, social justice, dignity and worth, relationships, integrity, competence) are foundational commitments defining social work
- Clients' interests are primary except when actions would cause serious, foreseeable, imminent harm to self or others
- Self-determination must be respected even when you disagree, limited only by serious, foreseeable, imminent risk
- Informed consent is ongoing process ensuring clear understanding of purpose, risks, costs, alternatives, and rights
- Practice only within boundaries of your competence; seek training, supervision, or refer when you lack needed expertise
- Cultural competence requires career-long learning, humility, self-examination, and adaptation to diverse clients
- Confidentiality is fundamental right broken only for serious, foreseeable, imminent harm or legal requirements
- Sexual relationships with current clients are absolutely prohibited; with former clients prohibited for two years and discouraged after
- Professional boundaries including appropriate physical contact, gifts, and multiple relationships require careful judgment
- When colleagues are impaired or act unethically, address directly when feasible then through appropriate channels
- Billing must accurately reflect services provided; fraud is unethical and illegal regardless of financial pressures
- When administrative demands conflict with ethics, advocate for change through proper channels without compromising client care
- Professional development and maintaining current knowledge are career-long ethical obligations, not one-time achievements
- Social justice work at individual, organizational, and policy levels is core professional commitment, not optional activity
- Ethical dilemmas involving conflicting values require systematic reasoning weighing competing considerations, not simple rule application

Chapter 14: Confidentiality and Privacy

Here's what they don't tell you clearly enough in school: confidentiality is both simpler and more complex than it seems. The simple part—you keep client information private. The complex part—everything else. When do you break confidentiality? How do you protect information in the digital age? What do you tell minors about privacy? How do you balance confidentiality with coordination of care?

Confidentiality isn't just legal requirement—it's foundation of trust. Clients tell you their deepest secrets, their shameful behaviors, their frightening thoughts. They share what they've never told anyone. That trust is precious and fragile. One breach can destroy it instantly.

But confidentiality isn't absolute. Sometimes you must break it to protect someone. Sometimes law requires disclosure. Sometimes sharing information helps clients get better care. Knowing when to maintain confidentiality and when to breach it is crucial clinical skill requiring judgment, knowledge of laws, and ethical reasoning.

You'll face situations where confidentiality obligations conflict with other values. A child tells you their parent hit them—you must report. A client mentions casually they've been using their dead parent's social security number—do you report? A client's partner calls demanding to know what was discussed in session—what do you say? These aren't hypothetical—they're Tuesday afternoon in clinical practice.

HIPAA Regulations

The Health Insurance Portability and Accountability Act (HIPAA) sets federal standards for protecting health information. If you work in healthcare setting or bill insurance, you're likely a "covered entity" required to comply with HIPAA. Even if you're not technically covered, HIPAA represents best practices for protecting client information.

Protected Health Information (PHI) is individually identifiable health information transmitted or maintained in any form or medium. This includes:

Demographic information: Name, address, birth date, Social Security number, medical record numbers, account numbers, email addresses, IP addresses, photographs, biometric identifiers.

Health information: Diagnoses, treatment information, medications, lab results, mental health notes, substance use history—anything related to past, present, or future physical or mental health or payment for care.

PHI must be protected whether it's written, electronic, or spoken. You can't leave records visible on your desk. You can't discuss clients where others might overhear. You can't send unencrypted emails containing PHI. You can't access records you don't need for legitimate work purposes.

The Privacy Rule establishes standards for how PHI can be used and disclosed:

Permitted uses without authorization:

Treatment: Sharing information with other providers involved in care. You can send records to client's psychiatrist, consult with client's primary care physician, or coordinate with their case manager—if they're providing treatment.

Payment: Using and disclosing information to obtain payment for services. You can submit claims to insurance, provide documentation for reimbursement, or discuss treatment with utilization reviewers.

Healthcare operations: Using information for quality improvement, training, credentialing, compliance. You can use de-identified information for program evaluation or include cases (with identifiers removed) in supervision.

Required disclosures:

To the individual: Clients have right to access their PHI. You must provide access with limited exceptions (likely to cause harm, compiled for legal proceedings, certain research situations).

To HHS for compliance review: Department of Health and Human Services can audit compliance. You must provide requested information.

Other permitted disclosures without authorization:

Public health activities: Reporting communicable diseases, vaccine reactions, FDA-regulated products problems, abuse or neglect.

Judicial and administrative proceedings: Court orders, subpoenas (with certain limitations), lawsuits involving client.

Law enforcement: Crimes on premises, emergencies, gunshot wounds, suspicious deaths.

To prevent serious threat: Disclosures to prevent or lessen serious and imminent threat to health or safety of person or public.

All other uses and disclosures require client authorization. You can't share information with family, friends, employers, schools, or anyone else without written authorization unless it falls under permitted or required uses.

Authorization must include:

- Description of information to be used or disclosed
- Who may use or disclose the information
- Who will receive the information
- Purpose of disclosure
- Expiration date or event

- Right to revoke authorization
- Potential for redisclosure by recipient
- Signature and date

Authorizations must be written in plain language clients can understand. Clients can revoke authorization at any time in writing.

Psychotherapy notes have special protection. These are notes documenting or analyzing conversation during private counseling session, kept separate from medical record. They don't include medication monitoring, session start and end times, diagnosis, treatment modality, or symptoms—those go in regular medical record.

Psychotherapy notes can be disclosed only with specific authorization for those notes or in limited circumstances (your own supervision, defending yourself in legal proceeding, preventing serious imminent threat, coroner investigation, HHS oversight).

Most settings don't maintain psychotherapy notes as defined by HIPAA because requirements are strict. Regular session documentation goes in medical record and can be disclosed for treatment, payment, and operations.

Minimum necessary standard: When using or disclosing PHI, use or disclose only minimum amount necessary to accomplish purpose. When sending records to another provider, you might send only recent treatment summary rather than entire file unless full file is necessary.

Exception: Minimum necessary doesn't apply to treatment disclosures. Providers can share whatever they determine necessary for treatment.

The Security Rule establishes standards for protecting electronic PHI:

Administrative safeguards: Security management processes, assigned security responsibility, workforce training, access management, security incident procedures.

Physical safeguards: Facility access controls, workstation and device security, media controls (disposal and reuse).

Technical safeguards: Access controls (unique user IDs, passwords), audit controls (tracking access), integrity controls (preventing unauthorized alterations), transmission security (encryption).

Practical implications:

Computers: Password-protected, auto-logout after period of inactivity, encrypted hard drives, secure disposal when discarded.

Emails: Use encrypted email for PHI. Don't send PHI via unsecured email. If you must use regular email, get client consent and include warning about lack of security.

Faxes: Cover sheet indicating confidential information, verify recipient fax number, fax machines in secure locations.

Phones: Don't leave detailed voicemails with PHI. "This is Maria from the clinic" is safer than "This is Maria calling about your depression medication."

Records storage: Locked file cabinets for paper records, restricted access to record rooms, secure cloud storage meeting HIPAA requirements.

Violations and penalties can be severe:

Tier 1 (unknowing violation): Up to $100 per violation, max $25,000 per year for identical violations.

Tier 2 (reasonable cause): $1,000-$50,000 per violation, max $100,000 per year.

Tier 3 (willful neglect, corrected): $10,000-$50,000 per violation, max $250,000 per year.

Tier 4 (willful neglect, not corrected): At least $50,000 per violation, max $1.5 million per year.

Criminal penalties for knowingly obtaining or disclosing PHI: fines up to $250,000 and imprisonment up to 10 years.

But penalties aren't the main concern. The main concern is trust. Violating confidentiality breaks trust with individual client and makes all clients less willing to share honestly.

Case Example: HIPAA Compliance - Dr. Chen's Practice

Dr. Chen, licensed clinical social worker in private practice, faces several HIPAA situations:

Situation 1: Client's partner calls

Maria's partner calls: "I'm worried about her. She seems depressed. What did you talk about in session yesterday?"

Proper response: "I can't confirm or deny whether Maria is my client without her written authorization. If she is someone I'm seeing, I couldn't discuss her treatment without her permission. I'd be happy to speak with you if Maria provides written authorization for me to do so."

Even confirming someone is a client violates HIPAA without authorization.

Situation 2: Coordination of care

Maria (who is Dr. Chen's client) is also seeing psychiatrist Dr. Patel for medication. Dr. Patel calls wanting to discuss Maria's progress.

Proper response: Dr. Chen checks whether Maria signed authorization for communication with Dr. Patel. She did—authorization allows release of treatment information to Dr. Patel for coordination of care purposes. Dr. Chen can discuss Maria's treatment with Dr. Patel.

If no authorization existed, Dr. Chen would need to obtain one before discussing Maria's case.

Situation 3: Subpoena

Dr. Chen receives subpoena demanding records for client John involved in custody battle.

Proper response: Dr. Chen consults attorney. Subpoena alone doesn't override HIPAA—usually requires court order or client authorization. Dr. Chen contacts John to inform him of subpoena and discuss options: John can authorize release, they can move to quash subpoena, or if court orders release, Dr. Chen must comply.

Situation 4: Insecure communication

Client texts: "Can we reschedule Tuesday's appointment? I'm having panic attacks again and can barely leave the house."

Proper response: Dr. Chen had client sign consent for text communication acknowledging lack of security. Response: "Yes, let's reschedule. Call the office or check the portal for available times." Dr. Chen doesn't text detailed clinical content even with consent—texts can be forwarded, phones can be stolen, and texting platforms generally aren't HIPAA-compliant.

Situation 5: Record storage

Dr. Chen's laptop with client files is stolen from car.

Proper response: Immediate breach notification—inform clients whose information was on laptop, document breach, report to HHS within 60 days, report to local media if breach affects 500+ individuals. Implement improved security—encrypted hard drive, never leaving devices in vehicles, cloud storage with automatic backup.

These examples show HIPAA isn't just bureaucracy—it's practical protection of client privacy requiring constant vigilance.

Mandatory Reporting Requirements

Confidentiality has limits. Laws require reporting certain situations regardless of client privacy. These mandated reporting requirements override confidentiality and require immediate action.

Child abuse and neglect reporting is mandated in all states. Social workers are mandated reporters—required by law to report suspected child abuse or neglect.

What triggers reporting:

Physical abuse: Non-accidental physical injury—bruises, burns, fractures, head injuries. Pattern of injuries, injuries inconsistent with explanation, or delay in seeking treatment raise concerns.

Sexual abuse: Sexual contact between adult and child, between children with significant age/power differential, exposure to pornography or sexual activity, exploitation.

Emotional/psychological abuse: Chronic pattern of behavior destroying child's self-worth—constant criticism, threats, rejection, isolation.

Neglect: Failure to provide basic needs—food, shelter, medical care, supervision, education. Neglect is most common form of maltreatment.

You report when you have reasonable suspicion, not proof. Reasonable suspicion means you have facts that would cause reasonable person to suspect abuse. You don't investigate—that's the job of child protective services. You report suspicions so trained investigators can assess.

How to report:

Most states require immediate verbal report (by phone) followed by written report within 24-48 hours. You report to state/county child protective services or law enforcement. Reports can be anonymous, but professional mandate means you typically identify yourself.

What to report:

- Child's name, age, address, location
- Parent/caregiver information
- Nature and extent of injuries or neglect
- Any information about prior abuse
- Your relationship to child (therapist, school counselor, etc.)
- What specifically raised your suspicion

Client notification: Inform client (or parents, if child is very young) that you're making report unless this would place child in immediate danger. "I'm concerned about what you've described. By law, I must report this to Child Protective Services. I'll help you through this process."

Documentation: Document what you observed/heard that triggered report, who you reported to, when, what information was provided, and how you informed client.

Immunity: Mandated reporters have immunity from liability for good-faith reports. You can't be sued for reporting suspected abuse even if investigation determines abuse didn't occur, as long as report was made in good faith.

Penalties for not reporting: Failure to report when mandated is crime in most states. Penalties include fines and potentially jail time. Professional licenses can be revoked.

Elder and dependent adult abuse reporting is mandated in most states. Similar to child abuse reporting, you must report suspected physical abuse, sexual abuse, emotional abuse, neglect, or financial exploitation of adults 65+ or dependent adults (those with physical or mental limitations preventing them from protecting themselves).

Triggers include:

- Unexplained injuries
- Poor hygiene or nutrition
- Over-sedation or under-medication
- Missing money or possessions

- Isolation from others
- Fearfulness around caregiver
- Caregiver preventing access to elder

You report to Adult Protective Services or law enforcement. Process similar to child abuse reporting—reasonable suspicion standard, immediate report, immunity for good-faith reports.

Danger to self reporting requirements vary by state. Some states require reporting suicidal ideation to specific authorities. More commonly, when client is imminent danger to self, you can breach confidentiality to prevent harm (calling emergency contacts, initiating involuntary hold) under duty to protect.

Danger to others may trigger reporting. The Tarasoff case (discussed next) established duty to warn or protect when client poses serious danger to identifiable victim. Some states have specific reporting requirements for threats of violence.

Case Example: Mandated Reporting - Child Abuse

Scenario 1: Clear abuse

You're seeing Emma, age 8, for anxiety. During session, she mentions daddy "gets mad and hits me hard" when she misbehaves. You see bruises on her arms and legs. Emma says daddy told her not to tell anyone or she'd get in more trouble.

Your response:

This triggers mandated reporting. Physical abuse is suspected—bruises plus child's statement about being hit hard.

"Emma, thank you for telling me. What you described—your dad hitting you hard—concerns me. That's not okay. I want you to be safe. By law, when I'm worried about a child's safety, I have to tell people whose job is to help keep children safe. I'm going to call Child Protective Services. They'll talk to you and your family to make sure you're safe."

You call CPS immediately, provide information, and follow up with written report. You document everything—what Emma said, what you observed, when and who you reported to.

CPS investigates. Possible outcomes: safety plan with family, services for family, temporary removal of child, criminal investigation of parent.

Scenario 2: Gray area

You're seeing Marcus, age 14. He mentions his mom "loses it sometimes" and "got physical" with him last week. Pressed for details, he says she grabbed his arm hard when he was being disrespectful. He's angry at her but doesn't seem afraid. You see no injuries.

Your response:

This is less clear. Single incident of grabbing arm during conflict, no injuries, no pattern. Is this reasonable parental discipline or abuse? Different professionals might assess differently.

Standard is reasonable suspicion. If facts would cause reasonable person to suspect abuse, you report. Grabbing arm forcefully could indicate physical abuse, or could be parent losing patience in discipline moment.

When uncertain, consult—with supervisor, with CPS hotline, with colleague—but err on side of reporting. It's CPS's job to investigate, not yours to determine if abuse occurred.

If you report: "Marcus, I'm concerned about what you described. When parents get physical even once, I worry about your safety. I need to report this to Child Protective Services so they can make sure you're safe and your family gets any help you might need."

If you don't report: Document thoroughly why you determined report wasn't warranted, what you observed and heard, your clinical reasoning, and that you'll monitor situation. If new information emerges or situation escalates, report then.

Scenario 3: Historical abuse

You're seeing Adult client Sarah, age 35. She discloses she was sexually abused by uncle ages 8-12. Uncle has been dead for 10 years. No children are currently at risk.

Your response:

This doesn't trigger mandated reporting. Reporting is about protecting children currently at risk. Historical abuse with no current child safety concerns doesn't require reporting.

You provide clinical response—processing trauma, supporting healing. You don't report to authorities.

Exception: If perpetrator is alive and has access to children (working with children, has grandchildren), then children may currently be at risk and reporting might be appropriate. Consult about specific circumstances.

Duty to Warn (Tarasoff)

The Tarasoff case established "duty to warn" or "duty to protect" when client poses serious danger to identifiable victim.

The case: Prosenjit Poddar, UC Berkeley student, told university psychologist he intended to kill woman who'd rejected him (Tatiana Tarasoff). Psychologist notified campus police, who briefly detained then released Poddar. No one warned Tarasoff or her family. Two months later, Poddar killed Tarasoff.

The ruling: California Supreme Court held that mental health professionals have duty to protect potential victims when client poses serious danger. "The protective privilege ends where public peril begins."

What Tarasoff requires:

Serious threat: Not vague anger or frustration. Specific threat or behavior indicating serious danger of violence.

Identifiable victim: Specific person or specific small group. "I hate everyone" doesn't trigger duty. "I'm going to kill my wife" does.

Credible capability: Person has means or capability to carry out threat. Threats from person with severe dementia or very young child are assessed differently than threats from capable adult.

When duty is triggered, you must take action:

Warn the victim: Contact intended victim directly to warn of danger. "I'm calling to inform you that X has made threats against you. I'm concerned for your safety and wanted you to be aware."

Notify law enforcement: Contact police so they can assess danger and take appropriate action—investigating, protective order, emergency detention.

Take other protective steps: Hospitalize client if criteria met, intensify treatment, involve family in safety planning.

Different states have different standards. Some require only warning potential victim. Some require reasonable efforts to protect (which might include warning, notifying police, hospitalizing, etc.). Some have immunity only if you warn; some have immunity for any reasonable protective action. Know your state law.

Documentation of Tarasoff situation:

- What client said or did that triggered concern
- Your assessment of seriousness and credibility
- Actions taken (who warned, when, how)
- Consultation obtained
- Client notification (if safe)
- Ongoing safety planning

Balancing act: Tarasoff requires breaching confidentiality to protect life. But unnecessary breaches harm therapeutic relationship. You carefully assess whether situation truly meets criteria before breaching.

Case Example: Duty to Warn - James's Threat

You're seeing James, 32, for anger management. During session, he's furious about recent breakup with girlfriend Lisa. "I can't believe she left me for that guy. I swear I'm going to kill her. She deserves to die for what she did."

Your assessment:

Is threat serious? James appears genuinely enraged. He has history of violence (assaulted previous girlfriend, has assault conviction). This isn't vague frustration—it's specific threat from someone with violent history.

Is victim identifiable? Yes. Specific person—Lisa, his ex-girlfriend.

Does he have capability? Yes. He's physically capable, knows where she lives, has history of violence.

Duty to warn is triggered.

Your immediate response in session:

"James, I hear you're extremely angry. But when you say you're going to kill Lisa, I take that seriously. I'm legally obligated to warn her and notify police. I know this feels like betrayal, but my first responsibility is preventing harm. Let's talk about this."

James could respond several ways:

Response 1: "I didn't mean it. I was just venting. I'd never actually hurt her."

You: "I understand you may not intend to act, but I heard specific threat from someone with capacity to carry it out. I still need to take protective action. Let's talk about what's happening for you that brought you to this point."

Response 2: "If you tell anyone, I'll deny it. This was confidential."

You: "Confidentiality has limits. When there's serious danger to someone, I must act to protect them. I'll document exactly what you said. Whether you deny it later doesn't change my obligation now."

Actions you take:

1. Warning Lisa: "This is [your name], James's therapist. I'm calling because James made threats against you during our session today. He stated he intends to kill you. I take this seriously given his history. I'm also notifying police. Please take precautions for your safety."

2. Notifying police: "I'm calling to report that my client James [full name and identifying info] made credible threats to kill his ex-girlfriend Lisa [identifying info]. He has history of violence and knows her location. I've warned her and wanted you to assess the danger."

3. Assessing hospitalization: Does James meet criteria for involuntary hold? If he's acutely dangerous and unwilling to contract for safety, yes. If threat seems to have de-escalated and he can commit to safety, intensive outpatient with frequent contact might be appropriate.

4. Documentation: Thorough notes: exact words James used, your assessment, who you contacted when, any actions taken.

Aftermath:

James might be angry about breach and terminate therapy. You accept this—protecting life takes priority over maintaining therapeutic relationship. He might understand you had no choice and continue treatment. Either way, you fulfilled legal and ethical duty.

Lisa is safer because she's warned and police are involved. They might seek restraining order, increase patrols near her home, or arrest James if threat meets criminal threshold.

False positive concern: What if James never would've acted and you damaged therapeutic relationship unnecessarily? You accept this risk. When serious threat to identifiable victim exists from capable person, you err on side of protection. Better to overreact than have someone die because you underreacted.

Confidentiality with Minors

Working with minors creates complex confidentiality issues. Who controls information—parent or child? How much privacy does adolescent deserve? When do you involve parents?

Legal framework:

Generally, parents have legal right to child's information because they're legal guardians. They consent to treatment on child's behalf and can access records. But states vary—some give minors rights to confidential treatment for specific issues (substance use, sexual health, mental health after certain age).

Clinical framework:

Even when parents have legal right to information, providing some confidentiality to minor serves clinical purposes. Adolescents won't be honest if everything goes to parents. Trust requires privacy.

Balancing approach:

At treatment outset, discuss confidentiality explicitly with parents and minor together:

"I want to talk about privacy. [To teen]: For you to feel safe being honest with me, you need to know I won't tell your parents everything you say. [To parents]: For therapy to work, your child needs space to talk privately about some things. Here's how I handle it:

"Most of what we discuss stays private. I won't give detailed session reports. But there are exceptions—things I must tell your parents:

- Safety issues: if you're in danger, being hurt, or thinking of hurting yourself
- Serious risk behaviors: drug use that's dangerous, sexual behavior putting you at risk
- Illegal activities that could have serious consequences
- When I need parent help to keep you safe or get you care

"For everything else, I'll encourage you to talk to your parents yourself, but I won't share without your permission.

"[To parents]: This may feel uncomfortable. You'll want to know everything. But your child needs some privacy to work through adolescent issues. I'll tell you general progress and involve you when necessary, but not every detail. Can you trust this process?"

Get explicit agreement from both. This prevents later conflict when parent demands information and you refuse.

During treatment:

Minor shares information requiring parent involvement (sexual abuse by family member, serious eating disorder, active self-harm):

"I'm glad you told me. This is one of those situations where I need to involve your parents. You're not safe handling this alone. Let's figure out together how to tell them. Would you like to tell them with me here? Or would you like me to tell them and you listen? Or should I tell them separately first?"

Involving minor in disclosure process respects their autonomy while ensuring parent is appropriately informed.

Minor shares concerning but not emergency information (experimented with marijuana once, had sex with boyfriend):

"Thank you for telling me. I know that took courage. This is something we can work on together without involving your parents right now. But I'd encourage you to think about talking to them at some point. They might be more understanding than you expect."

You maintain confidentiality because it's not safety emergency, but you encourage family communication.

Parent demands information:

"I pay for this therapy and I have a right to know what's discussed."

Your response: "I understand your concern. You do have legal right to information. But as we discussed at the start, detailed session content stays private to protect the therapeutic relationship. I can tell you [teen's name] is working on [general issue] and making progress. If I had serious safety concerns, I'd tell you immediately. Can you trust the process we agreed to?"

If parent insists, you're caught between clinical judgment (disclosure harms treatment) and legal right (parent controls minor's information). Consult supervisor and potentially attorney. You might decide to share information to preserve treatment—better to have parents involved in continuing treatment than lose ability to help teen entirely.

Emancipated minors and mature minors: Some states recognize emancipated minors (married, in military, financially independent) or mature minors (can consent to their own treatment after certain age for certain issues) as having adult rights to confidentiality. Know your state laws.

Case Example: Minor Confidentiality - Emma's Dilemma

Emma, 15, has been in therapy for anxiety. Her parents agreed to confidentiality framework at intake. During session, Emma discloses she's been cutting herself—superficial cuts on her arms, not requiring medical attention, no suicidal intent. She begs you not to tell her parents: "They'll freak out and make everything worse."

Your assessment:

Self-harm is concerning and potentially dangerous, but Emma's cutting appears to be coping mechanism, not suicide attempt. Cuts are superficial, she's managing emotions better through therapy, and frequency is decreasing. This falls in gray area—concerning but not immediate safety emergency.

Options:

Option 1: Maintain confidentiality

"I'm concerned about the cutting, but I understand you're using it to cope with overwhelming feelings. Let's work on developing other coping strategies. I won't tell your parents right now, but if the cutting gets worse or becomes medically dangerous, I'll need to involve them. Also, I strongly encourage you to tell them yourself when you're ready."

Risk: Cutting escalates and you missed opportunity for parent support. Parents find out independently and are furious they weren't told.

Benefit: Emma continues trusting you and engaging in treatment. You have opportunity to help her develop better coping before involving parents.

Option 2: Involve parents

"I know you don't want to tell your parents, but self-harm is serious. You need support you can't get in one therapy hour per week. Your parents care about you and want to help. Let's figure out together how to tell them."

Risk: Emma feels betrayed, stops trusting you, might terminate therapy.

Benefit: Parents can provide support, monitor Emma, potentially remove cutting implements, increase overall safety.

Option 3: Conditional confidentiality

"Here's what I can agree to: I won't tell your parents right now, but only if the cutting stops or decreases, you use other coping skills we develop, and you keep me informed. If cutting increases or becomes dangerous, I'll need to tell them. Also, I want you working toward telling them yourself. They deserve to know you're struggling so they can support you."

This balances Emma's privacy with safety. You maintain confidentiality conditionally, requiring Emma to work on the problem and move toward family disclosure.

What actually happens:

You choose Option 3. Over four weeks, Emma's cutting decreases. She's using other coping strategies—cold water on wrists, drawing on herself instead of cutting, calling crisis line when overwhelmed. Progress is real.

After six weeks, Emma decides to tell her parents with you present. Session goes better than she feared—parents are concerned but supportive, not punitive. They ask how to help. You provide guidance. Emma feels relieved having support.

This demonstrates that respecting minor privacy while maintaining safety can work. By not immediately breaching confidentiality, you preserved trust allowing Emma to address the problem and eventually involve parents on her own terms.

If cutting had escalated, you would've involved parents immediately regardless of Emma's wishes. Safety always supersedes privacy.

Limits of Confidentiality

Confidentiality has boundaries every client should understand. You explain limits clearly at treatment outset and remind them when relevant.

When you must break confidentiality:

1. Danger to self: When client is imminent danger to self through suicide or serious self-harm, you breach confidentiality to prevent harm—calling emergency contacts, initiating involuntary hold, coordinating with other providers.

2. Danger to others: Tarasoff situations where client poses serious threat to identifiable victim require warning victim and notifying authorities.

3. Child abuse or neglect: Mandated reporting requires disclosure when you suspect child abuse or neglect.

4. Elder/dependent adult abuse: Required reporting when you suspect abuse or neglect of vulnerable adults.

5. Court order: Legitimate court orders (not just subpoenas) require disclosure. You provide only information ordered, nothing more.

6. Client waiver: When client provides written authorization, you can share information as specified in authorization.

When you may break confidentiality:

7. Consultation and supervision: You can discuss cases in consultation and supervision for professional purposes, but you minimize identifying information and consult only with professionals bound by confidentiality.

8. Treatment team: When multiple providers treat same client, you can share information for coordination of care (though HIPAA authorization is best practice).

9. Insurance/payment: You can share information necessary for billing and utilization review.

10. Emergencies: When client is incapacitated (unconscious, psychotic), you may disclose information necessary for emergency treatment.

When confidentiality limits are unclear:

Third-party payment: When insurance pays, they receive some information—diagnosis, sometimes treatment plans and progress notes. Client should know this. Some clients choose to pay out-of-pocket specifically to avoid insurance company access to records.

Family involvement: How much to share with family members when client is adult but significantly impaired? Client with schizophrenia doesn't want parents to know about medication changes, but parents provide housing and support. You balance client autonomy with practical need for family involvement.

Group therapy: Confidentiality in groups requires all members to maintain privacy, but you can't guarantee they will. You explain this limitation: "I expect everyone to keep what's discussed here private, but I can't control what others do outside this room. Be thoughtful about what you share."

Technology: Phone calls, texts, emails, video sessions all have privacy limitations. Phone calls can be overheard. Texts can be forwarded. Emails can be hacked. Video platforms may not be fully secure. You inform clients of limitations and get consent for technology use.

How to explain limits:

Don't wait for crisis. At first session:

"I want to explain confidentiality—what I keep private and when I might need to share information. Generally, what you tell me stays between us. I don't share with family, friends, employers, anyone without your written permission.

"But there are exceptions—times when I'm required to share information or when it's necessary to keep someone safe:

"If you tell me you're planning to seriously hurt or kill yourself, I'll take action to keep you safe—that might mean calling emergency contacts, taking you to hospital, or calling 911.

"If you tell me you're planning to hurt someone else, I have to warn that person and notify police.

"If you tell me about child abuse or neglect, I'm required by law to report to Child Protective Services.

"If a judge orders me to provide information, I must comply.

"For everything else, I keep things confidential. But these safety situations require me to break confidentiality. Do you have questions about this?"

Getting explicit acknowledgment: "Do you understand the limits of confidentiality I've explained?"

Document that you explained limits and client acknowledged understanding.

When you must breach:

Tell client when possible: "I need to tell you that based on what you've shared, I'm required to report this to authorities. Here's what's going to happen..." Unless telling client creates immediate danger (they'll flee, destroy evidence, harm someone), inform them before breaching.

Breach minimally: Share only information necessary for the purpose. When warning Tarasoff victim, you don't share client's entire history—just the specific threat and necessary context.

Document thoroughly: What information was shared, with whom, when, why, and how you informed client.

Case Example: Explaining Limits

Scenario 1: Client didn't understand limits

Karen, your client for three months, discovers you sent session notes to her insurance company for utilization review. She's furious: "I never said you could share my private information!"

You check intake documents. Confidentiality explanation is there, including insurance company access, and Karen signed acknowledging she understood.

Response: "Karen, I understand you're upset. At our first session, I explained that because insurance is paying, they receive some information about treatment to determine coverage. You signed this form acknowledging that. I know it feels invasive. Let's talk about your concerns and what information they receive."

You review specifically what insurance received (diagnosis, dates of service, general treatment focus—not detailed session content). You discuss options: continue with insurance understanding they'll receive necessary information, or pay out-of-pocket for complete privacy.

This shows why clear initial explanation matters. When client understands limits from the start, later breaches don't feel like betrayals.

Scenario 2: Client tests limits

Marcus asks: "If I told you I smoked weed last night, would you tell my probation officer?"

Response: "Let's talk about confidentiality with probation. What I discuss with your probation officer depends on our agreement. If I have agreement to share information about substance use, then yes, I'd have to tell them. If I don't have that agreement, it stays confidential unless you're in danger or someone else is. Do we have an agreement about what I share with probation?"

If you have release of information: "Yes, we signed a release saying I update probation on your progress including substance use. So if you tell me about using, I'll need to report it."

If you don't have release: "No, we don't have an agreement for me to share with probation. What you tell me about drug use stays confidential unless it's creating safety issues."

Understanding your agreements and explaining them clearly prevents confusion.

Scenario 3: Parent demands information about adult child

Mother calls about her 25-year-old daughter Maria (your client): "I'm very worried about Maria. I think her depression is getting worse. What's happening in therapy?"

Response: "I understand your concern, but Maria is an adult. I can't confirm or deny whether she's my client without her permission. If she is someone I'm seeing, I couldn't discuss her treatment without her written authorization. I'd be happy to speak with you if Maria provides that authorization."

Mother pushes: "But I'm her mother! I have a right to know!"

Response: "I know this is frustrating. Adult children can make their own healthcare decisions including controlling their health information. The best thing is to talk directly with Maria about your concerns. If she wants me to speak with you, she can sign an authorization."

Even when family is genuinely concerned and would be helpful, you can't breach without client permission unless emergency exceptions apply (client is danger to self/others and family involvement is necessary for safety).

Practice Questions

1. HIPAA applies to:

A. Only hospitals
B. Covered entities including most healthcare providers and insurance
C. Only psychiatrists
D. No one really

2. Protected Health Information includes:

A. Only diagnosis
B. Any individually identifiable health information in any form
C. Only written records
D. Nothing specific

3. Psychotherapy notes:

A. Are part of medical record
B. Have special protection, kept separate, require specific authorization
C. Can be shared freely
D. Don't exist

4. The minimum necessary standard means:

A. Share everything
B. Use or disclose only minimum needed to accomplish purpose
C. Share nothing
D. Doesn't apply to anything

5. Mandated reporting of child abuse requires:

A. Proof of abuse
B. Reasonable suspicion
C. Certainty
D. Client permission

6. You should report child abuse:

A. Only if child tells you directly
B. When you have reasonable suspicion based on facts
C. Only if you witness it
D. Never

7. Immunity for mandated reporters means:

A. You can't be sued for good-faith reports even if abuse didn't occur
B. You'll never face consequences
C. Reports are always correct
D. Nothing

8. Tarasoff duty is triggered when:

A. Client is generally angry
B. Client poses serious danger to identifiable victim
C. You're curious
D. Client disagrees with someone

9. Tarasoff requires:

A. Just documenting the threat
B. Warning victim and/or taking protective steps
C. Only hospitalization
D. Nothing

10. With minors, confidentiality:

A. Is absolute
B. Requires balancing minor's privacy with parents' legal rights and safety
C. Belongs entirely to parents
D. Doesn't matter

11. At treatment outset with minors, you should:

A. Promise complete secrecy
B. Explicitly discuss confidentiality limits with parents and minor
C. Avoid the topic
D. Guarantee you'll tell parents everything

12. HIPAA violations can result in:

A. No consequences
B. Fines up to $1.5 million per year and imprisonment
C. Only warnings
D. Nothing serious

13. You can share PHI without authorization for:

A. Gossip
B. Treatment, payment, healthcare operations
C. Curiosity
D. Entertainment

14. Court orders require:

A. Ignoring them
B. Providing ordered information
C. Destroying records
D. Lying

15. Subpoenas:

A. Always require immediate disclosure
B. Often require additional steps; consult attorney
C. Should be ignored
D. Are the same as authorization

16. The Privacy Rule establishes:

A. Nothing useful
B. Standards for how PHI can be used and disclosed
C. That privacy doesn't matter
D. Only suggestions

17. The Security Rule addresses:

A. Building security
B. Electronic PHI protection through administrative, physical, technical safeguards
C. Nothing specific
D. Only passwords

18. Encrypted email is:

A. Unnecessary
B. Required for sending PHI electronically
C. Optional
D. Illegal

19. When client authorizes disclosure, authorization must include:

A. Just a signature
B. Description of info, purpose, recipients, expiration, revocation rights
C. Nothing specific
D. Only verbal agreement

20. Elder abuse reporting:

A. Is optional
B. Is mandated in most states for physical, sexual, emotional abuse, neglect, exploitation
C. Doesn't exist
D. Only applies to children

21. Failure to report mandated abuse can result in:

A. Nothing
B. Criminal penalties, fines, license revocation
C. Only suggestions to report next time
D. Rewards

22. Confidentiality in group therapy:

A. Is guaranteed
B. Requires all members maintain privacy but can't be guaranteed
C. Doesn't matter
D. Is only leader's responsibility

23. When you're unsure if situation triggers Tarasoff:

A. Ignore it
B. Consult and err on side of protection
C. Just wait
D. Never act

24. "Reasonable suspicion" for abuse reporting means:

A. Absolute proof
B. Facts that would cause reasonable person to suspect abuse
C. Just a feeling
D. Certainty

25. Technology in practice (texts, emails, video):

A. Is completely secure
B. Has privacy limitations requiring informed consent
C. Should never be used
D. Requires no consideration

26. Access to records:

A. Can be completely denied always
B. Must be provided with limited exceptions for serious harm
C. Requires court order always
D. Is never appropriate

27. Medical record documentation:

A. Can be vague
B. Should be accurate, timely, comprehensive
C. Doesn't matter
D. Is optional

28. When insurance pays for treatment:

A. They receive no information
B. They receive diagnosis and treatment information for authorization
C. Client has complete privacy
D. Share everything

29. In emergencies when client is incapacitated:

A. Never share information
B. May disclose information necessary for emergency treatment
C. Call family first always
D. Wait for authorization

30. Explaining confidentiality limits should occur:

A. Never
B. At treatment outset with clear explanation and documentation
C. Only if asked
D. After breach

31. Minimum information when warning Tarasoff victim:

A. Entire client history
B. Only specific threat and necessary context
C. Everything you know
D. Nothing

32. When parent of adult client demands information:

A. Provide it freely
B. Can't confirm client status without authorization
C. Tell them everything
D. Parents always have rights

33. Self-harm by minor:

A. Always requires parent notification
B. Requires judgment about severity and safety
C. Never tell parents
D. Isn't concerning

34. Historical child abuse disclosed by adult:

A. Must be reported immediately
B. Doesn't trigger reporting unless current child is at risk
C. Always requires police notification
D. Must tell perpetrator

35. Consultation about cases:

A. Should include identifying details publicly
B. Should minimize identifying information, only with those bound by confidentiality
C. Isn't allowed
D. Requires no precautions

36. When breaching confidentiality is necessary:

A. Never tell client
B. Inform client when possible unless doing so creates immediate danger
C. Surprise them
D. Lie about it

37. Documentation of breach should include:

A. Nothing
B. What was shared, with whom, when, why, how client was informed
C. Only that you called someone
D. Vague notes

38. Emancipated minors:

A. Have same rights as minors
B. May have adult rights to confidentiality in some states
C. Don't exist
D. Have no rights

39. Duty to protect:

A. Only means warning
B. May include warning, notifying police, hospitalizing, other protective steps
C. Is only one specific action
D. Doesn't exist

40. Third-party payment limitations:

A. Should be hidden from clients
B. Should be explained so clients know payer receives information
C. Don't exist
D. Give complete privacy

41. Treatment team coordination:

A. Doesn't need client permission
B. Ideally has client authorization for information sharing
C. Never happens
D. Requires no consideration

42. Voicemail messages should:

A. Include detailed clinical information
B. Be minimal without PHI ("This is Maria calling")
C. Share diagnosis
D. Tell everything

43. Faxing PHI requires:

A. No precautions
B. Confidential cover sheet, verified number, secure location
C. Broadcasting
D. Public posting

44. Disposal of records:

A. Trash them
B. Secure destruction (shredding, certified disposal service)
C. Leave in parking lot
D. Doesn't matter

45. Computer security includes:

A. No passwords
B. Passwords, auto-logout, encryption, secure disposal
C. Public access
D. Sharing logins

46. When minor shares concerning but not emergency information:

A. Immediately tell parents
B. Maintain confidentiality, work on issue, encourage family communication
C. Never address it
D. Ignore it

47. Laws requiring disclosure:

A. Can be ignored
B. Override confidentiality (mandated reporting, court orders)
C. Are just suggestions
D. Don't exist

48. Credible threat:

A. Any statement of anger
B. Specific threat from capable person with identifiable victim
C. Vague frustration
D. Doesn't trigger duty

49. When client refuses to authorize needed disclosure:

A. Share anyway without permission
B. Respect refusal unless emergency exception applies
C. Force them
D. Lie to them

50. Benefit of explaining limits clearly at outset:

A. Nothing
B. Prevents later feelings of betrayal when limits apply
C. Wastes time
D. Scares clients away

Answer Key with Detailed Explanations

1. B. Covered entities including most healthcare providers and insurance
HIPAA applies to "covered entities" which include most healthcare providers (physicians, hospitals, clinics, therapists who bill insurance), health plans, and healthcare clearinghouses. If you provide healthcare services and transmit health information electronically (billing insurance electronically), you're likely covered. Even if not technically covered, HIPAA represents best practices for protecting client information.

2. B. Any individually identifiable health information in any form
Protected Health Information (PHI) is any individually identifiable health information transmitted or maintained in any form or medium—written, electronic, or spoken. This includes demographic information (name, address, SSN, dates, emails, photos), health information (diagnoses, treatments, medications, mental health, substance use), and payment information. PHI must be protected regardless of format.

3. B. Have special protection, kept separate, require specific authorization
Psychotherapy notes have special protection under HIPAA. They're notes documenting or analyzing conversation during private counseling session, kept separate from medical record. They require specific authorization for disclosure (can't be disclosed for treatment, payment, operations like other medical information). Most settings don't maintain psychotherapy notes as defined by HIPAA because requirements are strict—regular session notes go in medical record.

4. B. Use or disclose only minimum needed to accomplish purpose
The minimum necessary standard requires using or disclosing only the minimum amount of PHI necessary to accomplish the intended purpose. When sending records to another provider, send only what's needed for their involvement, not the entire file unless full file is necessary. Exception: Minimum necessary doesn't apply to treatment disclosures—providers can share whatever they determine necessary for care.

5. B. Reasonable suspicion
Mandated reporting of child abuse requires reasonable suspicion, not proof or certainty. Reasonable suspicion means you have facts that would cause a reasonable person to suspect abuse. You don't investigate to gather proof—that's CPS's job. You report suspicions based on what you observe or hear so trained investigators can assess and determine what actually occurred.

6. B. When you have reasonable suspicion based on facts
You should report child abuse when you have reasonable suspicion based on facts—child's disclosure, observed injuries, pattern of indicators, or other concrete information raising concern. You don't need to witness abuse directly or have child tell you explicitly. If facts would cause reasonable person to suspect abuse, you report. Don't wait for certainty or permission—report when threshold of reasonable suspicion is met.

7. A. You can't be sued for good-faith reports even if abuse didn't occur
Immunity for mandated reporters means you can't be sued for reporting suspected abuse in good faith, even if investigation determines abuse didn't occur. As long as report was made based on reasonable suspicion in good faith (not maliciously or recklessly), you're protected from civil and criminal liability. This immunity encourages reporting by removing fear of lawsuits.

8. B. Client poses serious danger to identifiable victim
Tarasoff duty is triggered when client poses serious danger (not vague anger or general frustration) to identifiable victim (specific person or specific small group, not general threats). The danger must be credible based on client's capability and circumstances. General statements like "I hate everyone" don't trigger duty. Specific threats like "I'm going to kill my supervisor" from capable person do trigger duty.

9. B. Warning victim and/or taking protective steps
Tarasoff requires taking action to protect potential victim—this may include warning the victim directly, notifying law enforcement, hospitalizing the client if criteria met, or taking other reasonable protective steps. Simply documenting the threat without protective action doesn't fulfill duty. States vary on specific requirements (some require warning, some require reasonable protective efforts), so know your state law.

10. B. Requires balancing minor's privacy with parents' legal rights and safety
Confidentiality with minors requires balancing minor's need for privacy (necessary for honest communication and trust) with parents' legal rights to their child's information and safety considerations. Parents generally have legal rights to information, but providing some confidentiality to adolescents serves important clinical purposes. You balance these considerations while maintaining safety as primary concern.

11. B. Explicitly discuss confidentiality limits with parents and minor
At treatment outset with minors, explicitly discuss confidentiality with both parents and minor present—what stays private, what gets shared with parents (safety issues, serious risk behaviors, illegal activities), encouraging minor to communicate with parents. Get explicit agreement from both parties. This prevents later conflict when parent demands information or minor feels betrayed by necessary disclosure.

12. B. Fines up to $1.5 million per year and imprisonment
HIPAA violations can result in significant civil penalties (up to $50,000 per violation with annual maximum up to $1.5 million) and criminal penalties for knowing violations (fines up to $250,000 and imprisonment up to 10 years). Severity depends on violation type—unknowing, reasonable cause, willful neglect corrected, or willful neglect not corrected. But main concern isn't penalties—it's protecting client privacy and trust.

13. B. Treatment, payment, healthcare operations
You can share PHI without client authorization for treatment (coordinating care with other providers), payment (billing, claims processing, utilization review), and healthcare operations (quality improvement, training, compliance). These are permitted uses under HIPAA Privacy Rule. All other uses and disclosures require client authorization unless another specific exception applies (mandated reporting, emergencies, court orders).

14. B. Providing ordered information
Court orders require providing ordered information—they're legal mandates you must follow. Provide only information specifically ordered, nothing more. Document what was provided, when, pursuant to what order. Distinguish court orders from subpoenas—subpoenas alone often don't override HIPAA without additional steps. When receiving subpoena, consult attorney about whether court order is needed or if client authorization is required.

15. B. Often require additional steps; consult attorney
Subpoenas often require additional steps before disclosure—they don't automatically override HIPAA like court orders do. You typically need either client authorization or court order to respond to subpoena. When receiving subpoena, consult attorney, notify client, and determine appropriate response. Never ignore subpoena, but don't automatically comply without ensuring legal requirements are met.

16. B. Standards for how PHI can be used and disclosed
The HIPAA Privacy Rule establishes national standards for how Protected Health Information can be used and disclosed, when client authorization is required, what permitted uses exist, and what rights clients have to access their information. It provides framework protecting health information privacy while allowing necessary uses for treatment, payment, and operations.

17. B. Electronic PHI protection through administrative, physical, technical safeguards
The HIPAA Security Rule addresses protection of electronic PHI through three types of safeguards: administrative (policies, training, access management), physical (facility access, workstation security, device controls), and technical (access controls, encryption, audit logs). These safeguards protect electronic information from unauthorized access, alteration, or destruction.

18. B. Required for sending PHI electronically
Encrypted email is required for sending PHI electronically to protect against interception. Regular unsecured email doesn't meet HIPAA security standards. If you must use regular email, obtain specific client consent acknowledging risks, include confidentiality warning, and minimize PHI included. Better practice: use secure, encrypted messaging systems or HIPAA-compliant platforms for any electronic PHI transmission.

19. B. Description of info, purpose, recipients, expiration, revocation rights
When client authorizes disclosure, authorization must include: description of information to be disclosed, who may use/disclose it, who will receive it, purpose of disclosure, expiration date or event, signature and date, and statement of client's right to revoke authorization. Authorization must be written in plain language client can understand. Simple signature without these elements doesn't constitute valid authorization.

20. B. Is mandated in most states for physical, sexual, emotional abuse, neglect, exploitation
Elder and dependent adult abuse reporting is mandated in most states for adults 65+ or dependent adults with limitations preventing self-protection. Mandated reporting applies to physical abuse, sexual abuse, emotional/psychological abuse, neglect, and financial exploitation. Process is similar to child abuse reporting—reasonable suspicion standard, report to Adult Protective Services or law enforcement, immunity for good-faith reports.

21. B. Criminal penalties, fines, license revocation
Failure to report mandated abuse when required can result in criminal penalties (misdemeanor charges), fines (amounts vary by state), and professional license discipline including revocation. More importantly, failure to report can result in continued harm to vulnerable individuals. Mandated reporting is serious legal and ethical obligation with real consequences for non-compliance.

22. B. Requires all members maintain privacy but can't be guaranteed
Confidentiality in group therapy requires all members to maintain privacy of what's discussed, but the leader can't guarantee they will. You explain this limitation to potential group members: "I expect everyone to keep discussions confidential, but I can't control what others do outside this room. Be thoughtful about what personal information you share." Group members agree to confidentiality but you can't enforce it the way you can with individual confidentiality.

23. B. Consult and err on side of protection
When you're unsure if situation triggers Tarasoff duty, consult with supervisor, colleague, or attorney, and err on side of protection. Better to overreact and preserve safety than underreact and have someone harmed. Carefully assess: Is threat serious? Is victim identifiable? Does client have capability? If answers suggest yes, take protective action even if some uncertainty remains. Document your reasoning and consultation.

24. B. Facts that would cause reasonable person to suspect abuse
"Reasonable suspicion" for abuse reporting means having facts that would cause a reasonable person in similar circumstances to suspect abuse occurred. It's not just a vague feeling or hunch, but it's not proof or certainty either. Specific indicators like unexplained injuries plus concerning explanation, or

child's disclosure, or pattern of concerning signs create reasonable suspicion triggering reporting obligation.

25. B. Has privacy limitations requiring informed consent
Technology in practice (phone calls, texts, emails, video sessions) has inherent privacy limitations—calls can be overheard, texts forwarded, emails hacked, video platforms potentially insecure. You must inform clients of these limitations and obtain informed consent for technology use, explaining risks and getting agreement to proceed despite limitations. Document consent and use most secure options available.

26. B. Must be provided with limited exceptions for serious harm
Access to records must be provided to clients with limited exceptions. You can deny or limit access only when: access is reasonably likely to cause substantial harm to client or another person, request is for psychotherapy notes (which have special protection), information was compiled for legal proceedings, or specific research protocols prohibit access. Even when limiting, you discuss rationale with client and assist with potential harmful effects.

27. B. Should be accurate, timely, comprehensive
Medical record documentation should be accurate (factual and truthful), timely (recorded promptly while information is fresh), and comprehensive (sufficient detail to support continuity of care, communication with other providers, and accountability). Vague, delayed, or incomplete documentation harms client care and creates legal liability. Professional documentation standards are both clinical best practice and legal requirement.

28. B. They receive diagnosis and treatment information for authorization
When insurance pays for treatment, they receive diagnosis and often treatment plan, progress notes, or other clinical information necessary to authorize and pay for services. Client should understand this at treatment outset—insurance payment means some loss of privacy. Some clients choose to pay out-of-pocket specifically to avoid insurance company access to their mental health information.

29. B. May disclose information necessary for emergency treatment
In emergencies when client is incapacitated (unconscious, acutely psychotic, severe medical crisis), you may disclose information necessary for emergency treatment without authorization. This is recognized exception to confidentiality—preventing harm takes priority when client can't consent. Disclose only information necessary for immediate emergency care, and document circumstances justifying disclosure without authorization.

30. B. At treatment outset with clear explanation and documentation
Explaining confidentiality limits should occur at treatment outset—first session—with clear explanation of what's confidential and what circumstances require disclosure. Use understandable language, check client understanding, provide written summary, and document that limits were explained and client acknowledged understanding. Early clear explanation prevents later feelings of betrayal when limits apply and provides informed basis for client to decide whether to share sensitive information.

31. B. Only specific threat and necessary context

When warning Tarasoff victim, provide minimum necessary information—specific threat and necessary context for victim to protect themselves. You don't share client's entire history, detailed diagnosis, or unrelated information. Example: "I'm calling because my client X has made threats to harm you. He stated intention to [specific threat]. I'm concerned for your safety and am also notifying police. Please take appropriate precautions." Provide enough information for protection without unnecessary privacy violation.

32. B. Can't confirm client status without authorization
When parent of adult client demands information, you can't even confirm or deny whether the person is your client without authorization. Adult clients control their own health information regardless of family relationships. Appropriate response: "I can't confirm or deny whether that person is my client without their permission. If they are someone I'm seeing, I couldn't discuss their treatment without written authorization. I'd be happy to speak with you if they provide authorization."

33. B. Requires judgment about severity and safety
Self-harm by minor requires clinical judgment about severity and safety, not automatic parent notification. Superficial cutting used as coping mechanism with decreasing frequency might be managed without immediate parent involvement while working toward eventual disclosure. Severe self-harm, medical danger, or escalating pattern requires parent involvement for safety. Balance minor's privacy with safety needs, and when in doubt, prioritize safety.

34. B. Doesn't trigger reporting unless current child is at risk
Historical child abuse disclosed by adult client generally doesn't trigger mandated reporting because reporting is about protecting children currently at risk. Abuse that occurred years ago with perpetrator deceased or no current child access doesn't create current risk. Exception: If perpetrator is alive and has access to children (works with children, has grandchildren), current children may be at risk and reporting becomes appropriate. Focus is always on preventing current/future harm.

35. B. Should minimize identifying information, only with those bound by confidentiality
Consultation about cases should minimize identifying information—use initials or pseudonyms, omit unnecessary identifying details, focus on clinical issues not identifying features. Consult only with professionals bound by confidentiality (supervisors, colleagues, consultants under professional ethics). Don't discuss cases publicly, at social events, or with people who don't have professional need to know and obligation to maintain confidentiality.

36. B. Inform client when possible unless doing so creates immediate danger
When breaching confidentiality is necessary, inform client when possible before disclosure: "Based on what you've shared, I'm required to [report to CPS/warn the person/notify police]. Here's what's going to happen..." Exception: If telling client creates immediate danger (they'll flee, destroy evidence, harm someone), you breach without informing them first. But whenever safe and feasible, notify client about breach before or as soon as possible after it occurs.

37. B. What was shared, with whom, when, why, how client was informed
Documentation of confidentiality breach should include: what specific information was shared, with whom (name, agency, position), when (date and time), why (what triggered the breach—legal requirement, danger to self/others, court order), how client was informed (what you told them, when),

and any actions taken afterward. Thorough documentation protects you legally and provides clear record of your decision-making process and compliance with laws/ethics.

38. B. May have adult rights to confidentiality in some states
Emancipated minors (married, in military, financially independent, declared emancipated by court) may have adult rights to confidentiality in some states, meaning they control their own health information without parent access. Mature minor laws in some states give minors after certain age (often 12-16) right to consent to their own mental health, substance use, or sexual health treatment, which may include confidentiality rights. Know your state laws regarding minor rights.

39. B. May include warning, notifying police, hospitalizing, other protective steps
Duty to protect may include multiple possible actions: warning intended victim directly, notifying law enforcement, hospitalizing client if criteria met, intensifying treatment, involving family in safety planning, or other reasonable steps to prevent harm. It's not limited to one specific action. Different states have different requirements—some mandate warning, some require reasonable protective efforts. The goal is preventing harm through appropriate intervention.

40. B. Should be explained so clients know payer receives information
Third-party payment limitations should be explained clearly to clients so they understand that when insurance/employer/government pays, the payer receives clinical information (diagnosis, treatment plans, sometimes session notes) for authorization and payment. Some clients value complete privacy highly enough to pay out-of-pocket despite financial hardship. Informed consent means understanding privacy trade-offs when third parties pay.

41. B. Ideally has client authorization for information sharing
Treatment team coordination ideally includes client authorization for information sharing among team members. While HIPAA permits sharing for treatment purposes without authorization, best practice is explicit client consent for coordination. This ensures client understands who's involved in their care and what information is shared. Authorization should specify team members and types of information that will be shared.

42. B. Be minimal without PHI ("This is Maria calling")
Voicemail messages should be minimal without Protected Health Information. You don't know who might hear the message—partner, parent, employer checking phone, someone who finds lost phone. Safe approach: "This is Maria from ABC Clinic calling for John. Please call me at [number]." Don't include clinical information, appointment reminders with specifics, or identifiers like "This is your therapist calling."

43. B. Confidential cover sheet, verified number, secure location
Faxing PHI requires: confidential cover sheet indicating sensitive information and intended recipient only, verified recipient fax number (confirm before sending), and fax machine in secure location (not public area where others can see received documents). Include instructions for what recipient should do if fax is received in error. Fax is considered secure under HIPAA but requires these precautions.

44. B. Secure destruction (shredding, certified disposal service)
Disposal of records requires secure destruction—cross-cut shredding for paper records, certified

disposal service for large volumes, or certified electronic media destruction for digital storage devices. Simply throwing records in trash, even torn up, violates HIPAA. Records contain sensitive information requiring destruction that makes reconstruction impossible. Document disposal (dates, method) per retention requirements.

45. B. Passwords, auto-logout, encryption, secure disposal
Computer security for PHI includes: unique passwords (never shared), automatic logout after period of inactivity, encrypted hard drives and portable devices, secure wireless networks, anti-virus/firewall protection, access controls limiting who can view records, and secure disposal of devices when discarded. Physical security matters too—locked offices, positioned screens away from public view, logging off when leaving workstation.

46. B. Maintain confidentiality, work on issue, encourage family communication
When minor shares concerning but not emergency information (experimented with marijuana once, consensual sexual activity with peer), maintain confidentiality, work on the issue in therapy, and encourage minor to communicate with parents over time. You don't immediately breach confidentiality for every concern—balance privacy (necessary for treatment) with safety. If situation escalates to emergency level, you involve parents. Meanwhile, you work therapeutically on the issue.

47. B. Override confidentiality (mandated reporting, court orders)
Laws requiring disclosure override confidentiality—you must comply regardless of client wishes or typical confidentiality obligations. Examples: mandated reporting laws (child/elder abuse), court orders, specific state laws (gunshot wounds, certain communicable diseases). These legal requirements supersede ethical confidentiality obligations. You explain to clients that legal mandates limit confidentiality in specific circumstances.

48. B. Specific threat from capable person with identifiable victim
Credible threat that triggers Tarasoff duty requires: specific threat (not vague anger like "I hate everyone"), from capable person (has means and ability to carry out threat), against identifiable victim (specific person or small specific group). Vague frustration ("I'm so angry I could kill someone") or impossible threats (person with dementia threatening to build bomb) don't meet criteria. Assessment requires professional judgment about seriousness and credibility.

49. B. Respect refusal unless emergency exception applies
When client refuses to authorize needed disclosure (to insurance for payment, to other providers for coordination), generally respect their refusal—it's their information to control. Exception: Emergency situations where disclosure is necessary to prevent serious harm may override client refusal. You can discuss with client why disclosure would help, problem-solve concerns, and explain consequences of not authorizing (no insurance payment, limited coordination), but ultimately, competent adult clients control their information.

50. B. Prevents later feelings of betrayal when limits apply
The main benefit of clearly explaining confidentiality limits at treatment outset is preventing later feelings of betrayal when limits must be applied. When client understands from the beginning that you must report child abuse, warn potential victims, or respond to court orders, later disclosure feels less

like betrayal. They knew the rules and chose to proceed. Surprises damage trust; clear upfront explanations preserve it even when breaches occur.

Navigating the Privacy Maze

Confidentiality isn't simple. Laws vary by state. Situations are complex. Competing obligations conflict. Technology creates new challenges. You'll face gray areas where the right answer isn't obvious.

What helps is returning to core principles: confidentiality protects clients and enables the trust necessary for effective treatment. Laws that require disclosure do so to protect vulnerable people (children, elders) or prevent serious harm (danger to self or others). These aren't arbitrary rules—they reflect careful balance between privacy and safety.

When facing confidentiality dilemmas, ask yourself: What does law require? What does ethics require? What serves client welfare? What prevents serious harm? Often these align. When they conflict, systematic ethical decision-making, consultation, and documentation of reasoning guide appropriate action.

You won't get it perfect. Everyone makes judgment errors—breaching when not necessary, not breaching when you should have. What matters is approaching each situation thoughtfully, knowing relevant laws and ethics, consulting when uncertain, documenting carefully, and learning from experience.

Technology will continue creating new challenges. Teletherapy, electronic records, texting, apps, artificial intelligence—each innovation brings privacy concerns. Stay current with regulations, use secure platforms, inform clients of limitations, obtain informed consent, and always prioritize protection of client information.

The foundation remains unchanged: clients trust us with their most private information. We honor that trust by maintaining confidentiality except when law, ethics, or safety require disclosure. That's the essential commitment underlying all the specific rules and regulations.

Core Privacy and Confidentiality Principles

- HIPAA establishes federal standards for PHI protection covering healthcare providers, plans, and clearinghouses with civil and criminal penalties for violations
- PHI includes any individually identifiable health information in any form requiring protection through Privacy and Security Rules
- Permitted uses without authorization include treatment, payment, healthcare operations; all others require written client authorization
- Psychotherapy notes have special protection requiring specific authorization separate from general medical record access
- Minimum necessary standard requires using or disclosing only information needed to accomplish specific purpose

- Mandated reporting of child and elder abuse requires reasonable suspicion, not proof, with immunity for good-faith reports
- Failure to report mandated abuse can result in criminal penalties, fines, and license revocation
- Tarasoff duty is triggered by serious threat from capable person to identifiable victim requiring warning and/or protective steps
- Confidentiality with minors requires balancing minor's privacy needs with parents' legal rights and safety considerations
- Explaining confidentiality limits clearly at treatment outset with both parents and minors prevents later betrayal feelings
- Court orders require disclosure; subpoenas often require additional steps including consultation with attorney
- Technology (email, text, video) has inherent privacy limitations requiring informed client consent acknowledging risks
- When breaching confidentiality, inform client when possible unless doing so creates immediate danger, and document thoroughly
- Consultation should minimize identifying information and occur only with professionals bound by confidentiality
- Access to records must be provided except when likely to cause substantial harm, with discussion of limitations

Chapter 15: Boundaries and Dual Relationships

Boundaries. The word sounds simple. It's not. Boundaries are invisible lines distinguishing professional relationships from personal ones, protecting clients from exploitation, and maintaining the therapeutic frame. Cross them and you risk harming clients, damaging the profession, and destroying your career. Maintain them rigidly without thought and you might be cold and ineffective.

Here's the complexity: boundaries aren't identical for everyone. What's appropriate with one client might be problematic with another. What's normal in one setting or culture might be boundary violation in another. Context matters. Judgment matters. Rigid rules can't cover every situation.

But some boundaries are absolute. Sexual relationships with current clients—prohibited, no exceptions. Financial exploitation—prohibited. Using client relationships for your own needs instead of their therapeutic benefit—prohibited. These aren't gray areas. They're clear violations.

The tricky part is everything else. Accepting a gift. Running into clients in community. Being Facebook friends. Self-disclosing personal information. These situations require judgment, not just rule-following. You need to understand why boundaries exist, what they protect, and how to navigate complex situations while maintaining appropriate professional relationship.

Professional Boundaries

Professional boundaries define and protect the therapeutic relationship. They distinguish professional relationships (exist for client benefit) from personal relationships (exist for mutual benefit). In professional relationships, client needs come first. Your needs, wants, and preferences are secondary.

Why boundaries matter:

Power differential: Therapeutic relationships involve inherent power imbalance. You have expertise, knowledge, and professional authority. Clients are vulnerable, seeking help, often in distress. This power differential makes exploitation possible even when both parties think the relationship is mutual and consensual. Boundaries protect against exploitation.

Therapeutic frame: Boundaries create safe container for therapeutic work. Predictable, boundaried relationships allow clients to be vulnerable, explore difficult material, and experience corrective emotional experiences. When boundaries are unclear or violated, the therapeutic frame collapses and therapeutic work becomes impossible.

Trust: Clients trust you with their most private information, feelings, and fears. Maintaining boundaries honors that trust. Violating boundaries—using client relationships for your own needs, exploiting their vulnerability, crossing from professional to personal—betrays trust and causes harm.

Transference and countertransference: Clients develop feelings toward you based partly on past relationships (transference). You develop feelings toward clients based partly on your own history (countertransference). These feelings are normal and clinically useful. But acting on them through boundary violations transforms helpful therapeutic phenomena into harmful exploitation.

Types of boundaries:

Role boundaries: You're the therapist, client is the client. You don't become friends, romantic partners, business partners, or social connections. The relationship exists for therapeutic purposes only. When therapy ends, the professional relationship and its inherent power differential continues to some degree—you don't immediately become social peers.

Physical boundaries: Appropriate physical contact is limited and purposeful—handshake, brief hug when client-initiated and culturally appropriate. Sexual or romantic physical contact is absolutely prohibited. Even non-sexual touch requires careful judgment about appropriateness, cultural meaning, and potential for misinterpretation or harm.

Emotional boundaries: You provide empathy and care, but you're not emotionally dependent on clients. You don't seek emotional support from clients. You don't burden them with your problems. Emotional investment flows toward client benefit, not toward meeting your needs.

Time and space boundaries: Sessions have set start and end times. You meet in professional setting, not personal spaces. You maintain appropriate availability—not on call 24/7 but available within professional parameters. Boundaries around time and space maintain therapeutic frame.

Financial boundaries: Fee arrangements are clear, fair, and maintained. You don't exploit clients financially through inappropriate fees, billing for services not rendered, or pressuring clients to purchase products or services. Money in therapeutic relationships requires careful attention to avoid exploitation.

Communication boundaries: Contact between sessions is limited and purposeful. You don't chat socially with clients. Communications serve therapeutic purposes. You don't text or email constantly. Clear boundaries around communication prevent relationship from becoming social rather than therapeutic.

Self-disclosure boundaries: What you share about yourself is limited and serves therapeutic purpose. You don't burden clients with your problems. Self-disclosure, when used, is thoughtful and client-focused, not meeting your needs for connection or validation.

Boundary crossings vs. boundary violations:

Boundary crossing: Minor deviation from typical practice that's not harmful and may be therapeutically beneficial. Example: Attending client's art show when this supports recovery and has been discussed and processed. Running into client at community event and saying hello. Brief appropriate self-disclosure serving therapeutic purpose.

Crossings are intentional, thoughtful, discussed, documented, and clearly in client's interest. They're temporary and specific, not pattern of boundary erosion.

Boundary violation: Harmful transgression exploiting power differential and serving professional's needs rather than client's. Examples: Sexual or romantic relationships, financial exploitation, using client relationships for emotional support, befriending clients on social media without therapeutic rationale.

Violations harm clients, damage therapeutic relationship, and violate ethics. They're self-serving rather than client-focused.

The slippery slope: Boundary violations rarely happen suddenly. They develop through gradual erosion—small crossings become bigger, rationalizations accumulate, self-awareness decreases. The therapist who ends up sexually involved with client usually started with seemingly minor boundary crossings that progressively escalated.

Preventing violations requires vigilance about crossings. Each crossing should be examined: Is this truly in client's interest? Could it lead somewhere harmful? Am I rationalizing meeting my own needs? Consultation and supervision help maintain perspective.

Cultural considerations:

Appropriate boundaries vary across cultures. In some cultures, declining food or gifts is deeply offensive. In others, physical touch in greeting is expected. In collectivist cultures, boundaries between professional and personal might be less rigid than in individualist cultures.

Cultural responsiveness doesn't mean abandoning boundaries—it means adapting them thoughtfully. You learn cultural norms, discuss boundary issues explicitly with clients from different backgrounds, adjust practices to be culturally appropriate while maintaining core protective functions of boundaries.

Case Example: Boundary Crossing vs. Violation

Scenario 1: Appropriate crossing

You've been working with Marcus, 28, for depression following job loss. After six months of good progress, Marcus mentions he's having small art show at local coffee shop showcasing photographs he's been taking as part of behavioral activation. He invites you to attend.

Your assessment:

Marcus isn't suggesting social relationship—he's proud of accomplishment and wants to share with someone who's supported his recovery. Attending might reinforce progress. But it could also blur boundaries or create discomfort.

Your response:

"I appreciate you thinking of me. I'm proud of your progress and that you're showcasing your art. Let me think about whether attending fits within our professional relationship. Can we discuss it more next session?"

Next session, you discuss:

"I've thought about your art show. I'm honored you want to share your accomplishment. I think attending could support your recovery by showing I value this important step. But I want to be thoughtful about boundaries. If I attend, I'll come briefly, stay professional, and we'll process the experience in our next session. How does that sound?"

If Marcus agrees, you attend briefly (15-20 minutes), congratulate him, view art, and leave. Next session, you process: "How was it for you having me at your show? Did it feel supportive or uncomfortable? How do we maintain our professional relationship after that?"

This is boundary crossing done thoughtfully—intentional, discussed, clearly serving therapeutic purpose, processed afterward, and with attention to potential impact on relationship.

Scenario 2: Boundary violation

You've been working with Jennifer, 32, for anxiety. Over time, you've found yourself looking forward to her sessions more than others, thinking about her between sessions, and sharing more personal information with her than other clients. Jennifer seems to enjoy these conversations.

Your supervisor notices during supervision that you talk about Jennifer differently—more personally, with more emotion. Supervisor asks about boundaries.

You realize you've been gradually crossing boundaries: sessions running over time consistently, occasional texts between sessions about non-urgent matters, sharing details about your own anxiety struggles, meeting for coffee once "to continue a conversation about anxiety techniques."

Recognition: These aren't thoughtful therapeutic crossings—they're gradual boundary erosion serving your needs for connection rather than Jennifer's therapeutic needs. You're developing personal relationship with client, not maintaining professional boundaries.

Immediate action:

With supervisor's help, you recognize you need to restore boundaries. You tell Jennifer in next session:

"I've realized through supervision that our relationship has drifted from professional boundaries. I've been sharing too much personal information and we've been connecting more socially than therapeutically. This is my responsibility to fix. We need to re-establish appropriate professional boundaries—sessions will end on time, communication between sessions will be only about urgent clinical matters, and I'll keep focus on your therapeutic needs. I apologize for allowing boundaries to blur."

Jennifer might feel rejected or confused. You acknowledge those feelings, take responsibility, and maintain the necessary boundaries. If you can't restore appropriate professional relationship, you might need to transfer Jennifer's care to another therapist.

Prevention: Supervision, consultation, self-awareness, and willingness to recognize when your needs are creeping into therapeutic relationship prevent boundary violations.

Multiple Relationships

Multiple relationships (also called dual relationships) occur when you have another significant relationship with client beyond the therapeutic one. You're both therapist and something else—teacher, supervisor, business associate, friend, family member, romantic partner.

Some multiple relationships are unavoidable (small communities, specific settings). Some are harmful and prohibited (sexual relationships, financial exploitation). Most fall somewhere in between, requiring careful judgment.

Problematic multiple relationships:

Sexual relationships: Absolutely prohibited with current clients. Prohibited for at least two years with former clients, and discouraged even after two years unless extraordinary circumstances demonstrate no exploitation. The power differential, vulnerability, and potential for harm make sexual relationships fundamentally incompatible with professional relationship.

Business relationships: Generally prohibited. You don't employ clients, enter business ventures with them, or create financial dependencies beyond therapeutic fees. Exception might be extremely limited transactions (client owns only bookstore in small town and you buy books there) when alternative isn't feasible, no exploitation exists, and relationship is discussed and monitored.

Social relationships: Generally problematic. You don't become friends with current clients. Casual social contact in small communities might be unavoidable, but deliberate social relationships undermine therapeutic relationship. Friendships create mutual expectations incompatible with one-way therapeutic focus.

Supervisory or evaluative relationships: Providing therapy to someone you supervise or evaluate creates problematic dual relationship. Power dynamics conflict—supervisor/employee plus therapist/client is too complex. If mental health services are needed, refer to another provider.

Less problematic but requiring attention:

Small community relationships: In rural or small communities, you might share church, shop at same stores, have children in same school as clients. These overlaps are unavoidable. You discuss them explicitly, establish how to handle community encounters, and monitor for impact on therapeutic relationship.

Professional relationships: You might treat colleague's family member, treat someone who works at your agency (but not in reporting relationship), or share professional organizations with clients. These require careful boundary attention but might not be avoidable or immediately harmful if well-managed.

Family relationships: Treating family members of someone you're already treating creates dual relationship. Seeing mother and daughter separately means you know things about each that might affect therapy with the other. Some family therapists navigate this, but individual therapists often refer family members to other providers.

Managing unavoidable multiple relationships:

Discuss explicitly: "I realize we see each other at church every Sunday. Let's talk about how we'll handle that—should we acknowledge each other? Would you prefer I not approach you in public? How will we maintain your privacy in these settings?"

Obtain consultation: Regularly discuss multiple relationships with supervisor. Outside perspective helps you recognize when relationships are becoming problematic.

Document thoroughly: Document the multiple relationship, why it's unavoidable, how you're managing it, and how you're monitoring for negative impact.

Monitor continuously: Regularly assess whether multiple relationship is affecting therapy. If it starts interfering, address directly and consider referral if it can't be managed.

Empower client choice: Give clients information about potential complications from multiple relationships and let them decide whether to proceed. "This creates some complexity—you might feel less free to share certain things knowing we're in same faith community. Would you prefer to work with someone you won't see in other contexts?"

Be prepared to refer: If multiple relationship becomes problematic or therapeutic relationship suffers, be willing to refer even if client wants to continue. "I've realized our overlapping relationships are interfering with therapy effectiveness. For your benefit, I think you'd be better served by working with a therapist you don't encounter in other contexts."

Case Example: Multiple Relationships in Small Community

Dr. Johnson is the only licensed clinical social worker in town of 3,000 people. She faces constant multiple relationships.

Situation 1: Church member

Sarah, active member of Dr. Johnson's church, seeks therapy for depression. They see each other every Sunday, serve on same committee, and their children are in same youth group.

Dr. Johnson's response:

"Sarah, I want to discuss how we'll handle the fact that we see each other regularly at church. This creates what we call a dual relationship—I'm both your therapist and your fellow church member. Let's talk about how to manage this:

"In therapy, you can talk about anything, including church-related issues. I won't let what I know from church influence therapy inappropriately.

"At church, how would you like me to interact with you? Would you prefer brief hellos or should I not approach you? How do we maintain your privacy?

"If our church relationship starts interfering with therapy—if you feel inhibited discussing certain things—we'll need to address that.

"You also have the option of driving to the next town (40 miles) to see a therapist you don't encounter elsewhere. What feels right for you?"

Sarah decides to proceed with Dr. Johnson. They establish that Dr. Johnson will say brief hello at church but not seek out conversations. They agree to monthly check-ins about whether church relationship is affecting therapy.

Situation 2: Son's teacher

Mrs. Martinez, Dr. Johnson's son's high school teacher, seeks therapy for marital problems. Dr. Johnson sees Mrs. Martinez at parent-teacher conferences and school events.

Dr. Johnson's response:

"I'm glad you reached out for help. But I need to discuss a complication. I'm [son's name]'s mother—you're his teacher. This creates dual relationship that could be problematic. For example, you might feel uncomfortable discussing frustrations about work if I'm parent of one of your students. Or I might have information about school situations from my son that affects how I hear what you tell me.

"I'm concerned this dual relationship could interfere with therapy effectiveness. I'd like to refer you to Dr. Smith in [next town]. I know it's inconvenient, but I think you'd be better served by someone without these overlapping relationships."

Mrs. Martinez insists she's comfortable with Dr. Johnson. Dr. Johnson refers anyway: "I appreciate your comfort with me, but professional guidelines suggest avoiding dual relationships when possible. I have responsibility to ensure you get best possible care, which means therapist without these complications."

Situation 3: Business relationship

Tom, who owns only grocery store in town, seeks therapy. Dr. Johnson shops there weekly and knows Tom in that context.

Dr. Johnson's response:

"Tom, I want you to get help, but I need to mention that we have existing relationship—I shop at your store weekly. This is less problematic than some dual relationships since it's limited commercial interaction, but we should discuss it.

"Would it feel uncomfortable for you knowing I'm in your store regularly? Would you feel inhibited discussing work frustrations knowing I'm a customer?

"We can manage this by keeping our therapy relationship completely separate from our customer-clerk relationship. At the store, we'll interact normally as we have been. In therapy, we focus entirely on your therapeutic needs.

"Alternatively, I can refer you to provider in next town if you'd prefer therapist you don't encounter in daily life."

Tom chooses to proceed. They establish clear boundaries—store interactions remain unchanged, therapy discussions can include store-related stress without affecting their commercial relationship, and they check regularly about whether dual relationship is problematic.

These examples show how to navigate unavoidable multiple relationships in small communities—explicit discussion, client choice, clear boundaries, regular monitoring, and willingness to refer when relationships become problematic.

Social Media and Technology Issues

Social media and technology create new boundary challenges. Traditional boundaries were designed for in-person therapy where professional and personal lives were more separate. Now, online presence makes information accessible, social connections visible, and boundaries more complex.

Social media connection with clients:

Facebook, Instagram, LinkedIn friendship requests from clients:

Generally, you should decline. Accepting friend/connection requests blurs boundaries. You see client's photos, posts, friend lists. They see yours. Information that should remain private becomes visible. The therapeutic relationship requires professional distance that social media friendship undermines.

How to decline:

When client sends request, don't ignore it (feels rejecting). Address it directly in session:

"I received your Facebook friend request. I appreciate you thinking of me, but I have policy of not connecting with clients on social media. This isn't about you personally—it's about maintaining professional boundaries that help therapy work effectively. When we're Facebook friends, it changes our relationship in ways that can interfere with therapy. I hope you understand."

Document that you explained policy and client's response.

Exceptions: Might be different in small communities where everyone is connected on social media. But even then, you might create professional-only accounts separate from personal social media, or explain to clients that your posts and theirs won't be private from each other.

Searching for clients online:

Should you Google clients? Check their social media?

Arguments against: Invades privacy. Information gathered outside therapeutic relationship affects how you see client. Client didn't consent to you accessing this information. Creates unfair power dynamic—you know about them from online searching but they don't know what you know.

Arguments for: Information is publicly available—it's not invading privacy to look at public posts. You might learn important safety information (suicidal posts, concerning statements). Understanding client's online presence helps you understand their world.

Middle ground: Have clear policy and communicate it. Some therapists never search clients online. Others search only for specific clinical reasons (safety concerns, verifying information) and inform clients: "I occasionally look at publicly available online information about clients when I have specific clinical concerns. I wanted you to know this is something I might do."

If you do search, document why you searched and what you found. Don't search out of curiosity or voyeurism—only for legitimate clinical purposes.

What if you accidentally see client information online?

You're scrolling Facebook and see mutual friend posted photo including your client at party. Client looks intoxicated. You weren't searching for information about client, but now you have it.

Address in next session: "I want to mention that I saw you in a mutual friend's Facebook post from last weekend. I wasn't looking for information about you, but I did see the post. I don't want information I acquire outside our sessions to affect our work without discussing it. How do you feel about me having seen that?"

Transparency about information you've gained helps maintain trust.

Client searches for you online:

Assume clients will Google you. They'll find your credentials, professional information, maybe personal information. This is normal and expected.

Managing your online presence:

Professional information: Having professional website, Psychology Today profile, agency bio is appropriate and helpful. Clients should be able to verify your credentials and learn about your approach.

Personal information: Decide what personal information you're comfortable with clients accessing. Completely private social media (truly private, not just "friends only") keeps personal life separate. Public social media means accepting that clients will see your posts, photos, and opinions.

Privacy settings: Use privacy settings to control what's visible. But assume anything online might eventually be seen by clients. Don't post things professionally or personally that would be problematic if clients saw them.

Professional boundaries online: Even in personal posts, you represent the profession. Discriminatory statements, unprofessional behavior, or content contradicting professional values damages credibility and potentially violates ethics.

Telehealth boundaries:

Virtual therapy creates unique boundary issues:

Home environments: Providing therapy from home (yours or client's) reveals personal information—decor, family members in background, pets, neighborhoods. You can't be completely private in home environment.

Managing home environment: Use neutral background or virtual background. Ensure privacy (no interruptions, soundproofing). Establish that home-based therapy doesn't mean casual relationship—professional boundaries still apply even when you're both in personal spaces.

Technology problems: Poor connection, frozen screens, disconnections create interruptions affecting therapeutic flow. Have plans for technical difficulties (phone backup number, how to reconnect, policy about missed time).

After-hours contact: Email and text create expectations about availability. Establish clear policies about when and how you'll respond to electronic communications. Don't create expectation of immediate response except for emergencies.

Case Example: Social Media Boundaries

Situation 1: Client finds personal post

You're treating Amanda for anxiety. You posted on your personal (but not private) Facebook page about political rally you attended, expressing strong views.

Amanda sees it and mentions in session: "I saw your Facebook post about the rally. I had no idea you felt so strongly about those issues."

Your response:

"Yes, I did post about that. I should mention that while I try to keep my personal views private from clients, I understand information online is accessible. How do you feel about having seen that post? Does it affect how comfortable you feel in therapy?"

Amanda: "A little. I voted differently than you. I worry you might judge me."

"I appreciate your honesty. My political views are my personal opinions and don't affect how I work with clients. I respect people across political spectrum and my job is to help you with your anxiety, not judge your beliefs. But if my post has made you uncomfortable, let's address that. Would it help to discuss this more, or would you prefer to work with someone whose personal views you don't know about?"

Amanda decides to continue. You're more careful about public posts knowing clients might see them, and you process how online information affects therapeutic relationship.

Situation 2: Client wants to connect professionally on LinkedIn

James, your client, sends LinkedIn connection request. LinkedIn is professional networking, not personal social media.

Your response:

Consider: LinkedIn connections are visible to others, connection implies professional relationship/endorsement, and you'll see James's professional posts and he'll see yours.

You might accept professional LinkedIn connections with clients since it's professional networking platform, not personal social media. Or you might decline all social media connections including LinkedIn to avoid any complications.

You address in session: "I received your LinkedIn request. I have policy about social media connections with clients. [Either: I don't connect with current clients on any platform to maintain clear boundaries. Or: I'm comfortable with LinkedIn since it's professional networking, not personal social media.] Here's my thinking about why..."

Situation 3: Concerning social media post

You happen to see (through mutual friend's share) that your client posted: "I can't do this anymore. Tonight's the night. Goodbye everyone."

This appears to be suicide note. Time-sensitive situation.

Your response:

Immediate action: Contact client immediately—call, text if you have permission. "I saw concerning post you made. I'm worried about your safety. Please contact me right away." If no response and you believe danger is imminent, call 911 for welfare check or contact emergency contacts.

After ensuring safety: "I want to talk about what happened. I saw your post that concerned me. I know you didn't post it for me to see, but once I saw it, I had to act. How are you doing now? Let's talk about what led to that post and how we prevent this from happening again."

Discuss boundaries: "This brings up question about social media. I don't routinely monitor your social media, but if I happen to see something concerning, I'll act on it. How do you feel about that? Would you prefer I never look at your social media even if concerning post is brought to my attention?"

Social media creates scenarios where boundaries and safety intersect. You can't ignore safety concerns just because information came through social media channel.

Self-Disclosure

Self-disclosure is sharing personal information about yourself with clients. Used skillfully, self-disclosure can build rapport, normalize experiences, model healthy behavior, and strengthen therapeutic alliance. Used poorly, it burdens clients, meets therapist's needs rather than client's, or undermines professional boundaries.

Types of self-disclosure:

Unavoidable disclosure: Some information is inherently available—your gender presentation, approximate age, name, credentials, office location, professional background. Clients observe your appearance, wedding ring, photographs in office. This information exists whether you intentionally share it or not.

Deliberate disclosure for therapeutic purpose: Intentionally sharing personal information to serve therapeutic goal. "I've also experienced loss of a parent. I know how profound that grief can be. While my experience was different from yours, I have some understanding of what you're facing."

Inappropriate disclosure for therapist's needs: Sharing personal problems, seeking support, burdening client with your issues. "I'm going through terrible divorce. My partner is being so unreasonable..." This reverses the helping relationship—client becomes supporter, which is role reversal and boundary violation.

When self-disclosure might be appropriate:

Normalizing: "Many people experience intrusive thoughts—even therapists. You're not alone in this."

Building rapport: In early sessions when client is uncertain about connecting, limited appropriate disclosure might help: "I grew up in similar neighborhood. I understand some of the culture you're describing."

Modeling: "When I struggled with public speaking anxiety, I found that preparation helped more than trying to eliminate nervousness. Let me tell you what worked for me..."

Demonstrating hope: "I've recovered from depression. I know from personal experience that the hopelessness you feel isn't permanent. Recovery is possible."

Creating authenticity: Brief appropriate disclosure can make you more human and relatable rather than blank screen. "I have two teenagers at home, so I understand some of parenting challenges you're describing."

Guidelines for appropriate self-disclosure:

Purpose: Ask yourself, "Who does this serve?" If it serves therapeutic purpose—normalizing, modeling, building rapport, offering hope—it might be appropriate. If it serves your needs—venting, seeking support, making yourself feel important—it's inappropriate.

Brevity: Keep it brief. The focus should quickly return to client. "I've experienced panic attacks, so I understand how frightening they are. Tell me more about what your panic attacks are like." You disclose enough to build connection, then refocus on client.

Relevance: Disclosure should relate directly to client's issue. Don't tangent into your own story. Stay connected to what client is working on.

Timing: Disclosure is generally more appropriate after therapeutic alliance is established. Early sessions focused on client, with minimal therapist disclosure. As trust builds and you understand client's needs, selective disclosure might help.

Frequency: Infrequent disclosure is more powerful. Constantly sharing personal experiences shifts focus from client to you. Save disclosure for moments when it will be genuinely helpful.

Depth: Share general information, not intimate details. "I've been through divorce" is different from "Let me tell you all the painful details of my divorce." Depth of disclosure should match therapeutic purpose—deeper disclosure requires stronger justification.

Invitation to respond: After disclosure, explicitly redirect to client. "I mention this because I think it relates to what you're experiencing. What are your thoughts?" You share, then immediately refocus on their experience.

Cultural considerations: Some cultures expect more personal relationship with helpers. Self-disclosure might be necessary for trust in cultures valuing personal connection over professional distance. Match disclosure to cultural expectations while maintaining appropriate boundaries.

When self-disclosure is problematic:

Burdening client: Sharing your problems, expecting client support, or making them worry about you reverses roles inappropriately.

Meeting your needs: Disclosing because you need to talk, need validation, or want attention from client.

Overshadowing client: Your story becomes focus instead of client's experience.

Creating obligation: Client feels they should support you or respond to your disclosure when they need to be supported themselves.

Damaging credibility: Sharing information that makes client doubt your competence or ability to help them.

What not to disclose:

Current personal crises ("I'm dealing with my own severe depression right now")
Controversial political or religious views (usually)
Intimate relationship details
Financial problems
Substance use
Legal problems
Information that would make client feel unsafe
Anything that serves your emotional needs rather than client's therapeutic needs

Case Example: Appropriate and Inappropriate Self-Disclosure

Appropriate disclosure:

You're working with Maria, 35, who's terrified to return to work after maternity leave. She worries she can't balance motherhood and career.

Maria: "You don't understand. You probably don't have kids. You don't know how impossible this feels."

You: "I do have children, actually. I remember the anxiety of returning to work after my first child was born. I worried about the same things—being a good mother and good professional. I won't pretend our situations are identical, but I have some understanding of that particular challenge. Tell me more about what specifically feels impossible to you."

Why this works: Brief, relevant, builds rapport, normalizes her experience, and quickly refocuses on her needs. You shared to help her feel understood, not to tell your story.

Inappropriate disclosure:

Same situation, but instead:

You: "Oh, I totally understand. When my first child was born, it was a nightmare. My partner was completely unhelpful with childcare. I felt like I was doing everything—all the nighttime feedings, all the housework, and trying to work full-time. I was exhausted and resentful. Let me tell you about this huge fight we had about division of labor..."

Why this doesn't work: Too much detail, too long, focused on you rather than client, burdens client with your relationship problems, shifts focus from her experience to yours. This meets your needs (venting about your partner) rather than her needs.

Another inappropriate example:

Different client, Tom, discussing stress at work.

You: "I'm actually dealing with huge stress right now myself. My supervisor is making my life miserable. I'm thinking about filing a complaint but I'm worried about retaliation. It's affecting my sleep and my anxiety is through the roof. I shouldn't burden you with this, but it's really getting to me."

Why this doesn't work: You're seeking support from client, burdening them with your problems, reversing roles, and potentially making them worry about your ability to help them. This is clear boundary violation.

Handling disclosure requests from clients:

Client: "Are you married?"

You have options:

Answer briefly then explore: "Yes, I am. I'm curious what prompted that question. What are you wondering about?"

Explore first: "I'm wondering what prompted that question. What are you thinking about or wanting to know?"

Set boundary: "I prefer to keep focus on you rather than my personal life. Can you tell me what you're wondering about that made you ask?"

Choose based on therapeutic alliance, client needs, and whether disclosure serves therapeutic purpose. Sometimes answering simple factual questions builds rapport. Sometimes exploring the question is more therapeutically useful.

Self-disclosure in supervision and consultation:

In supervision or consultation (when you're the supervisee/consultee), appropriate self-disclosure helps learning. Sharing mistakes, uncertainties, and countertransference reactions allows supervisor to help you grow. This is different from therapy—supervision serves your professional development, making disclosure about your work appropriate and necessary.

But even in supervision, some boundaries exist. You don't burden supervisor with extensive personal problems unrelated to your work, though brief mention of life stressors affecting work performance is appropriate.

Practice Questions

1. Professional boundaries exist to:

A. Make therapists' lives easier
B. Protect clients from exploitation and maintain therapeutic frame
C. Create distance from clients
D. Follow arbitrary rules

2. The power differential in therapy means:

A. Therapists are superior people
B. Inherent imbalance makes exploitation possible even when relationship seems mutual
C. Clients have no power
D. Nothing significant

3. Sexual relationships with current clients are:

A. Acceptable if both consent
B. Absolutely prohibited with no exceptions
C. Fine after sufficient time
D. Therapist's choice

4. Boundary crossing differs from boundary violation in that crossing:

A. Is always harmful
B. Is minor, therapeutic deviation while violation is harmful exploitation
C. Is the same as violation
D. Doesn't matter

5. Multiple relationships are:

A. Always prohibited
B. Sometimes unavoidable; require careful management
C. Always fine
D. Only about sexual relationships

6. Social relationships with current clients:

A. Build rapport nicely
B. Generally undermine therapeutic relationship
C. Are encouraged
D. Don't affect therapy

7. In small communities, unavoidable multiple relationships require:

A. Immediate referral
B. Explicit discussion, clear boundaries, regular monitoring
C. Ignoring the issue
D. Treating everyone regardless

8. Accepting Facebook friend requests from clients:

A. Builds alliance
B. Generally should be declined to maintain boundaries
C. Is encouraged
D. Doesn't matter

9. If you accidentally see client information online:

A. Ignore it
B. Address it in session to maintain transparency
C. Use it therapeutically without mentioning
D. Punish the client

10. Searching for clients online:

A. Is always appropriate
B. Requires clear policy and clinical justification
C. Should be done constantly
D. Is always wrong

11. Your personal social media should:

A. Be completely uncensored
B. Consider that clients might see posts and maintain professionalism
C. Include all your opinions
D. Definitely connect with clients

12. Telehealth from home environments:

A. Eliminates all boundaries
B. Still requires professional boundaries despite personal spaces
C. Means casual relationships
D. Changes nothing

13. Self-disclosure is appropriate when:

A. You need support
B. It serves therapeutic purpose—normalizing, modeling, building rapport
C. You want to talk about yourself
D. Always

14. Appropriate self-disclosure is:

A. Long and detailed
B. Brief, relevant, focused on therapeutic purpose, then refocused on client
C. All about you
D. Constant

15. Inappropriate self-disclosure:

A. Serves client needs
B. Burdens client, meets therapist needs, overshadows client experience
C. Is brief
D. Never happens

16. Physical boundaries include:

A. No touch ever
B. Appropriate limited contact; sexual/romantic contact prohibited
C. Touch whenever
D. Only sexual contact limitations

17. Financial boundaries require:

A. Exploiting clients for money
B. Clear, fair fee arrangements without exploitation
C. Charging whatever you want
D. Free services always

18. Time and space boundaries:

A. Are flexible based on your needs
B. Maintain therapeutic frame through set times and professional spaces
C. Don't matter
D. Mean seeing clients anywhere

19. Emotional boundaries mean:

A. Being cold and distant
B. Providing empathy without becoming emotionally dependent on clients
C. No emotions allowed
D. Seeking support from clients

20. Role boundaries mean:

A. You can be friends after termination
B. Relationship exists for therapeutic purposes; you're not friends/partners/social connections
C. Multiple roles are fine
D. Roles don't matter

21. Transference and countertransference:

A. Should be acted on
B. Are normal and therapeutically useful but shouldn't be enacted through boundary violations
C. Mean you should date clients
D. Don't exist

22. The slippery slope of boundary violations means:

A. One violation means many
B. Violations develop through gradual erosion of boundaries
C. Slopes are dangerous
D. Nothing significant

23. Cultural considerations for boundaries:

A. Mean abandoning all boundaries
B. Require thoughtful adaptation while maintaining core protective functions
C. Don't matter
D. Mean identical boundaries for everyone

24. Business relationships with clients:

A. Are encouraged
B. Are generally prohibited due to conflicting interests
C. Build rapport
D. Don't affect therapy

25. Treating family members of current client:

A. Is ideal
B. Creates dual relationship requiring referral of family member usually
C. Helps everyone
D. Is required

26. Providing therapy to someone you supervise:

A. Is efficient
B. Creates problematic dual relationship; should refer
C. Is encouraged
D. Doesn't matter

27. When declining client's social media request:

A. Ignore it
B. Address directly in session explaining boundary policy
C. Accept then unfriend
D. Be angry

28. If client sees your controversial personal post:

A. Delete it quickly
B. Process how it affects therapeutic relationship
C. Blame the client
D. Ignore it

29. Concerning social media posts by client:

A. Are private; ignore them
B. Require action if you see them and they indicate danger
C. Are entertainment
D. Mean nothing

30. Managing your online presence means:

A. Never being online
B. Using privacy settings and being thoughtful about professional image
C. Posting whatever you want
D. Hiding everything

31. When client asks personal question:

A. Always answer
B. Consider therapeutic purpose; explore question or answer briefly
C. Never answer
D. Get angry

32. Burdening clients with your problems:

A. Builds rapport
B. Is inappropriate role reversal
C. Is helpful
D. Shows authenticity

33. Frequency of self-disclosure should be:

A. Constant
B. Infrequent and purposeful
C. Every session
D. Never

34. Depth of self-disclosure:

A. Should be very intimate
B. Should match therapeutic purpose; general not intimate
C. Doesn't matter
D. Should be extensive

35. After self-disclosing:

A. Keep talking about yourself
B. Explicitly redirect focus to client
C. Wait for client to support you
D. Change topics

36. Treating colleague's family member:

A. Is ideal—you know the family
B. Requires careful boundaries and might warrant referral
C. Should always be done
D. Is prohibited

37. What information is unavoidably disclosed:

A. Everything
B. Appearance, gender, approximate age, credentials, office setting
C. Nothing
D. Only name

38. Legitimate reason for self-disclosure includes:

A. Needing to vent
B. Modeling, normalizing, building rapport, offering hope
C. Making yourself feel important
D. Avoiding client's issues

39. "Who does this serve?" question helps determine:

A. Who pays
B. Whether disclosure serves therapeutic purpose or therapist needs
C. Who's in charge
D. Nothing useful

40. Clients will likely:

A. Never search for you online
B. Google you; assume online presence might be seen
C. Not care about you
D. Never use technology

Answer Key with Detailed Explanations

1. B. Protect clients from exploitation and maintain therapeutic frame
Professional boundaries exist to protect clients from exploitation given inherent power differential and to maintain therapeutic frame that allows vulnerable therapeutic work. They're not arbitrary rules or just for therapists' convenience—they serve essential protective and therapeutic functions. Boundaries create safe container where clients can be vulnerable, explore difficult material, and trust that relationship serves their needs.

2. B. Inherent imbalance makes exploitation possible even when relationship seems mutual
The power differential means therapist has expertise, authority, and knowledge while client is vulnerable and seeking help. This inherent imbalance makes exploitation possible even when both parties believe relationship is mutual and consensual. Clients' feelings toward therapists (transference) and vulnerable state mean true equality and mutuality aren't possible, which is why boundaries protecting against exploitation are essential.

3. B. Absolutely prohibited with no exceptions
Sexual relationships with current clients are absolutely prohibited with no exceptions regardless of consent, mutual attraction, or belief in "true love." The power differential, vulnerability, and transference make genuine consent impossible. This is among the clearest, most absolute ethical prohibitions. With former clients, prohibited for at least two years and discouraged even after.

4. B. Is minor, therapeutic deviation while violation is harmful exploitation
Boundary crossing is minor deviation from typical practice that's not harmful and may be therapeutically beneficial (attending client's art show when discussed and serving recovery). Boundary violation is harmful transgression exploiting power differential and serving therapist's needs (sexual relationship, financial exploitation). Crossings are intentional, therapeutic, and temporary; violations are harmful and self-serving.

5. B. Sometimes unavoidable; require careful management
Multiple relationships are sometimes unavoidable, particularly in small communities or specific settings. They require careful management—explicit discussion, clear boundaries, consultation, monitoring, and willingness to refer if problematic. Some multiple relationships are prohibited (sexual, exploitative business relationships). Others are unavoidable but manageable with thoughtful attention.

6. B. Generally undermine therapeutic relationship
Social relationships with current clients generally undermine therapeutic relationship by creating mutual expectations incompatible with one-way therapeutic focus. Friendships involve reciprocity, shared experiences, and mutual support—all conflicting with professional relationship that exists solely for client benefit. Professional relationship requires distance that social friendship undermines, making therapy less effective.

7. B. Explicit discussion, clear boundaries, regular monitoring
In small communities where some multiple relationships are unavoidable (same church, children in same school, shopping at same stores), manage through explicit discussion of how to handle encounters, clear boundaries about interactions in different contexts, regular monitoring of impact on therapy, and documentation. Referral might not be feasible if you're only provider. Management, not avoidance, becomes strategy.

8. B. Generally should be declined to maintain boundaries
Accepting Facebook friend requests from clients generally should be declined to maintain professional boundaries. Social media friendship means seeing each other's posts, photos, and personal lives, blurring boundaries necessary for effective therapy. Address requests directly in

session: "I appreciate you thinking of me, but I have policy of not connecting with clients on social media to maintain boundaries that help therapy work."

9. B. Address it in session to maintain transparency
If you accidentally see client information online (mutual friend's post showing client), address it in session to maintain transparency: "I want to mention I saw you in a friend's Facebook post. I wasn't looking for information about you, but I did see it. I don't want information I acquire outside sessions to affect our work without discussing it. How do you feel about my having seen that?" Transparency maintains trust.

10. B. Requires clear policy and clinical justification
Searching for clients online requires clear policy (do you do this? when? why?) and clinical justification (specific safety concerns, verification of information). Some therapists never search; others search only for legitimate clinical reasons and inform clients. Don't search out of curiosity or voyeurism. If you search, document clinical justification and what you found. Have consistent policy you communicate to clients.

11. B. Consider that clients might see posts and maintain professionalism
Your personal social media should consider that clients might see your posts (they will Google you and might find personal accounts). Maintain professionalism—even in personal posts, you represent the profession. Don't post discriminatory statements, unprofessional behavior, or content contradicting professional values. Use privacy settings, but assume anything online might be seen by clients.

12. B. Still requires professional boundaries despite personal spaces
Telehealth from home environments still requires professional boundaries despite both parties being in personal spaces. Use neutral backgrounds, ensure privacy, establish that home-based therapy doesn't mean casual relationship. Professional boundaries apply regardless of setting—virtual therapy is professional service, not casual video chat with friend.

13. B. It serves therapeutic purpose—normalizing, modeling, building rapport
Self-disclosure is appropriate when it serves therapeutic purpose: normalizing client's experience ("Many people experience this—even therapists"), modeling healthy behavior, building rapport, or offering hope. It's inappropriate when it meets therapist's needs (venting, seeking support), burdens client, or overshadows client's experience. Ask "Who does this serve?" to determine appropriateness.

14. B. Brief, relevant, focused on therapeutic purpose, then refocused on client
Appropriate self-disclosure is brief (not long detailed stories), relevant to client's issue (directly connected to what they're working on), focused on therapeutic purpose (serves their needs), and quickly refocused on client ("I mention this because it relates to your experience. What are your thoughts?"). Focus should remain primarily on client, with disclosure as brief therapeutic tool.

15. B. Burdens client, meets therapist needs, overshadows client experience
Inappropriate self-disclosure burdens client with therapist's problems, meets therapist's needs for support or validation, overshadows client's experience by making therapist the focus, creates obligation for client to respond supportively, or damages therapist's credibility. Any disclosure serving therapist's emotional needs rather than client's therapeutic needs is inappropriate boundary violation.

16. B. Appropriate limited contact; sexual/romantic contact prohibited
Physical boundaries allow appropriate limited contact (handshake, brief appropriate hug when client-initiated and culturally appropriate) while prohibiting sexual or romantic contact. Never-touch-ever is too rigid and culturally insensitive. But contact requires careful judgment about appropriateness, cultural meaning, potential for misinterpretation, and harm. Sexual/romantic contact is absolutely prohibited.

17. B. Clear, fair fee arrangements without exploitation
Financial boundaries require clear, fair fee arrangements without exploitation. You don't charge excessive fees, bill for services not rendered, pressure clients to purchase products, or create financial dependencies. Money in therapeutic relationships requires careful attention to power differential and potential exploitation. Fees should be transparent, fair, and consistently maintained.

18. B. Maintain therapeutic frame through set times and professional spaces
Time and space boundaries maintain therapeutic frame through set session times (start and end), professional spaces (office, not personal homes typically), and appropriate availability (within professional parameters, not 24/7 personal availability). These boundaries create predictable, safe structure for therapeutic work and distinguish professional relationship from personal ones.

19. B. Providing empathy without becoming emotionally dependent on clients
Emotional boundaries mean providing empathy and care without becoming emotionally dependent on clients or seeking emotional support from them. Emotional investment flows toward client benefit, not toward meeting your needs. You don't burden clients with your feelings or problems. You maintain professional emotional distance while offering genuine empathy and therapeutic care.

20. B. Relationship exists for therapeutic purposes; you're not friends/partners/social connections
Role boundaries mean the relationship exists solely for therapeutic purposes—you're therapist, client is client. You don't become friends, romantic partners, business associates, or social connections. Professional role continues even after therapy ends to some degree (power differential persists). The relationship serves client's therapeutic needs exclusively.

21. B. Are normal and therapeutically useful but shouldn't be enacted through boundary violations
Transference (client's feelings toward you based on past relationships) and countertransference (your feelings toward client based on your history) are normal therapeutic phenomena that provide useful clinical information. But acting on these feelings through boundary violations (sexual relationship, seeking personal connection) transforms helpful therapeutic dynamics into harmful exploitation. You work with these feelings therapeutically, not enact them.

22. B. Violations develop through gradual erosion of boundaries
The slippery slope means boundary violations rarely happen suddenly—they develop through gradual erosion. Small crossings become bigger, rationalizations accumulate, self-awareness decreases. Therapist who ends up sexually involved with client usually started with seemingly minor boundary crossings that progressively escalated. Preventing violations requires vigilance about each crossing and consulting about boundary decisions.

23. B. Require thoughtful adaptation while maintaining core protective functions
Cultural considerations require thoughtful adaptation of boundaries while maintaining core protective functions. Appropriate boundaries vary across cultures (gift-giving, physical touch, personal-professional separation). Cultural responsiveness doesn't mean abandoning boundaries—it means learning cultural norms, discussing boundaries explicitly with clients from different backgrounds, and adapting practices to be culturally appropriate while protecting clients.

24. B. Are generally prohibited due to conflicting interests
Business relationships with clients are generally prohibited because financial interests conflict with therapeutic relationship. You don't employ clients, enter business ventures with them, or create financial dependencies beyond therapeutic fees. Exception might be extremely limited unavoidable transactions in small communities when no exploitation exists and relationship is monitored, but business relationships generally violate boundaries.

25. B. Creates dual relationship requiring referral of family member usually
Treating family members of current client creates dual relationship—you know things about each that affect therapy with the other, loyalty conflicts arise, confidentiality becomes complex. Generally, refer family members to other providers. Some family therapists navigate this intentionally, but individual therapists typically avoid treating multiple family members.

26. B. Creates problematic dual relationship; should refer
Providing therapy to someone you supervise creates problematic dual relationship—power dynamics conflict (supervisor/employee and therapist/client), supervisee can't be vulnerable in therapy with supervisor, evaluation responsibility conflicts with therapeutic relationship. If supervisee needs mental health services, refer to another provider. Don't combine supervisory and therapeutic roles.

27. B. Address directly in session explaining boundary policy
When declining client's social media request, address it directly in session rather than ignoring (feels rejecting): "I received your friend request. I appreciate you thinking of me, but I have policy of not connecting with clients on social media to maintain boundaries that help therapy work effectively. This isn't about you personally—it's professional policy. I hope you understand." Document explanation and response.

28. B. Process how it affects therapeutic relationship
If client sees your controversial personal post, process how it affects therapeutic relationship: "I understand you saw my post about [topic]. My personal views are my opinions and don't affect how I work with clients. But if seeing that post has made you uncomfortable or affected how safe you feel in therapy, let's address that. Would you prefer working with someone whose personal views you don't know about?" Address impact on therapeutic relationship directly.

29. B. Require action if you see them and they indicate danger
Concerning social media posts by clients (appearing to be suicide note, threats of violence) require action if you see them and they indicate danger. You can't ignore safety concerns just because information came through social media. Contact client immediately, ensure safety, potentially initiate emergency intervention. Then discuss boundaries around social media and how you'll handle concerning posts you happen to see.

30. B. Using privacy settings and being thoughtful about professional image
Managing your online presence means using privacy settings to control visibility, being thoughtful about professional image (remembering you represent the profession even in personal posts), and recognizing that clients will Google you and might find your social media. Completely private social media keeps personal separate. Public social media means accepting clients will see posts. Be intentional about online presence.

31. B. Consider therapeutic purpose; explore question or answer briefly
When client asks personal question, consider therapeutic purpose. You might explore first ("What prompts that question?"), answer briefly then explore ("Yes, I'm married. What made you wonder about that?"), or set boundary ("I prefer to keep focus on you. What are you wondering about?"). Choose based on alliance, client needs, and whether disclosure serves therapeutic purpose. Not all personal questions require answers.

32. B. Is inappropriate role reversal
Burdening clients with your problems ("I'm dealing with terrible divorce," "My anxiety is through the roof") is inappropriate role reversal where client becomes your supporter. This meets your needs rather than serving client's therapy, violates boundaries by making them responsible for your emotional state, and damages therapeutic relationship. Clients are there to be helped, not to help you.

33. B. Infrequent and purposeful
Frequency of self-disclosure should be infrequent and purposeful. Constantly sharing personal experiences shifts focus from client to you. Save disclosure for moments when it will genuinely help—normalizing, modeling, building rapport. Infrequent disclosure is more powerful because it stands out and clearly serves therapeutic purpose rather than being routine chat about yourself.

34. B. Should match therapeutic purpose; general not intimate
Depth of self-disclosure should match therapeutic purpose—share general information, not intimate details. "I've experienced anxiety" serves normalizing purpose. Detailed account of your anxiety episodes and personal struggles is excessive. Depth should be minimal necessary to achieve therapeutic goal. Deeper disclosure requires stronger justification of therapeutic benefit.

35. B. Explicitly redirect focus to client
After self-disclosing, explicitly redirect focus to client: "I mention this because I think it relates to your experience. What are your thoughts?" or "That's my experience, but I want to hear more about yours." You share briefly, then immediately return focus to client. Don't wait for them to support you or continue discussing your experience—proactively shift back to their needs.

36. B. Requires careful boundaries and might warrant referral
Treating colleague's family member requires careful boundaries—separate professional relationship from colleague relationship, manage information carefully, avoid dual loyalty conflicts. Often warrants referral to avoid complications. If you proceed, discuss explicitly how you'll manage the dual relationship, obtain clear consent, and monitor carefully for problems. When feasible, referral is cleaner solution.

37. B. Appearance, gender, approximate age, credentials, office setting
Information unavoidably disclosed includes observable characteristics—your appearance, gender presentation, approximate age, name, credentials displayed in office, office location and setting, professional background, photographs or objects in office. Clients observe this information whether you intentionally share it or not. This is different from deliberate disclosure of personal experiences or intimate information.

38. B. Modeling, normalizing, building rapport, offering hope
Legitimate therapeutic reasons for self-disclosure include: modeling healthy behavior, normalizing client's experience, building rapport when alliance is weak, offering hope through shared recovery experience, or demonstrating understanding. These serve client's therapeutic needs. Needing to vent, making yourself feel important, or avoiding client's issues are inappropriate reasons serving your needs.

39. B. Whether disclosure serves therapeutic purpose or therapist needs
"Who does this serve?" question helps determine whether disclosure serves therapeutic purpose (client's needs—normalizing, modeling, rapport) or therapist needs (venting, seeking support, validation). If answer is "this serves my need to talk about myself" or "this makes me feel important," disclosure is inappropriate. If answer is "this helps client feel less alone" or "this models healthy coping," it might be appropriate.

40. B. Google you; assume online presence might be seen
Clients will likely Google you—this is normal and expected. Assume your online presence (professional website, social media with inadequate privacy settings, public posts) might be seen by clients. Manage online presence accordingly—privacy settings for personal accounts, professional boundaries maintained even in personal posts, recognition that anything online might eventually be accessed by clients. Don't post things you'd be uncomfortable with clients seeing.

The Art of Appropriate Distance

Boundaries aren't walls—they're membranes. They allow appropriate connection while maintaining necessary distance. Too rigid and you're cold, disconnected, unable to build rapport. Too loose and you risk exploitation, role confusion, and therapeutic ineffectiveness.

The art is finding the right distance for each client, each situation, each cultural context. Some clients need more formal boundaries to feel safe. Others need warmer, more personally engaged relationships to trust. You adapt while maintaining core protective functions.

What helps is understanding why boundaries exist. They're not about being rigid or unfriendly. They're about keeping clients safe from exploitation, maintaining the therapeutic frame that allows vulnerable work, and ensuring the relationship serves client needs rather than yours.

When you're uncertain about boundaries—whether to accept a gift, how to handle running into client at community event, whether specific self-disclosure is appropriate—consultation helps. Outside perspective from supervisor or colleague provides clarity when you're too close to the situation to judge objectively.

Technology creates ongoing challenges. New platforms, new ways of connecting, new information accessible—each requires thoughtful consideration of boundary implications. The core principles remain constant: maintain professional relationship, protect clients, serve therapeutic purposes. How you apply these principles evolves with changing technology.

You'll make mistakes. Everyone does. When you recognize boundary error—disclosed too much, accepted invitation you shouldn't have, let relationship drift toward social rather than professional—acknowledge it, repair what you can, restore appropriate boundaries, learn from experience, and get consultation.

Boundaries ultimately serve love for clients. Not romantic love—professional love that says "Your welfare matters more than my comfort, my needs, my preferences." That love requires distance, limits, and sometimes disappointing clients by maintaining boundaries they wish you'd cross. It's love that protects rather than gratifies. That's the heart of appropriate professional boundaries.

Essential Boundary Understanding

- Professional boundaries protect clients from exploitation and maintain therapeutic frame, not arbitrary rules but essential protective functions
- Power differential makes exploitation possible even when relationship seems mutual, requiring clear boundaries preventing harm
- Sexual relationships with current clients absolutely prohibited; with former clients prohibited minimum two years and discouraged after
- Boundary crossings are minor therapeutic deviations; violations are harmful exploitations serving therapist rather than client needs
- Multiple relationships sometimes unavoidable requiring explicit discussion, clear boundaries, monitoring, and willingness to refer if problematic
- Social media connections with clients generally should be declined; have clear policy about online presence and client access
- Searching for clients online requires clinical justification and clear policy; address information you accidentally encounter
- Self-disclosure appropriate when serving therapeutic purpose (normalizing, modeling, rapport) not when meeting therapist's needs
- Appropriate disclosure is brief, relevant, quickly refocused on client; inappropriate disclosure burdens client or overshadows their experience
- Cultural considerations require adapting boundaries thoughtfully while maintaining core protective functions
- Role boundaries mean relationship exists for therapeutic purposes; you're not friends, partners, or social connections

- Transference and countertransference are therapeutically useful but shouldn't be enacted through boundary violations
- Small community multiple relationships managed through explicit discussion, clear encounter guidelines, and regular monitoring
- Technology requires ongoing boundary attention as new platforms create new connection opportunities and information access
- When uncertain about boundaries, consultation provides outside perspective for objective judgment and ethical decision-making

Chapter 16: Professional Development and Self-Care

Nobody tells you this in school: this work will change you. You'll carry pieces of clients' stories home. You'll lie awake thinking about the teenager who disclosed abuse today. You'll feel the weight of someone's suicidal crisis on your shoulders. You'll absorb trauma, witness suffering, and hold pain that isn't yours but affects you nonetheless.

And here's the other thing they don't emphasize enough: you can't pour from an empty cup. Burned-out, traumatized, exhausted therapists can't help anyone. Self-care isn't luxury or selfishness—it's ethical obligation. You owe it to your clients to be well enough to serve them effectively.

Professional development and self-care aren't separate concerns—they're intertwined. Ongoing learning keeps you competent and engaged. Supervision provides support and perspective. Cultural competence ensures you serve diverse clients effectively. Burnout prevention protects your capacity to continue this work. Your professional identity evolves throughout your career, shaped by experiences, learning, and intentional growth.

This chapter is about sustaining yourself for the long haul. Because this work is marathon, not sprint. The clients who need you ten years from now deserve a therapist who's still well, still learning, still capable. That requires intentional attention to development and care starting now.

Supervision and Consultation

Supervision isn't just for students and new professionals. It's career-long resource for learning, support, ethical guidance, and maintaining perspective. Even experienced practitioners benefit from outside perspective on complex cases, ethical dilemmas, and their own blind spots.

Types of supervision:

Administrative supervision: Focuses on job performance, productivity, adherence to agency policies, and employment-related issues. Your administrative supervisor evaluates your work, assigns cases, and addresses personnel matters. Required in most employment settings.

Clinical supervision: Focuses on clinical skill development, case conceptualization, intervention strategies, and professional growth. Clinical supervisor helps you become more effective therapist through teaching, feedback, and support. May be same person as administrative supervisor or separate.

Licensure supervision: Required for licensure in most states. Specified number of hours (typically 2000-4000) under qualified supervisor meeting state requirements. Focuses on developing competencies required for independent practice. Structured, documented, and must meet specific regulatory standards.

Peer supervision: Consultation among colleagues at similar experience level. No hierarchical evaluative relationship—mutual support and learning. Group of peers meets regularly to discuss cases, share resources, and provide perspective. Valuable throughout career.

Functions of supervision:

Education and skill development: Supervisor teaches theory, techniques, and interventions. You learn through instruction, demonstration, observation, and feedback. Supervision fills gaps in your knowledge and builds specific competencies.

Support and encouragement: This work is hard. Supervision provides space to process difficult feelings, celebrate successes, and receive encouragement. Supervisor validates struggles while helping you develop resilience.

Case consultation: Discussing cases provides fresh perspective. When you're stuck, supervisor helps you see options you've missed. Complex cases benefit from collaborative thinking.

Ethical guidance: Supervisors help navigate ethical dilemmas, identify ethical issues you might miss, and think through appropriate responses. They provide ethical reasoning models and support ethical decision-making.

Quality assurance: Supervisors monitor quality of care clients receive. They identify problems early, provide corrective feedback, and ensure clients are well-served. This protects clients and helps you improve.

Professional socialization: Supervisors model professional behavior, help you develop professional identity, and guide you through professional culture and expectations.

What makes supervision effective:

Regular, consistent meetings: Weekly or biweekly sessions scheduled consistently. Not just crisis management—regular contact allows ongoing learning and relationship building.

Clear expectations: Both parties understand supervision purpose, what will be discussed, how feedback will be given, evaluation criteria, and documentation requirements. Written supervision contract clarifies expectations.

Safe environment: You can discuss mistakes, uncertainties, and struggles without fear of punishment. Supervisor creates atmosphere where vulnerability and learning are possible.

Appropriate boundaries: Supervision isn't therapy. While personal issues affecting work are discussed, supervision focuses on professional development. If your personal issues require therapeutic attention, supervisor helps you access appropriate resources.

Constructive feedback: Balance of affirmation and correction. Strengths are recognized, areas for growth identified clearly. Feedback is specific, behavioral, and actionable—not vague criticism.

Cultural humility: Supervisor acknowledges limits of their cultural knowledge, learns from supervisee's experiences, and helps develop cultural competence without imposing supervisor's cultural values.

Theoretical framework: Supervisor articulates their theoretical orientation and helps you develop yours. May be similar approaches or intentionally different to broaden perspective.

Your responsibilities as supervisee:

Preparation: Come prepared with cases to discuss, questions formulated, and relevant documentation. Don't waste supervision time being disorganized.

Honesty: Disclose mistakes, uncertainties, and concerns. Hiding problems prevents learning and potentially harms clients. Supervision only works if you're honest.

Openness to feedback: Receive feedback non-defensively. Consider supervisor's perspective even when it's uncomfortable. You don't have to agree with everything, but remain open to learning.

Implementation: Try suggestions and interventions supervisor recommends. Report back on results. Learning happens through doing, not just discussing.

Self-awareness: Reflect on your reactions, patterns, and areas for growth. Bring observations about yourself to supervision for exploration.

Ethical practice: Adhere to ethical standards, discuss ethical concerns, and seek guidance on dilemmas. Take ethics seriously.

When supervision isn't working:

Incompatibility: Sometimes personalities, styles, or approaches don't mesh. If relationship is unproductive despite good-faith efforts, discuss openly. Consider whether different supervisor would serve better.

Inadequate supervision: Supervisor cancels frequently, provides vague unhelpful feedback, or doesn't address your learning needs. Document concerns and raise them with supervisor or administrator.

Unethical supervision: Supervisor violates boundaries, provides inadequate supervision while documenting adequate hours, or behaves unethically. Report through appropriate channels—licensing board, professional organization, agency administration.

Beyond required supervision:

Voluntary consultation: Seek consultation beyond required supervision. Consult about complex cases, ethical dilemmas, new populations, or unfamiliar situations. Consultation is strength, not weakness.

Peer consultation groups: Join or form group of colleagues meeting regularly for mutual consultation. Rich learning happens through peer discussion. Different perspectives expand thinking.

Specialized consultation: For specialized issues (trauma, eating disorders, specific populations), consult with experts. Brief consultation with specialist provides guidance for cases outside your typical expertise.

Case Example: Effective Supervision - Sarah's Development

Sarah, newly licensed social worker in community mental health, meets weekly with clinical supervisor Dr. Martinez.

Week 1 - Establishing relationship:

Dr. Martinez: "Let's talk about how we'll structure our supervision. I see my role as helping you develop clinical skills, providing support, ensuring quality care for clients, and helping you navigate ethical issues. What do you hope to get from supervision?"

Sarah: "I want to get better at case conceptualization. I struggle to see patterns and formulate treatment plans. I also want support with difficult cases—I carry them home sometimes."

Dr. Martinez: "Good goals. We'll focus on both skill development and support. Bring cases you're struggling with, and we'll work through conceptualization together. We'll also discuss how you're managing emotionally. I'll give direct feedback—both strengths and areas to develop. I want this to feel safe for you to discuss mistakes and uncertainties. Questions?"

They establish structure: Sarah brings two cases weekly, they review one video-recorded session monthly, they discuss professional development goals quarterly. Clear expectations are set.

Week 4 - Working with difficult case:

Sarah presents Marcus, client with paranoid thinking making treatment challenging.

Sarah: "I don't know what to do with Marcus. He thinks I'm conspiring with his family against him. Nothing I say helps."

Dr. Martinez: "Tell me more about the pattern. What happens specifically?"

Sarah describes interactions. Dr. Martinez helps her see: Sarah's reassurance increases Marcus's suspicion because it mirrors what conspirators would say. Alternative approach—validation without reassurance.

Dr. Martinez: "What if instead of reassuring him you're not conspiring, you validated: 'When you're worried people are working against you, that must feel frightening. Let's talk about what would help you feel safer here.' You're not confirming or denying—you're validating the feeling and problem-solving."

Sarah tries this. Next week, she reports it helped. Marcus was less suspicious when she validated rather than reassured. This small success builds Sarah's confidence and skills.

Week 8 - Addressing mistake:

Sarah discloses she forgot to file mandated abuse report for 48 hours after hearing concerning information.

Sarah: "I messed up. Client disclosed her boyfriend hit her child two days ago. I documented it but forgot to call CPS. I just called this morning. I'm worried I'll get in trouble."

Dr. Martinez: "I appreciate your honesty in telling me. Let's address this. First, you've now made the report—good. Document exactly when you learned the information, when you reported, and why there was delay. Second, let's understand what happened. How did you forget something this important?"

Sarah: "I was overwhelmed. I had crisis with another client right after that session. Then I got caught up in documentation and it slipped my mind."

Dr. Martinez: "This tells us you need better systems for tracking mandated reports. Let's develop a protocol—maybe flagging these in your notes immediately, setting reminder on your phone, telling supervisor same day. We also need to address your being overwhelmed. How can you manage crises without forgetting critical responsibilities?"

They problem-solve systems for tracking reports and managing overwhelming days. Dr. Martinez documents the incident but frames it as learning opportunity, not punitive action. Sarah develops better systems and learns from the mistake.

Week 15 - Recognizing burnout signs:

Dr. Martinez notices Sarah seems exhausted and disengaged.

Dr. Martinez: "I'm concerned about you. You seem tired, you're less engaged in supervision, and you mentioned feeling numb with clients. What's happening?"

Sarah: "I don't know. I just feel depleted. I'm dreading work. Clients' stories all blend together. I know I should care but I feel nothing."

Dr. Martinez: "Those are burnout warning signs. Let's address this seriously. What's your self-care like?"

Sarah admits she's not exercising, eating poorly, sleeping poorly, and bringing work home constantly. No boundaries between work and personal life.

Dr. Martinez: "We need to rebuild your capacity. First, immediate changes: no work at home for two weeks. Use your PTO—take long weekend. Restart exercise even if brief. Second, let's look at your caseload. Are you seeing too many high-acuity clients? Third, we'll discuss your emotional processing. How are you managing what you hear in sessions?"

They develop plan for recovering from burnout. Dr. Martinez reduces Sarah's caseload temporarily, helps her set boundaries, and works with her on emotional processing strategies. Over weeks, Sarah's engagement returns.

Month 9 - Professional growth:

Sarah has developed significantly. Dr. Martinez notices improved case conceptualization, better boundaries, more confidence.

Dr. Martinez: "I want to give you feedback on your growth. Nine months ago, you struggled with conceptualization and carried too much home. Now you're formulating cases well, setting appropriate boundaries, and managing emotional impact better. I see real development. Where do you see yourself?"

Sarah: "I feel more competent. I still have lots to learn, but I trust my judgment more. I can recognize when I need help. I'm managing the work better."

Dr. Martinez: "That self-awareness is professional maturity. What's your next learning edge?"

Sarah: "I want to develop trauma-focused skills. I'm seeing more trauma cases and I feel underprepared."

Dr. Martinez: "Good goal. Let's plan training in evidence-based trauma treatment. Meanwhile, I can teach you some basics, and you can start with less complex trauma cases with close supervision."

This supervision relationship demonstrates key elements: regular consistent meetings, clear structure, safety for vulnerability, constructive feedback, support through difficulties, skill development, and attention to both clinical growth and personal well-being.

Cultural Competence in Practice

Cultural competence isn't achieved through single training or reading books about different cultures. It's ongoing process of learning, self-examination, humility, and adaptation. You never fully arrive—you continuously develop cultural responsiveness.

Dimensions of culture:

Culture extends beyond race and ethnicity. It includes:

Race and ethnicity: Shared ancestry, physical characteristics, cultural traditions, historical experiences. Racism and discrimination affect mental health and help-seeking.

National origin and immigration status: Where people are from, immigration experiences, acculturation stress, language barriers, documentation concerns.

Religion and spirituality: Beliefs, practices, values, community, meaning-making systems, views of suffering and healing.

Socioeconomic status: Income, education, occupation, access to resources. Class affects worldview, opportunities, and stressors.

Gender identity and expression: How people understand and express gender. Transgender, non-binary, gender-nonconforming individuals face unique stressors and discrimination.

Sexual orientation: Lesbian, gay, bisexual, pansexual, asexual orientations. LGBTQ+ individuals experience minority stress and discrimination.

Disability: Physical, sensory, cognitive, psychiatric disabilities. Disability culture, ableism, accessibility issues.

Age: Developmental stage, generational experiences, cohort effects. Ageism affects older and younger individuals differently.

Geographic region: Urban, rural, regional differences in culture, values, and resources.

Professional culture: Healthcare culture, academic culture, corporate culture—each has norms and values.

People hold multiple cultural identities simultaneously. A Black lesbian woman with disability experiences intersection of racism, homophobia, sexism, and ableism. Intersectionality means cultural identities interact in complex ways.

Cultural humility:

Cultural humility is more realistic goal than cultural competence. Humility recognizes:

You can't know everything: Cultures are diverse, individuals vary within cultures, and cultural knowledge constantly evolves. You can't become expert on every culture.

Clients are experts on their experience: They know their culture, their identity, their experience better than you ever will. Learn from them.

Self-examination is ongoing: Your cultural values, biases, and assumptions affect your work. Continuous self-reflection helps you recognize and address them.

Power imbalances exist: Therapist-client relationship involves power differential often compounded by racial, class, or other cultural power differences. Acknowledge and address power dynamics.

Lifelong learning: Cultural competence is never complete. Each client teaches you something. Each experience expands understanding.

Developing cultural competence:

Self-awareness: Examine your cultural identity—what groups you belong to, what values you hold, what privileges or disadvantages you experience, what biases you carry. How does your culture shape your worldview? What assumptions do you make?

Reflection questions:

- What is my cultural background and how has it shaped me?
- What privileges do I have? What experiences of marginalization?
- What stereotypes or biases do I hold about groups different from mine?
- How do my values about family, communication, independence, emotional expression come from my culture?
- What makes me uncomfortable or defensive when discussing culture?

Knowledge acquisition: Learn about cultures you work with—history, values, traditions, communication styles, help-seeking patterns, experiences of discrimination. Read books written by people from these cultures, attend cultural events, engage with diverse communities.

But avoid stereotyping. Knowledge about cultures provides general understanding—individuals vary enormously within cultures. Don't assume.

Skill development: Adapt assessment and intervention to be culturally responsive. This might include:

- Using interpreters effectively when language barriers exist
- Adapting communication style (direct vs. indirect, formal vs. informal)
- Involving family appropriately given cultural values
- Understanding different expressions of distress

- Adapting evidence-based treatments to cultural context
- Addressing experiences of discrimination and oppression
- Recognizing cultural strengths and resilience

Culturally adapted interventions: Research shows culturally adapted interventions are more effective than standard treatments for some populations. Adaptations might include:

- Surface structure changes (language, images, examples that reflect client's culture)
- Deep structure changes (cultural values, worldview, explanatory models of illness incorporated into treatment)
- Involving cultural healers or community resources
- Addressing culturally specific stressors (immigration, discrimination, acculturation)

Addressing microaggressions: Microaggressions are brief, commonplace indignities communicating hostile or derogatory messages to people from marginalized groups. Examples:

"Where are you really from?" (assumes non-white person isn't American)
"You're so articulate" (surprise that person of color is articulate)
"I don't see color" (denial of racial identity and experiences)
Clutching purse when Black man approaches (assumption of criminality)
"That's so gay" as insult (homophobia)

In therapy, microaggressions from you harm clients and damage trust. If you commit microaggression:

1. **Acknowledge it**: "I realize what I just said was problematic."
2. **Apologize genuinely**: "I apologize. That was hurtful."
3. **Learn**: "Help me understand how that affected you."
4. **Change behavior**: Don't repeat the microaggression.

Organizational cultural competence: Individual competence isn't enough. Agencies must be culturally responsive:

- Diverse staff reflecting communities served
- Multilingual services and materials
- Culturally appropriate assessment tools
- Policies addressing discrimination
- Cultural competence training for all staff

- Community partnerships with cultural organizations
- Accessible locations and hours
- Culturally responsive treatment models

Advocate for organizational changes supporting cultural competence.

Case Example: Cultural Humility - Dr. Thompson's Learning

Dr. Thompson, white therapist in urban clinic, works with Fatima, 24-year-old Muslim woman of Somali heritage, for anxiety and depression.

Session 3 - Recognizing cultural assumptions:

Dr. Thompson asks about Fatima's support system.

Dr. Thompson: "You mentioned you live with your parents. At 24, have you thought about moving out and establishing independence?"

Fatima looks uncomfortable: "In my culture, women typically live with family until marriage. Moving out alone wouldn't be appropriate."

Dr. Thompson realizes her question reflected Western individualist values assuming independence means living alone. In Fatima's collectivist culture, living with family is normative and valued, not sign of dependence.

Dr. Thompson: "I apologize. I made assumption based on my cultural values about independence. In your culture, how is young adulthood typically navigated? I want to understand your experience, not impose my values."

Fatima explains cultural norms. Dr. Thompson learns and adjusts her understanding of Fatima's situation. The assumed "problem" (living with parents) isn't a problem—it's cultural norm.

Session 5 - Addressing discrimination experiences:

Fatima describes constant experiences of Islamophobia—being followed in stores, having hijab pulled by stranger, hearing anti-Muslim comments.

Dr. Thompson: "That must be exhausting and frightening. How does this affect your anxiety?"

Fatima: "It's part of why I'm anxious. I'm always alert, always worried. But I feel like I shouldn't complain. Other people have it worse."

Dr. Thompson: "The constant vigilance required to stay safe in face of discrimination absolutely contributes to anxiety. This isn't you being oversensitive—it's rational response to real danger. Your anxiety makes sense given what you face. How can we address both the anxiety symptoms and the discrimination causing them?"

They discuss coping with discrimination, connecting to Muslim community for support, and whether political advocacy might provide sense of control. Dr. Thompson recognizes that treating Fatima's anxiety without acknowledging discrimination context would be incomplete.

Session 8 - Adapting treatment:

Dr. Thompson planned to use standard CBT for anxiety. She realizes adaptations are needed.

Dr. Thompson: "I'm thinking about treatment approach. Standard anxiety treatment might include gradually facing feared situations. But some of your fears are realistic—you really might face Islamophobia in certain places. How do we distinguish realistic caution from excessive anxiety?"

Fatima: "Exactly. I worry about that too."

Dr. Thompson: "Let's work on this together. We'll identify situations where anxiety is disproportionate to actual risk versus situations where caution is warranted. We'll develop skills for managing unavoidable discrimination while also reducing unnecessary anxiety. Does that fit for you?"

This adapted approach acknowledges that safety concerns for Muslim woman are different from general anxiety—treatment must account for realistic discrimination while addressing symptoms that interfere with functioning.

Session 12 - Consulting with cultural resource:

Dr. Thompson realizes she doesn't understand Islamic views on mental health well enough to work effectively with Fatima.

Dr. Thompson: "I want to provide best care for you. I realize I don't fully understand how Islamic faith and Somali culture view mental health and healing. Would you be open to me consulting with Imam or cultural consultant to better understand? With your permission, of course."

Fatima appreciates this. Dr. Thompson (with Fatima's written consent) consults with Imam familiar with mental health issues. She learns about Islamic perspectives on suffering, healing, and the role of faith in recovery. This deepens her understanding and helps her integrate Fatima's faith into treatment.

Session 16 - Involving family:

Dr. Thompson learns that in Fatima's culture, involving family in important decisions is expected. Individual therapy without family involvement might seem strange or inappropriate.

Dr. Thompson: "Would it be helpful to include your family in some sessions? In your culture, how is healing typically approached—individually or with family involvement?"

Fatima: "Family is important. But I don't want them to know everything we discuss."

Dr. Thompson: "We can involve family in ways that work for you. Maybe one or two sessions where we discuss general treatment goals and how they can support you, without sharing everything we talk about privately. What feels right?"

They involve Fatima's mother and sister in two family sessions focused on psychoeducation about anxiety and family support strategies. This honors cultural values while maintaining appropriate individual therapy space.

Outcome:

Through cultural humility—recognizing her limitations, learning from Fatima, consulting with cultural resources, adapting treatment—Dr. Thompson provides more effective culturally responsive care. Fatima's anxiety improves, and she feels understood in her cultural context, not judged by Western individualist standards.

This example demonstrates cultural humility in action: acknowledging assumptions, apologizing for microaggressions, learning from client, consulting with cultural resources, adapting treatment, involving family appropriately, and addressing discrimination as mental health factor.

Vicarious Trauma and Burnout Prevention

This work extracts a toll. Hearing traumatic stories day after day affects you. Witnessing human suffering, absorbing others' pain, carrying the weight of responsibility—these change you. Without attention to self-care and trauma exposure, you risk vicarious trauma and burnout.

Vicarious trauma (also called secondary traumatic stress or compassion fatigue) is trauma resulting from exposure to others' traumatic experiences. Through empathic engagement with clients' trauma, you experience trauma symptoms yourself even though traumatic events didn't happen to you directly.

Symptoms of vicarious trauma:

Intrusion: Intrusive thoughts about clients' trauma, nightmares featuring clients' experiences, difficulty separating your life from clients' lives, preoccupation with trauma stories.

Avoidance: Avoiding trauma clients, emotional numbing during sessions, disconnecting from clients' emotions, avoiding your own emotions.

Hyperarousal: Increased anxiety, startle response, difficulty sleeping, irritability, difficulty concentrating.

Cognitive changes: Changed worldview (believing world is dangerous, people can't be trusted), loss of hope, difficulty maintaining relationships, questioning meaning and purpose.

Emotional changes: Sadness, grief, anger, guilt (about your privileges, about not doing enough), helplessness, decreased empathy.

Behavioral changes: Increased substance use, social withdrawal, difficulty maintaining boundaries, risky behaviors, compulsive behaviors.

Burnout differs from vicarious trauma. Burnout is physical, emotional, and mental exhaustion resulting from prolonged stress. Not specific to trauma work—any high-stress helping profession risks burnout.

Components of burnout:

Emotional exhaustion: Feeling drained, depleted, unable to give more. Compassion fatigue—difficulty mustering empathy.

Depersonalization: Cynical, detached, negative attitudes toward clients. Seeing clients as objects or problems rather than people. Dark humor, callousness.

Reduced personal accomplishment: Feeling ineffective, questioning competence, doubting whether your work makes difference.

Risk factors for vicarious trauma and burnout:

Work factors:

- High caseload, especially trauma-heavy caseload
- Lack of control over work conditions
- Inadequate support and supervision
- Vicarious traumatization of colleagues (organizational trauma)
- Unclear expectations and role ambiguity
- Limited resources

Personal factors:

- Personal trauma history (not necessarily disqualifying but increases vulnerability)
- Difficulty setting boundaries
- Perfectionism and self-criticism
- Isolation—limited social support
- Poor self-care
- Over-identification with clients

Protective factors:

Professional:

- Regular supervision providing support and perspective
- Peer support and consultation
- Balanced caseload (not all high-acuity or trauma cases)
- Sense of control over work
- Clear role expectations
- Adequate resources
- Work-life balance with clear boundaries

Personal:

- Strong social support network
- Healthy relationships
- Activities outside work providing meaning and joy
- Self-awareness and willingness to address personal issues
- Realistic expectations (can't save everyone, can't eliminate all suffering)
- Spirituality or meaning-making framework
- Good physical health and self-care

Preventing vicarious trauma and burnout:

Professional boundaries: Leave work at work. No charts at home. Limited after-hours availability. Separate work and personal life physically and mentally.

Supervision and consultation: Process difficult cases. Discuss emotional impact. Get support. Supervision isn't just about skills—it's about processing what you carry.

Balanced caseload: Don't see only trauma cases or highest-acuity clients. Mix of client types and severity provides balance. If you specialize in trauma, ensure breaks and diversity.

Peer support: Talk with colleagues who understand. Shared experience validates struggles and reduces isolation.

Personal therapy: Many therapists benefit from their own therapy. Processing your reactions, addressing personal issues, and experiencing being a client enhances both well-being and clinical skills.

Physical self-care:

- Adequate sleep (7-9 hours)

- Regular exercise (proven to reduce stress and improve mood)
- Healthy nutrition
- Limit substance use
- Medical care when needed

Emotional and spiritual self-care:

- Activities bringing joy (hobbies, creative pursuits, time in nature)
- Connection with others (friends, family, community)
- Meaning-making practices (spirituality, religion, philosophy, activism)
- Mindfulness and meditation
- Gratitude practices

Cognitive self-care:

- Continuing education keeping you engaged
- Reading for pleasure
- Intellectual stimulation outside work
- Creative expression
- Limiting exposure to additional trauma (media, disturbing content)

Organizational responsibility: Organizations should support worker well-being through:

- Manageable caseloads
- Adequate supervision
- Trauma-informed organizational practices
- Mental health resources for staff
- Work-life balance policies
- Cultural appreciation not just accommodation

When you're experiencing vicarious trauma or burnout:

Recognize it early: Don't wait until you're completely depleted. Notice warning signs—increased cynicism, difficulty sleeping, dreading work, emotional numbing, withdrawal.

Take it seriously: Vicarious trauma and burnout aren't weakness. They're occupational hazards requiring intervention.

Seek help: Consult supervisor, seek personal therapy, talk to physician, access EAP. Don't tough it out alone.

Make changes: Reduce caseload, take time off, set better boundaries, increase self-care. Temporary adjustments allow recovery.

Consider leave: If seriously impaired, take medical or personal leave. Better to step away temporarily than harm clients or destroy yourself.

Reassess career fit: Sometimes burnout signals wrong setting, wrong population, or wrong career. It's okay to make changes. Better to find sustainable path than suffer indefinitely.

Case Example: Recognizing and Addressing Burnout

Michael, therapist at rape crisis center, has worked with sexual assault survivors for five years. Recently, he notices changes:

- Dreading work each morning
- Feeling numb during sessions
- Irritability with partner and friends
- Intrusive thoughts about clients' assaults
- Nightmares featuring assault scenarios
- Increased drinking to relax
- Questioning whether his work helps anyone
- Cynical comments about clients to colleagues

His supervisor, noticing changes in supervision, raises concern.

Supervisor: "Michael, I'm concerned. You seem exhausted, you're making cynical comments about clients, and you mentioned drinking more. What's happening?"

Michael: "I don't know. I just feel done. I can't listen to another rape story. I look at my schedule and feel nothing. I know I should care but I'm empty."

Supervisor: "Those are clear burnout signs, possibly vicarious trauma. We need to address this seriously. Let's talk about what's contributing and what changes we can make."

Assessment reveals:

- Michael's entire caseload is trauma (30+ sexual assault survivors)
- He hasn't taken vacation in 18 months
- He works 50+ hours weekly, takes work home

- Personal life is minimal—work dominates everything
- He stopped exercising and socializing
- His own history of childhood abuse (unaddressed) is activated by client stories

Intervention plan:

Immediate changes:

- Reduce caseload to 20 clients
- Mix of clients—not all active trauma work
- No work at home—leave charts at office
- Mandatory two-week vacation

Ongoing support:

- Weekly individual supervision focusing on emotional processing
- Peer support group with other trauma therapists
- Personal therapy to address vicarious trauma and personal history
- Monthly consultation with trauma specialist

Self-care plan:

- Exercise 3x weekly (rejoins gym)
- Weekly social time with friends
- Daily 20-minute mindfulness practice
- Alcohol limit (no more than 2 drinks, not daily)
- Hobby time (photography he's neglected)

Organizational changes (supervisor advocates):

- Policy limiting trauma caseload to 60% for any therapist
- Monthly trauma-specific supervision group
- Training on vicarious trauma and self-care
- Expanded EAP access for staff

Progress:

After two weeks vacation, Michael returns somewhat refreshed but still depleted. Over three months with reduced caseload, therapy, and self-care, he improves gradually. Numbness decreases. He reconnects with why he does this work. Energy returns.

Six months later, Michael functions well. He's learned to recognize burnout signs early, maintains better boundaries, prioritizes self-care, and accepts that sustainable career requires ongoing attention to well-being.

He also recognizes this setting might not be sustainable long-term. After another year, he transitions to more general mental health work where trauma is one issue among many, not exclusive focus. This isn't failure—it's realistic recognition of his limits and needs.

Lessons: Vicarious trauma and burnout are real occupational hazards requiring serious response. Early recognition, multiple interventions, organizational support, and sometimes job changes are necessary for long-term sustainability.

Continuing Education

Learning doesn't end with degrees and licensure. The field evolves—new research, new treatments, new understanding of problems. Staying current is ethical obligation ensuring you provide competent care based on best available evidence.

Why continuing education matters:

Competence: Knowledge and skills erode without reinforcement. Continuing education maintains and enhances competence.

Evidence-based practice: Research produces new findings constantly. CE keeps you current with evidence.

Licensure requirement: Most states require CE hours for license renewal (typically 20-40 hours every 2 years).

Professional development: Learning engages you intellectually, prevents stagnation, and expands capabilities.

Client welfare: Clients deserve therapists who use current best practices, not outdated or disproven methods.

Types of continuing education:

Formal training: Workshops, conferences, intensive training programs. Often focused on specific treatment modalities (EMDR training, DBT training) or populations (older adults, eating disorders).

Online courses: Convenient, self-paced, accessible. Range from brief webinars to extensive courses. Quality varies—choose accredited providers.

Reading: Professional journals, books, treatment manuals. Free or low-cost. Requires self-discipline to stay current.

Supervision and consultation: Learning through case discussion and feedback. Counts as CE in some states.

Teaching: Teaching others deepens your own understanding. Preparing presentations requires mastering material thoroughly.

Research participation: Participating in studies, collaborating on research, or conducting research provides cutting-edge knowledge.

Peer learning groups: Colleagues presenting to each other, discussing readings, watching videos together. Mutual learning.

Choosing continuing education:

Match to practice: Choose CE relevant to your population and problems you treat. If you work with children, pursue child-focused CE. If you rarely see eating disorders, extensive eating disorder training might not be priority.

Fill gaps: Identify areas where you lack knowledge or confidence. Target CE to fill those gaps.

Depth vs. breadth: Balance deep training in specific areas with broad overview of many topics. Don't just stick to what you know—expand capabilities while developing expertise.

Quality: Choose reputable providers. Look for evidence-based content, qualified instructors, accreditation by professional organizations.

Application: Best CE provides practical skills you can implement immediately. Pure theory without application is less useful.

Cost-benefit: Expensive isn't always better. Free or low-cost options (journal articles, webinars, peer learning) can be excellent. But sometimes significant investment in quality training is worthwhile.

Ethics and cultural competence: Include ethics CE regularly. Most states require ethics hours specifically. Pursue cultural competence training continuously.

Documentation: Track CE carefully. Keep certificates, note hours, dates, topics. You'll need documentation for license renewal and potentially for audits.

Barriers to continuing education:

Cost: CE can be expensive. Strategies: free or low-cost options (webinars, journal articles, peer groups), employer-sponsored CE, tax deductions for professional development, prioritize most valuable learning.

Time: Busy schedules make CE difficult. Strategies: online self-paced courses, lunch-and-learn sessions, incorporating reading into routine, using commute time for podcasts or audiobooks.

Accessibility: Geographic isolation, disability, caregiving responsibilities limit access. Strategies: online options, recorded webinars, reading materials, phone consultation groups.

Quality concerns: Not all CE is equally valuable. Strategies: research providers, read reviews, ask colleagues for recommendations, try brief affordable offerings before committing to expensive trainings.

Applying learning to practice:

Learning without application is wasted. After CE:

Review and consolidate: Summarize key points, create reference materials, discuss with colleagues.

Plan implementation: Identify specific ways to apply learning. Which clients could benefit? What changes to make?

Start small: Don't try to implement everything at once. Choose one or two new techniques or concepts to integrate.

Seek consultation: Discuss application with supervisor or consultant. Get support implementing new skills.

Evaluate results: Monitor whether new approaches help. Stay with what works, adjust what doesn't.

Share learning: Teaching others reinforces your learning. Present to colleagues, write about applications, supervise others.

Case Example: Strategic Continuing Education - Dr. Lee's Plan

Dr. Lee, licensed 8 years ago, works in group practice seeing adults with depression and anxiety. She's comfortable with CBT but recognizes limitations. She develops strategic CE plan.

Year 1 Goals:

Primary focus: Develop trauma-informed approach

Rationale: Many clients describe childhood trauma, but Dr. Lee has limited trauma-specific training. She often feels stuck with these clients.

CE activities:

- 2-day workshop on trauma-informed CBT (16 hours)
- 6-week online course on ACT for trauma (12 hours)

- Monthly trauma consultation group with colleagues (12 hours over year)
- Reading: *The Body Keeps the Score*, *Trauma-Focused CBT manuals* (10 hours)

Total: 50 hours (exceeds 40-hour requirement)

Application: Begins using trauma-informed approaches with 5 clients. Brings cases to consultation group monthly. Notices improved engagement and progress with trauma clients.

Year 2 Goals:

Primary focus: Cultural competence and health equity

Rationale: Dr. Lee's practice increasingly includes clients of color, immigrants, and LGBTQ+ clients. She recognizes cultural gaps in her understanding.

CE activities:

- Conference on multicultural counseling (20 hours)
- Webinar series on LGBTQ+-affirmative therapy (8 hours)
- Reading: *Cultural Psychotherapy* and articles on health disparities (10 hours)
- Ethics course including cultural considerations (6 hours)

Total: 44 hours

Application: Implements culturally adapted assessment and interventions. Seeks consultation from culturally diverse colleagues. Examines own biases through personal therapy and supervision.

Year 3 Goals:

Primary focus: Specialized certification in DBT

Rationale: Dr. Lee sees clients with emotion dysregulation. Standard CBT isn't sufficient. DBT skills would enhance effectiveness.

CE activities:

- Intensive DBT training (40 hours over two weeks)
- DBT consultation team (bi-weekly for year, 24 hours)
- Advanced DBT modules training (20 hours)
- Self-study of DBT manual and research (20 hours)

Total: 104 hours (pursuing certification requiring 100+ hours)

Application: Begins DBT skills group. Integrates DBT approaches in individual therapy. Joins DBT consultation team for ongoing support and adherence to model.

Ongoing throughout all years:

- State and national conference attendance (annual)
- Journal article reading (monthly)
- Peer supervision group (monthly)
- Ethics updates (biannual)

Outcomes: Over three years, Dr. Lee develops expertise in trauma-informed care, cultural competence, and DBT. Her practice expands to include more complex clients. She's more effective, engaged, and confident. She's invited to present at conferences and provide training to others based on her expertise.

Key principles demonstrated: Strategic planning targeting practice needs, balance of depth (DBT certification) and breadth (trauma, culture, ethics), multiple learning modalities, consistent application of learning, and documentation of hours for licensure.

Professional Identity

Who are you as a professional? What values guide your work? What's your theoretical orientation? How do you understand the helping process? These questions define professional identity—your sense of yourself as social worker, your approach to the work, and your place in the profession.

Professional identity develops throughout career. Students begin with broad, idealistic visions. New professionals often adhere rigidly to one approach, seeking certainty. Experienced professionals develop more nuanced, integrated identities incorporating diverse influences.

Components of professional identity:

Theoretical orientation: What theory or theories guide your understanding of human behavior and change? CBT? Psychodynamic? Person-centered? Eclectic integration? Your theoretical lens shapes how you conceptualize problems and intervene.

Early career: Often adopt supervisor's orientation or school's emphasis. Might rigidly adhere to one approach.

Mid-career: Recognize limitations of single approach. Begin integrating multiple perspectives.

Later career: Develop personal integration—coherent approach drawing from multiple theories in way unique to you.

Professional values: What matters most in your work? Social justice? Evidence-based practice? Client empowerment? Relationship quality? Values guide decision-making, especially in ethical dilemmas.

Examine your values explicitly. When values conflict (client autonomy vs. protection from harm, fidelity to evidence vs. cultural adaptation), which takes priority?

Role conception: How do you see your role? Expert providing solutions? Collaborator working alongside clients? Advocate challenging systems? Teacher imparting skills? Guide accompanying journey? Your role conception affects intervention style.

Professional boundaries: How do you define professional relationship? What boundaries do you maintain? How do you balance warmth and distance? Your boundaries reflect values and theoretical orientation.

Specialty and niche: What populations, problems, or settings do you focus on? Generalist or specialist? Your specialty shapes identity—"I'm a trauma therapist," "I work with LGBTQ+ youth," "I specialize in couples therapy."

Relationship to profession: How do you engage with social work profession? Active in professional organizations? Contribute to literature? Mentor students? Advocate for policy? Teach? Your professional engagement shapes identity.

Developing professional identity:

Reflection: Regularly reflect on your work—What theories guide me? What values drive decisions? What kind of therapist am I? What kind do I want to be? Reflection deepens self-understanding.

Supervision and mentorship: Supervisors and mentors model professional identity. They teach not just techniques but ways of being professional. Choose mentors whose identity resonates with your aspirations.

Professional experiences: Each client, each success and failure, each challenge shapes identity. Difficult cases teach you limits and strengths. Populations you work with influence specialty development.

Training and education: Formal training, workshops, readings shape your theoretical knowledge and approach. Seek training consistent with identity you're developing.

Professional community: Colleagues, professional organizations, conferences connect you to broader profession. These connections shape how you see yourself and your work.

Personal values and experiences: Your personal values, life experiences, and identity (cultural, gender, sexual orientation, etc.) inform professional identity. Integration of personal and professional selves creates authentic practice.

Stages of professional development:

Stage 1: Beginning student/professional (0-2 years)

Focus: Learning basics, managing anxiety, developing minimal competence

Identity: Uncertain, anxious, dependent on supervisors, seeking right answers, often rigid application of theories

Needs: Structure, clear guidance, reassurance, basic skill development

Stage 2: Advanced beginner (2-5 years)

Focus: Developing confidence, recognizing patterns, beginning to integrate learning

Identity: Growing confidence, less rigid, beginning to develop personal style, still looking to external authorities

Needs: Continued supervision, exposure to diverse approaches, beginning specialization

Stage 3: Competent professional (5-10 years)

Focus: Consolidating skills, developing efficiency, taking responsibility for outcomes

Identity: Clear sense of professional self, theoretical integration beginning, comfort with uncertainty, recognition of limits

Needs: Specialized training, peer consultation, mentorship of others

Stage 4: Proficient/Expert professional (10+ years)

Focus: Intuitive practice, pattern recognition, handling complexity, contributing to field

Identity: Integrated theoretical approach, comfort with ambiguity, personal style well-developed, mentorship and teaching

Needs: Intellectual stimulation, prevention of stagnation, passing knowledge to next generation

Challenges to professional identity:

Imposter syndrome: Feeling like fraud despite competence. Common especially early career. Addressed through: normalizing (everyone feels this sometimes), documenting competence (what you've learned and accomplished), supervision providing perspective.

Compassion fatigue: Losing connection to why you do this work. Addressed through: reconnecting to values, self-care, reducing trauma exposure, varying caseload.

Ethical violations: Serious boundary violations or ethical breaches damage professional identity. Prevention through: supervision, consultation, self-awareness, addressing warning signs early.

Burnout: Can lead to questioning career choice. Addressed through: self-care, work-life balance, possible job change, potentially leaving field if truly unsustainable.

Theoretical confusion: Trying to integrate too much leads to incoherence. Addressed through: focused study, choosing primary orientation with selective integration, supervision helping clarify approach.

Maintaining vital professional identity:

Continuous learning: Intellectual engagement prevents stagnation. Stay curious.

Connection to purpose: Remember why you do this work. What drew you to profession? What sustains you?

Work-life balance: Professional identity is one part of full identity. Maintain other roles, relationships, interests.

Self-compassion: You'll make mistakes, have limits, sometimes fail. Treat yourself with compassion you'd offer clients.

Evolution: Allow identity to evolve. Who you are as professional 20 years in differs from who you are starting out. Growth and change are healthy.

Case Example: Identity Development - Maria's Journey

Year 1 (grad student): Maria enters social work program with passion for social justice. She's idealistic, certain she'll change the world, drawn to macro practice and policy.

Identity: "I'm going to fight systemic oppression. Clinical work is Band-Aid on structural problems."

Theoretical orientation: None yet—learning everything.

Challenge: Required clinical internship feels like betrayal of social justice values.

Turning point: Client Rosa, undocumented immigrant, describes how therapy helped her cope with deportation fears. Maria realizes clinical work and social justice aren't opposed—helping individuals survive oppression is justice work.

Years 2-3 (new professional): Maria works at immigrant services organization providing therapy and case management. She's anxious about competence, relies heavily on CBT manual, seeks constant reassurance from supervisor.

Identity: "I'm a clinical social worker serving immigrant communities."

Theoretical orientation: CBT (only approach she feels comfortable with)

Challenge: CBT manual doesn't address immigration trauma, acculturation stress, or collective trauma. Clients improve modestly but she feels something's missing.

Turning point: Training in narrative therapy resonates—understanding how oppression shapes life stories and reclaiming narratives feels more fitting for her clients.

Years 4-7 (developing confidence): Maria pursues training in trauma-informed care, narrative therapy, and liberation psychology. She begins integrating approaches.

Identity: "I'm a trauma therapist working with immigrants and refugees, integrating clinical work with advocacy."

Theoretical orientation: Integration of CBT, narrative therapy, and trauma-informed approaches with social justice lens

Development: Starts advocacy work—testifying about mental health impact of detention, training other providers on immigrant mental health, writing op-eds. Realizes she can do both clinical and macro work.

Years 8-12 (consolidation): Maria develops expertise in immigration-related trauma. She's invited to present at conferences, supervises interns, consults with other agencies.

Identity: "I'm specialist in immigration trauma, integrating therapy, advocacy, and training. I bridge clinical and macro practice."

Theoretical orientation: Coherent personal integration—trauma-informed narrative therapy with emphasis on resilience and resistance, grounded in liberation psychology

Contribution: Publishes articles on culturally responsive trauma treatment, develops training curriculum, mentors Latino/a students.

Years 13+ (expert/mentor): Maria is recognized expert. She maintains clinical practice (preventing disconnection from direct service) while doing training, consultation, advocacy, and supervision.

Identity: "I'm clinical social worker, trainer, advocate. My work addresses individual healing and systemic change. I develop next generation of practitioners committed to justice."

Theoretical orientation: Mature integration—she's developed her own model synthesizing multiple approaches, tested through research collaboration

Evolution: Considers doctorate to contribute to research and teach at university level. Recognizes identity continues evolving—she's not finished developing.

Key themes in Maria's development:

- Initial idealism evolves into nuanced understanding
- Rigid theory application becomes flexible integration
- Either/or thinking (clinical vs. macro) becomes both/and

- Anxiety and dependence become confidence and independence
- Focus on self becomes mentorship of others
- Single approach becomes personal theoretical integration
- Professional identity expands while staying rooted in core values

This journey illustrates normal professional identity development—beginning with idealism and uncertainty, progressing through learning and integration, arriving at mature professional self while recognizing ongoing growth.

Practice Questions

1. Supervision functions include:

A. Only evaluation
B. Education, support, case consultation, ethical guidance, quality assurance
C. Just documentation
D. Punishment

2. Effective supervision requires:

A. Punishment for mistakes
B. Regular meetings, clear expectations, safety, constructive feedback
C. Secrecy
D. No structure

3. As supervisee, you should:

A. Hide mistakes
B. Be honest, open to feedback, implement suggestions
C. Be defensive
D. Ignore supervision

4. Licensure supervision:

A. Is same as any supervision
B. Must meet specific state requirements for hours and supervisor qualifications
C. Doesn't matter
D. Is optional

5. Cultural humility means:

A. Knowing everything about all cultures
B. Recognizing limits, learning from clients, ongoing self-examination
C. Ignoring culture
D. Cultural superiority

6. Cultural competence includes:

A. Only race and ethnicity
B. Multiple dimensions—race, ethnicity, religion, SES, gender, orientation, disability, age
C. Just language
D. Nothing specific

7. Microaggressions are:

A. Not real
B. Brief indignities communicating hostile messages to marginalized groups
C. Acceptable
D. Compliments

8. When you commit microaggression:

A. Deny it
B. Acknowledge, apologize, learn, change behavior
C. Blame the client
D. Ignore it

9. Culturally adapted interventions:

A. Aren't necessary
B. Are more effective than standard treatments for some populations
C. Reduce effectiveness
D. Insult clients

10. Vicarious trauma results from:

A. Direct trauma to you
B. Exposure to others' traumatic experiences through empathic engagement
C. Nothing
D. Weak character

11. Vicarious trauma symptoms include:

A. Only happiness
B. Intrusion, avoidance, hyperarousal, worldview changes
C. Nothing observable
D. Increased energy

12. Burnout components include:

A. Increased energy
B. Emotional exhaustion, depersonalization, reduced accomplishment

C. Enthusiasm
D. Better boundaries

13. Risk factors for burnout include:

A. Good self-care
B. High caseload, lack of support, poor boundaries, trauma-heavy work
C. Excellent supervision
D. Regular vacations

14. Preventing vicarious trauma requires:

A. Ignoring feelings
B. Boundaries, supervision, balanced caseload, self-care, peer support
C. Working more
D. Avoiding all support

15. If experiencing vicarious trauma:

A. Ignore it
B. Recognize early, take seriously, seek help, make changes
C. Work harder
D. It will pass on its own

16. Continuing education serves:

A. Just license requirement
B. Maintaining competence, staying current, professional development
C. Wasting time
D. Entertainment only

17. Choosing CE should consider:

A. Only cost
B. Relevance to practice, gaps in knowledge, quality, application
C. Whatever is easiest
D. Only what you already know

18. Applying CE learning requires:

A. Forgetting it immediately
B. Review, implementation plan, start small, consultation, evaluation
C. Trying everything at once
D. Never using it

19. Professional identity includes:

A. Only job title
B. Theoretical orientation, values, role conception, specialty, relationship to profession
C. Nothing specific
D. What others tell you

20. Theoretical orientation:

A. Doesn't matter
B. Guides understanding of behavior and change; evolves toward integration
C. Must stay rigid forever
D. Is chosen randomly

21. Beginning professionals often:

A. Are immediately expert
B. Experience anxiety, depend on supervisors, apply theories rigidly
C. Know everything
D. Need no support

22. Expert professionals typically:

A. Stop learning
B. Practice intuitively, handle complexity, contribute to field, mentor others
C. Know everything already
D. Don't need supervision

23. Imposter syndrome:

A. Means you're fraud
B. Is common; feeling like fraud despite competence
C. Only affects beginners
D. Is permanent

24. Self-care is:

A. Selfish
B. Ethical obligation ensuring capacity to serve clients
C. Optional
D. Weakness

25. Physical self-care includes:

A. Ignoring health
B. Sleep, exercise, nutrition, medical care, limiting substances
C. Only sleep
D. Nothing specific

26. Emotional self-care includes:

A. Isolation
B. Joy activities, connection, meaning-making, mindfulness, gratitude
C. Only therapy
D. Suppressing feelings

27. Work-life boundaries require:

A. Working constantly
B. Leaving work at work, clear separation, limited after-hours availability
C. No separation
D. Taking all work home

28. Personal therapy for therapists:

A. Is shameful
B. Enhances well-being and clinical skills; many therapists benefit
C. Means you're incompetent
D. Should be avoided

29. Balanced caseload means:

A. Only trauma cases
B. Mix of client types and severity providing variety
C. All high-acuity
D. Only easy cases

30. Peer support provides:

A. Competition
B. Shared experience, validation, reduced isolation, different perspectives
C. Judgment
D. Nothing useful

31. Cultural self-awareness involves:

A. Ignoring your culture
B. Examining your cultural identity, values, privileges, biases
C. Assuming you're unbiased
D. Cultural superiority

32. Learning about cultures requires:

A. Stereotyping
B. Reading, attending events, engaging communities while avoiding stereotypes

C. One workshop
D. Nothing

33. Intersectionality means:

A. Street corners
B. Cultural identities interact in complex ways
C. Only one identity matters
D. Categories are separate

34. When supervision isn't working:

A. Suffer silently
B. Discuss openly, consider different supervisor if needed
C. Quit immediately
D. Complain to everyone except supervisor

35. Licensure CE requirements:

A. Are optional
B. Must be met for license renewal; typically 20-40 hours every 2 years
C. Don't exist
D. Are just suggestions

36. Ethics CE:

A. Isn't necessary
B. Is required specifically in most states; should be pursued regularly
C. Is one-time
D. Doesn't matter

37. Barriers to CE include:

A. Nothing
B. Cost, time, accessibility, quality concerns
C. Only cost
D. Too much availability

38. Documentation of CE:

A. Isn't necessary
B. Should be tracked carefully with certificates, hours, dates for license renewal
C. Can be vague
D. Memory is enough

39. Professional values:

A. Are assigned
B. Guide decision-making, especially in ethical dilemmas
C. Don't matter
D. Are universal

40. Professional community connection:

A. Wastes time
B. Shapes identity through colleagues, organizations, conferences
C. Isn't important
D. Creates competition only

Answer Key with Detailed Explanations

1. B. Education, support, case consultation, ethical guidance, quality assurance
Supervision serves multiple functions: education and skill development (teaching theory and techniques), support and encouragement (processing difficult feelings), case consultation (providing fresh perspective), ethical guidance (navigating dilemmas), and quality assurance (monitoring care quality). It's not just evaluation or punishment—supervision is comprehensive professional support and development.

2. B. Regular meetings, clear expectations, safety, constructive feedback
Effective supervision requires: regular consistent meetings (weekly or biweekly), clear expectations (both parties understand purpose and process), safe environment (can discuss mistakes without fear), and constructive feedback (balance of affirmation and correction). Structure, safety, and clarity make supervision productive. Punishment, secrecy, and lack of structure undermine supervision.

3. B. Be honest, open to feedback, implement suggestions
As supervisee, you should: prepare for sessions, be honest about mistakes and uncertainties (hiding prevents learning), receive feedback non-defensively, implement suggested interventions, report results, reflect on your patterns, and practice ethically. Hiding mistakes, being defensive, or ignoring supervision wastes opportunity for growth and potentially harms clients.

4. B. Must meet specific state requirements for hours and supervisor qualifications
Licensure supervision must meet specific state requirements regarding: number of supervised hours (typically 2000-4000), supervisor qualifications (licensed, experienced, meets state requirements), supervision frequency and format, and documentation. It's structured, regulated, and documented to ensure quality. Not same as informal supervision or optional—it's required for licensure.

5. B. Recognizing limits, learning from clients, ongoing self-examination
Cultural humility involves: recognizing you can't know everything about all cultures,

understanding clients are experts on their experience, engaging in ongoing self-examination of biases, acknowledging power imbalances, and committing to lifelong learning. It's more realistic and appropriate than claiming cultural "competence" or mastery. Humility means ongoing learning, not expertise.

6. B. Multiple dimensions—race, ethnicity, religion, SES, gender, orientation, disability, age
Cultural competence includes multiple dimensions beyond race/ethnicity: religion/spirituality, socioeconomic status, gender identity/expression, sexual orientation, disability, age, national origin/immigration status, geographic region. Culture is multifaceted. People hold multiple cultural identities simultaneously that intersect in complex ways. Comprehensive cultural competence addresses all dimensions.

7. B. Brief indignities communicating hostile messages to marginalized groups
Microaggressions are brief, commonplace indignities—verbal, behavioral, or environmental—that communicate hostile, derogatory, or negative messages to people from marginalized groups. Examples: "Where are you really from?" (assumes non-white person isn't American), "You're so articulate" (surprise that person of color is articulate). They're real, harmful, cumulative stressors, not compliments or acceptable.

8. B. Acknowledge, apologize, learn, change behavior
When you commit microaggression: acknowledge it ("I realize what I said was problematic"), apologize genuinely ("I apologize. That was hurtful"), learn ("Help me understand how that affected you"), and change behavior (don't repeat it). Don't deny, become defensive, blame the client, or ignore it. Take responsibility and grow from the mistake.

9. B. Are more effective than standard treatments for some populations
Research shows culturally adapted interventions are more effective than standard treatments for some populations. Adaptations include: surface structure changes (language, images reflecting culture) and deep structure changes (cultural values, worldview, explanatory models incorporated). Cultural adaptation isn't insulting or unnecessary—it enhances effectiveness by making treatment relevant and responsive to cultural context.

10. B. Exposure to others' traumatic experiences through empathic engagement
Vicarious trauma (secondary traumatic stress, compassion fatigue) results from exposure to others' traumatic experiences through empathic engagement with their trauma stories. Through repeatedly hearing trauma accounts and empathizing with clients' pain, you experience trauma symptoms yourself even though events didn't happen to you directly. It's not weak character or direct trauma to you—it's occupational hazard of trauma work.

11. B. Intrusion, avoidance, hyperarousal, worldview changes
Vicarious trauma symptoms include: intrusion (intrusive thoughts about clients' trauma, nightmares, preoccupation), avoidance (emotional numbing, avoiding trauma clients), hyperarousal (anxiety, startle response, sleep problems, irritability), and cognitive/worldview

changes (believing world is dangerous, people can't be trusted, loss of hope). These mirror PTSD symptoms but result from exposure to others' trauma.

12. B. Emotional exhaustion, depersonalization, reduced accomplishment
Burnout components include: emotional exhaustion (feeling drained, depleted, unable to give more), depersonalization (cynical, detached, negative attitudes toward clients, seeing them as objects), and reduced personal accomplishment (feeling ineffective, questioning competence, doubting impact). Not increased energy or enthusiasm—burnout is depletion and disengagement.

13. B. High caseload, lack of support, poor boundaries, trauma-heavy work
Risk factors for burnout include: high or trauma-heavy caseload, lack of control over work, inadequate support/supervision, unclear expectations, limited resources, personal trauma history, difficulty with boundaries, perfectionism, isolation, poor self-care, over-identification with clients. Good self-care, excellent supervision, and regular vacations are protective factors that reduce burnout risk.

14. B. Boundaries, supervision, balanced caseload, self-care, peer support
Preventing vicarious trauma requires: professional boundaries (leave work at work), supervision/consultation (process emotional impact), balanced caseload (not all trauma cases), personal therapy when helpful, physical self-care (sleep, exercise, nutrition), emotional/spiritual self-care (joy activities, connection, meaning-making), peer support, organizational support, and limiting additional trauma exposure. Multiple strategies needed.

15. B. Recognize early, take seriously, seek help, make changes
If experiencing vicarious trauma: recognize warning signs early (don't wait until depleted), take it seriously (it's occupational hazard requiring intervention), seek help (supervision, therapy, medical care, EAP), and make changes (reduce caseload, take time off, increase self-care, set better boundaries). Don't ignore, work harder, or tough it out alone. Early intervention prevents severe impairment.

16. B. Maintaining competence, staying current, professional development
Continuing education serves: maintaining and enhancing competence (knowledge erodes without reinforcement), staying current with evidence and best practices, meeting licensure requirements, professional development (intellectual engagement, expanding capabilities), and ensuring client welfare (providing current best care). It's not just license requirement or time-wasting—it's professional obligation.

17. B. Relevance to practice, gaps in knowledge, quality, application
Choosing CE should consider: relevance to your practice (populations and problems you treat), filling knowledge gaps (targeting areas of uncertainty), quality (reputable providers, evidence-based content, qualified instructors), practical application (skills you can implement immediately), cost-benefit analysis, and including ethics and cultural competence regularly. Strategic choice maximizes learning value.

18. B. Review, implementation plan, start small, consultation, evaluation
Applying CE learning requires: reviewing and consolidating key points, developing implementation plan (how to use in practice), starting small (one or two techniques initially, not everything at once), seeking consultation about application, and evaluating results (monitoring whether approaches help). Learning without application is wasted. Intentional implementation creates practice change.

19. B. Theoretical orientation, values, role conception, specialty, relationship to profession
Professional identity includes: theoretical orientation (theories guiding understanding and intervention), professional values (what matters most in work), role conception (how you see your role), specialty/niche (populations or problems you focus on), and relationship to profession (engagement with social work profession through organizations, literature, mentorship, advocacy). Not just job title—it's comprehensive professional self-concept.

20. B. Guides understanding of behavior and change; evolves toward integration
Theoretical orientation guides your understanding of human behavior and change processes, shapes how you conceptualize problems and intervene. Early career often involves rigid adherence to one approach. Mid-to-late career typically involves integration of multiple perspectives in coherent personal approach. Orientation matters (influences all clinical work), evolves over time, and is chosen thoughtfully not randomly.

21. B. Experience anxiety, depend on supervisors, apply theories rigidly
Beginning professionals (0-2 years) typically: experience significant anxiety about competence, depend heavily on supervisors for direction, seek right answers, apply theories rigidly (need structure and certainty), focus on learning basics and developing minimal competence. This is normal developmental stage. They're not immediately expert, don't know everything, and definitely need support.

22. B. Practice intuitively, handle complexity, contribute to field, mentor others
Expert professionals (10+ years typically): practice intuitively drawing on pattern recognition, handle complexity comfortably, contribute to field (teaching, writing, presenting), mentor next generation, have integrated theoretical approach, are comfortable with ambiguity. But they don't stop learning or cease needing consultation—even experts benefit from ongoing development and outside perspective.

23. B. Is common; feeling like fraud despite competence
Imposter syndrome is feeling like fraud despite actual competence—believing you'll be "found out" as not knowing enough or being good enough. It's extremely common, especially early career but can persist. Doesn't mean you're actually fraud. Addressed through: normalizing (everyone feels this sometimes), documenting actual competence (reviewing what you've learned and accomplished), and supervision/therapy providing perspective.

24. B. Ethical obligation ensuring capacity to serve clients
Self-care is ethical obligation, not selfishness or optional luxury. Burned-out, depleted,

traumatized therapists can't help clients effectively. You owe clients your well-being—maintaining capacity to serve them requires intentional self-care. It's professional responsibility ensuring you're healthy enough to do the work. Not weakness—it's strength and professionalism.

25. B. Sleep, exercise, nutrition, medical care, limiting substances
Physical self-care includes: adequate sleep (7-9 hours), regular exercise (proven to reduce stress and improve mood), healthy nutrition, medical care when needed, limiting substance use, and attending to physical health. Physical well-being affects mental and emotional capacity. Neglecting physical health impairs professional functioning. Basic physical care is foundation for sustainable practice.

26. B. Joy activities, connection, meaning-making, mindfulness, gratitude
Emotional self-care includes: activities bringing joy (hobbies, creative pursuits, nature time), connection with others (friends, family, community), meaning-making practices (spirituality, religion, philosophy, activism), mindfulness and meditation, and gratitude practices. Not just therapy (though that helps some therapists), and not suppressing feelings. Emotional self-care nourishes inner life.

27. B. Leaving work at work, clear separation, limited after-hours availability
Work-life boundaries require: leaving work at work (no charts at home when possible), clear separation between professional and personal time, limited after-hours availability (not on call 24/7, clear emergency protocols), and protecting personal time. Don't work constantly or take all work home. Boundaries between work and life sustain you for long career.

28. B. Enhances well-being and clinical skills; many therapists benefit
Personal therapy for therapists enhances well-being and clinical skills. Many therapists benefit from their own therapy—processing reactions to work, addressing personal issues, experiencing being client, deepening self-awareness. It's not shameful, doesn't mean you're incompetent, and shouldn't be avoided. It's often valuable professional and personal development tool.

29. B. Mix of client types and severity providing variety
Balanced caseload includes mix of: client types (not all trauma, not all same diagnosis), severity levels (not all high-acuity or crisis, not all easy cases), and variety of issues. Balance prevents burnout, maintains engagement, and allows recovery between intense sessions. If you specialize in trauma, ensure you're not seeing only trauma all day every day—variation sustains you.

30. B. Shared experience, validation, reduced isolation, different perspectives
Peer support provides: shared experience with colleagues who understand the work, validation of struggles and successes, reduced isolation (knowing you're not alone), different perspectives on cases and challenges, mutual learning, and professional connection. Not competition or judgment—peer support is collegial mutual aid among people doing similar work.

31. B. Examining your cultural identity, values, privileges, biases
Cultural self-awareness involves examining: your cultural identity and what groups you belong to, values you hold and where they come from, privileges and disadvantages you experience, biases and stereotypes you carry, assumptions you make, and how your culture shapes your worldview and practice. Not ignoring culture or assuming you're unbiased—it's intentional examination of how culture influences you.

32. B. Reading, attending events, engaging communities while avoiding stereotypes
Learning about cultures requires: reading (especially books by people from those cultures), attending cultural events, engaging with diverse communities, consultation with cultural insiders, and ongoing education. But avoid stereotyping—knowledge about cultures provides general understanding while recognizing individuals vary enormously within cultures. Don't assume individual matches cultural generalizations.

33. B. Cultural identities interact in complex ways
Intersectionality means multiple cultural identities (race, gender, sexual orientation, class, disability, etc.) interact and intersect in complex ways creating unique experiences. Black lesbian woman experiences intersection of racism, sexism, and homophobia simultaneously—not separate additive categories but interactive intersection. Identities aren't separate—they're interwoven creating unique social positions.

34. B. Discuss openly, consider different supervisor if needed
When supervision isn't working: discuss concerns openly with supervisor when safe, attempt to resolve issues through communication, document concerns if serious, and if incompatibility persists despite good-faith efforts or if supervision is inadequate/unethical, seek different supervisor or report through appropriate channels. Don't suffer silently or quit immediately without attempting resolution. Address problems professionally.

35. B. Must be met for license renewal; typically 20-40 hours every 2 years
Licensure continuing education requirements must be met for license renewal—they're mandatory, not optional. Most states require 20-40 hours every 2 years, often with specific ethics hours required. Track hours carefully, keep certificates, and ensure CE meets state requirements (approved providers, relevant topics). Failure to meet CE requirements results in license lapse or non-renewal.

36. B. Is required specifically in most states; should be pursued regularly
Ethics CE is required specifically in most states (typically 2-6 hours per renewal period), separate from general CE hours. Beyond meeting requirements, pursue ethics training regularly throughout career—ethical dilemmas are common, laws and standards evolve, and ongoing ethics education supports ethical practice. It's not one-time learning—ethics requires continuous attention.

37. B. Cost, time, accessibility, quality concerns
Barriers to continuing education include: cost (expensive trainings), time constraints (busy

schedules make CE difficult), accessibility issues (geographic isolation, disability, caregiving responsibilities), and quality concerns (not all CE is equally valuable). Strategies to overcome barriers: free/low-cost options, online self-paced courses, employer-sponsored CE, research providers for quality, prioritize most valuable learning.

38. B. Should be tracked carefully with certificates, hours, dates for license renewal
Documentation of CE should be tracked carefully: keep certificates of completion, note hours earned, record dates and topics, maintain organized file for license renewal, and retain documentation for audit period (often 4-6 years). Don't rely on memory or vague records. Many states audit CE compliance—detailed documentation protects you and ensures you can verify compliance.

39. B. Guide decision-making, especially in ethical dilemmas
Professional values guide decision-making throughout practice, especially in ethical dilemmas where competing considerations conflict. When client autonomy conflicts with protection from harm, when evidence-based practice conflicts with cultural adaptation, when multiple "right" answers exist—values guide choices. They're not assigned or universal—they're personally held commitments developed through reflection, experience, and professional socialization.

40. B. Shapes identity through colleagues, organizations, conferences
Professional community connection shapes identity through: relationships with colleagues providing models and support, participation in professional organizations (NASW, specialty organizations) connecting you to broader profession, conference attendance exposing you to cutting-edge work and diverse practitioners, collaborative projects, and professional networks. Community connection creates sense of belonging to profession larger than individual practice.

Sustaining Yourself for the Long Haul

This work is marathon, not sprint. The clients who need you five years from now, ten years from now, twenty years from now deserve a therapist who's still well, still learning, still capable. Creating that sustainable practice requires intentional ongoing attention.

You can't do this work well if you're depleted. The airplane oxygen mask principle applies—secure your own mask before helping others. Self-care isn't selfish—it's prerequisite for serving others. This isn't optional self-indulgence. It's professional responsibility.

Professional development keeps you engaged. Learning new approaches, developing expertise, contributing to the field—these create meaning beyond daily clinical work. Stagnation breeds burnout. Growth sustains interest and competence.

Cultural competence ensures you serve all clients well. Without ongoing learning about diverse populations, examining your biases, adapting practice to be responsive—you'll inadvertently harm clients from backgrounds different from yours. Cultural work is never complete. It's lifelong commitment.

Supervision and consultation provide perspective. Even experienced therapists benefit from outside eyes on their work. Complex cases, ethical dilemmas, countertransference reactions—all benefit from collaborative thinking. Isolation is dangerous. Connection to colleagues sustains you.

Your professional identity evolves throughout career. Early rigidity gives way to integration. Anxiety transforms into confidence. Dependence on external authorities becomes internal wisdom. But evolution requires reflection, mentorship, diverse experiences, and willingness to change.

The work will affect you. You'll carry stories. You'll absorb pain. You'll witness suffering that changes you. But you can do this work sustainably if you:

- Maintain boundaries between work and life
- Engage in regular supervision and consultation
- Pursue ongoing learning and development
- Practice comprehensive self-care (physical, emotional, spiritual, cognitive)
- Build strong support systems personal and professional
- Develop cultural humility and competence
- Find meaning in the work beyond individual sessions
- Allow your professional identity to evolve
- Recognize warning signs of burnout and vicarious trauma early
- Take action when you're struggling—seek help, make changes, take time off when needed

The profession needs committed, competent, healthy practitioners for the long term. Be one of them. This work is too important, and the need too great, for you to burn out in five years. Sustain yourself intentionally, develop yourself continuously, and you can do this work for decades—growing, contributing, serving, and finding meaning in helping others build better lives.

Core Principles for Professional Sustainability

- Supervision provides education, support, case consultation, ethical guidance, and quality assurance throughout your career, not just for beginners
- Effective supervision requires regular meetings, clear expectations, psychological safety for vulnerability, and constructive balanced feedback

- Cultural humility involves recognizing knowledge limits, learning from clients, ongoing self-examination, and lifelong learning, not cultural mastery
- Cultural competence addresses multiple intersecting dimensions including race, ethnicity, religion, SES, gender, orientation, disability, and age
- Microaggressions are harmful brief indignities requiring acknowledgment, genuine apology, learning, and behavior change when committed
- Vicarious trauma results from empathic exposure to clients' trauma causing secondary traumatic stress symptoms in the therapist
- Burnout involves emotional exhaustion, depersonalization, and reduced sense of accomplishment from prolonged occupational stress
- Preventing vicarious trauma and burnout requires boundaries, supervision, balanced caseload, comprehensive self-care, and peer support
- Self-care is ethical obligation ensuring capacity to serve clients, not selfishness or optional luxury—you can't pour from empty cup
- Continuing education maintains competence, keeps you current with evidence, meets licensure requirements, and sustains professional engagement
- Professional identity includes theoretical orientation, values, role conception, specialty, and evolves from anxiety and rigidity toward integration and wisdom
- Beginning professionals experience anxiety and dependence; expert professionals practice intuitively, handle complexity, and mentor others
- Balanced caseload includes mix of client types and severity preventing burnout through variety and allowing recovery between intense sessions
- Work-life boundaries requiring leaving work at work, clear time separation, and limited after-hours availability sustain long-term practice
- Professional development through learning, supervision, cultural competence work, and identity evolution creates sustainable, meaningful, effective practice across career span

Chapter 17: LCSW Clinical Exam

Practice Exam 1 (170 Questions)

Mixed Content from All Domains - Full-Length Simulated Exam

Question 1: According to Erikson's psychosocial development theory, a 45-year-old client struggling to find meaning in their career is most likely experiencing which developmental crisis? A. Identity vs. Role Confusion, B. Intimacy vs. Isolation, C. Generativity vs. Stagnation, D. Integrity vs. Despair

Answer: C. Generativity vs. Stagnation.

This stage occurs during middle adulthood (40-65 years) where individuals focus on contributing to society and helping guide future generations, or they experience stagnation.

Question 2: A social worker discovers their client is also a member of their church congregation. What is the MOST appropriate action according to the NASW Code of Ethics? A. Continue treatment and avoid discussing the dual relationship, B. Terminate services immediately, C. Discuss the dual relationship with the client and consider referral, D. Seek supervision only if the client raises concerns

Answer: C. Discuss the dual relationship with the client and consider referral

The NASW Code requires social workers to address dual relationships proactively, discuss potential conflicts with clients, and make referrals when necessary to avoid harm.

Question 3: A client presents with persistent sadness, loss of interest in activities, significant weight loss, and insomnia for the past 3 weeks. Which DSM-5-TR diagnosis is MOST appropriate? A. Major Depressive Disorder, B. Persistent Depressive Disorder, C. Adjustment Disorder with Depressed Mood, D. Unspecified Depressive Disorder

Answer: D. Unspecified Depressive Disorder

While symptoms suggest depression, Major Depressive Disorder requires at least 2 weeks of symptoms, but the question states 3 weeks. However, without confirmation of meeting all criteria, Unspecified is most appropriate until full assessment is completed.

Question 4: When using Motivational Interviewing with a client ambivalent about quitting smoking, which technique is MOST effective? A. Confronting the client about health risks, B. Exploring discrepancies between values and behaviors, C. Providing educational materials about smoking cessation, D. Setting a quit date for the client

Answer: B. Exploring discrepancies between values and behaviors

Motivational Interviewing focuses on resolving ambivalence by helping clients identify discrepancies between their current behaviors and personal values or goals.

Question 5: A 7-year-old child demonstrates difficulty sitting still, frequently interrupts others, and has trouble waiting their turn. According to Piaget's theory, this child is in which developmental stage? A. Sensorimotor, B. Preoperational, C. Concrete Operational, D. Formal Operational

Answer: C. Concrete Operational

Children ages 7-11 are in the Concrete Operational stage, characterized by logical thinking about concrete events. The described behaviors suggest possible ADHD symptoms but don't affect developmental stage classification.

Question 6: A client threatens to harm their ex-partner. What is the social worker's PRIMARY ethical obligation? A. Maintain confidentiality unless client signs a release, B. Warn the intended victim and notify authorities, C. Document the threat in the clinical record only, D. Explore the client's feelings about the relationship

Answer: B. Warn the intended victim and notify authorities

The Tarasoff duty to warn/protect requires social workers to breach confidentiality when there is a credible threat to an identifiable victim.

Question 7: In family systems therapy, triangulation refers to: A. A three-generation pattern of dysfunction, B. Involving a third person to reduce anxiety between two people, C. The relationship between three siblings, D. A treatment approach involving three therapists

Answer: B. Involving a third person to reduce anxiety between two people

Triangulation occurs when two people in conflict involve a third party to stabilize their relationship and reduce anxiety, a key concept in Bowen's family systems theory.

Question 8: A client diagnosed with Borderline Personality Disorder calls the social worker at 2 AM reporting suicidal thoughts. The MOST appropriate response is to: A. Tell the client to call back during business hours, B. Assess lethality and safety plan or refer to crisis services, C. Ignore the call to avoid reinforcing attention-seeking behavior, D. Schedule an emergency session for the next morning

Answer: B. Assess lethality and safety plan or refer to crisis services

Safety always takes priority. The social worker must assess suicide risk and ensure client safety through crisis intervention or appropriate referral.

Question 9: Which defense mechanism involves attributing one's own unacceptable thoughts to others? A. Displacement, B. Projection, C. Rationalization, D. Sublimation

Answer: B. Projection

Projection is attributing one's own unacceptable thoughts, feelings, or motives to another person as a way to avoid acknowledging them in oneself.

Question 10: A social worker learns that a colleague has been billing for sessions not provided. The FIRST step should be to: A. Report the colleague to the licensing board immediately, B. Discuss concerns directly with the colleague, C. Document the observations and wait for more evidence, D. Report to local law enforcement

Answer: B. Discuss concerns directly with the colleague

The NASW Code encourages addressing ethical concerns directly with the colleague first, unless immediate harm is occurring or the situation requires mandatory reporting.

Question 11: Cognitive-Behavioral Therapy (CBT) is MOST effective for treating: A. Schizophrenia, B. Anxiety and Depression, C. Intellectual Disability, D. Dementia

Answer: B. Anxiety and Depression

CBT has the strongest evidence base for treating anxiety disorders and depression by addressing maladaptive thought patterns and behaviors.

Question 12: A 65-year-old client reflects on their life with satisfaction and acceptance of past choices. According to Erikson, this represents: A. Generativity, B. Integrity, C. Intimacy, D. Industry

Answer: B. Integrity

Integrity vs. Despair is Erikson's final stage (65+ years) where individuals reflect on life with either satisfaction (integrity) or regret (despair).

Question 13: When working with a client from a different cultural background, cultural competence requires the social worker to: A. Treat all clients exactly the same regardless of culture, B. Learn everything about the client's culture before beginning treatment, C. Recognize their own biases and seek to understand the client's worldview, D. Refer the client to a therapist from their own culture

Answer: C. Recognize their own biases and seek to understand the client's worldview

Cultural competence involves self-awareness, recognizing one's own biases, and actively working to understand each client's unique cultural perspective.

Question 14: A client diagnosed with Major Depressive Disorder shows no improvement after 8 weeks of weekly therapy. The social worker should: A. Continue the same approach for another 8 weeks, B. Terminate services due to lack of progress, C. Reassess the treatment plan and consider modifications or referral, D. Increase sessions to twice weekly automatically

Answer: C. Reassess the treatment plan and consider modifications or referral

When treatment is ineffective, ethical practice requires reassessment, consultation, and modification of approach or appropriate referral.

Question 15: Dialectical Behavior Therapy (DBT) was originally developed to treat: A. Schizophrenia, B. Borderline Personality Disorder, C. Obsessive-Compulsive Disorder, D. Autism Spectrum Disorder

Answer: B. Borderline Personality Disorder

DBT was developed by Marsha Linehan specifically to treat Borderline Personality Disorder and focuses on emotion regulation, distress tolerance, mindfulness, and interpersonal effectiveness.

Question 16: A mandated reporter must report suspected child abuse: A. Only when there is definitive proof, B. When there is reasonable suspicion, C. Only if the child discloses abuse directly, D. After consulting with a supervisor

Answer: B. When there is reasonable suspicion

Mandated reporters must report when they have reasonable suspicion or cause to believe abuse or neglect has occurred, not when they have proof.

Question 17: In crisis intervention, the PRIMARY goal is to: A. Resolve all underlying psychological issues, B. Restore the client to pre-crisis functioning, C. Provide long-term psychotherapy, D. Diagnose mental disorders

Answer: B. Restore the client to pre-crisis functioning

Crisis intervention is time-limited and focuses on stabilization and returning the client to their previous level of functioning.

Question 18: A client asks the social worker personal questions about their marriage. The BEST response is to: A. Answer honestly to build rapport, B. Explore the client's reasons for asking and redirect to therapeutic goals, C. Refuse to answer and tell the client it's inappropriate, D. Share limited personal information

Answer: B. Explore the client's reasons for asking and redirect to therapeutic goals

This maintains professional boundaries while exploring the therapeutic meaning behind the question and keeping focus on the client's needs.

Question 19: Transference occurs when: A. The therapist projects feelings onto the client, B. The client projects feelings from past relationships onto the therapist, C. The therapist refers the client to another provider, D. The client transfers to a new therapist

Answer: B. The client projects feelings from past relationships onto the therapist

Transference is when a client unconsciously redirects feelings and attitudes from past relationships onto the therapist.

Question 20: A social worker must obtain informed consent that includes: A. Only the fee structure, B. Nature of services, risks, benefits, alternatives, and limits of confidentiality, C. Only the treatment goals, D. A guarantee of positive outcomes

Answer: B. Nature of services, risks, benefits, alternatives, and limits of confidentiality

Informed consent requires comprehensive information about all aspects of treatment to ensure clients can make knowledgeable decisions.

Question 21: Solution-Focused Brief Therapy emphasizes: A. Exploring childhood trauma, B. Analyzing unconscious conflicts, C. Identifying and building on client strengths and solutions, D. Confronting defense mechanisms

Answer: C. Identifying and building on client strengths and solutions

Solution-Focused Brief Therapy focuses on client strengths, resources, and solutions rather than problems and pathology.

Question 22: A client exhibits flight of ideas, decreased need for sleep, and grandiosity for 10 days. This MOST likely indicates: A. Major Depressive Episode, B. Manic Episode, C. Panic Attack, D. Generalized Anxiety Disorder

Answer: B. Manic Episode

These symptoms (flight of ideas, decreased sleep, grandiosity) lasting at least one week indicate a manic episode characteristic of Bipolar I Disorder.

Question 23: When terminating services with a client, the social worker should: A. Stop sessions immediately when goals are met, B. Process the termination, review progress, and provide referrals if needed, C. Continue sessions indefinitely to prevent relapse, D. Terminate by letter to avoid emotional reactions

Answer: B. Process the termination, review progress, and provide referrals if needed

Ethical termination involves preparation, processing feelings, reviewing gains, and ensuring continuity of care through appropriate referrals.

Question 24: A biopsychosocial assessment includes: A. Only psychological factors, B. Biological, psychological, and social factors, C. Only medical history, D. Only family dynamics

Answer: B. Biological, psychological, and social factors

The biopsychosocial model comprehensively assesses biological, psychological, and social factors contributing to the client's presenting concerns.

Question 25: Attachment theory was developed by: A. Sigmund Freud, B. Carl Rogers, C. John Bowlby, D. B.F. Skinner

Answer: C. John Bowlby

John Bowlby developed attachment theory, which examines the importance of early caregiver-child bonds on later development and relationships.

Question 26: A client reports hearing voices commanding them to harm themselves. The IMMEDIATE priority is: A. Exploring the content of the voices, B. Assessing suicide risk and ensuring safety, C. Diagnosing the psychotic disorder, D. Referring to a psychiatrist

Answer: B. Assessing suicide risk and ensuring safety

Command hallucinations to self-harm require immediate safety assessment and intervention to prevent harm.

Question 27: Countertransference refers to: A. The client's feelings toward the therapist, B. The therapist's emotional reactions to the client, C. Transferring a client to another therapist, D. The client changing therapists

Answer: B. The therapist's emotional reactions to the client

Countertransference involves the therapist's own emotional reactions and projections toward the client, often stemming from the therapist's past experiences.

Question 28: HIPAA regulations require: A. Unlimited sharing of client information with all healthcare providers, B. Protection of client health information privacy and security, C. That all records be kept indefinitely, D. Disclosure of all client information to family members

Answer: B. Protection of client health information privacy and security

HIPAA (Health Insurance Portability and Accountability Act) mandates protection of client health information privacy and security with specific guidelines for disclosure.

Question 29: A SMART goal is: A. Vague and open-ended, B. Specific, Measurable, Achievable, Relevant, and Time-bound, C. Only focused on long-term outcomes, D. Created solely by the therapist

Answer: B. Specific, Measurable, Achievable, Relevant, and Time-bound

SMART goals are Specific, Measurable, Achievable, Relevant, and Time-bound, providing clear treatment targets and progress measurement.

Question 30: Piaget's concept of conservation typically develops during: A. Sensorimotor stage, B. Preoperational stage, C. Concrete Operational stage, D. Formal Operational stage

Answer: C. Concrete Operational stage

Conservation (understanding that quantity remains the same despite changes in appearance) develops during the Concrete Operational stage (ages 7-11).

Question 31: A social worker's client is also their child's teacher. This represents: A. An unavoidable situation requiring no action, B. A dual relationship requiring discussion and likely referral, C. An acceptable relationship if kept separate, D. A minor boundary issue

Answer: B. A dual relationship requiring discussion and likely referral

This dual relationship creates multiple roles that could impair professional judgment and requires addressing, likely through referral.

Question 32: Group therapy is MOST effective for: A. Acute psychosis, B. Building interpersonal skills and receiving peer support, C. Clients who refuse individual therapy, D. Emergency crisis situations

Answer: B. Building interpersonal skills and receiving peer support

Group therapy provides unique opportunities for interpersonal learning, peer feedback, universality, and social skill development.

Question 33: A client with Generalized Anxiety Disorder would MOST likely present with: A. Excessive worry about multiple areas for at least 6 months, B. Intense fear of a specific object, C. Flashbacks to a traumatic event, D. Compulsive handwashing

Answer: A. Excessive worry about multiple areas for at least 6 months

GAD is characterized by excessive, difficult-to-control worry about various events or activities occurring most days for at least 6 months.

Question 34: The ecological perspective in social work emphasizes: A. Only individual factors, B. The interaction between individuals and their environment, C. Biological determinants only, D. Unconscious motivations

Answer: B. The interaction between individuals and their environment

The ecological perspective examines the reciprocal interactions between individuals and their multiple environmental systems.

Question 35: When a client misses three consecutive appointments without notice, the social worker should: A. Terminate services immediately, B. Attempt to contact the client and document efforts, C. Assume the client has dropped out and close the case, D. Wait for the client to contact them

Answer: B. Attempt to contact the client and document efforts

Professional responsibility includes reasonable efforts to re-engage clients and proper documentation before termination.

Question 36: Negative reinforcement in behavioral therapy involves: A. Punishing unwanted behavior, B. Removing an aversive stimulus to increase behavior, C. Ignoring inappropriate behavior, D. Adding a pleasant stimulus

Answer: B. Removing an aversive stimulus to increase behavior

Negative reinforcement increases behavior by removing an unpleasant stimulus, strengthening the desired response.

Question 37: A client reports flashbacks, nightmares, and hypervigilance following a car accident 2 months ago. The MOST likely diagnosis is: A. Adjustment Disorder, B. Acute Stress Disorder, C. Post-Traumatic Stress Disorder, D. Generalized Anxiety Disorder

Answer: C. Post-Traumatic Stress Disorder

Symptoms lasting more than one month following trauma indicate PTSD (Acute Stress Disorder is diagnosed within the first month).

Question 38: Informed consent must be obtained: A. Only at the first session, B. Only when required by law, C. Initially and updated as treatment evolves, D. Only for medication management

Answer: C. Initially and updated as treatment evolves

Informed consent is an ongoing process that must be obtained initially and updated as treatment circumstances change.

Question 39: A social worker discovers they have unresolved feelings about a client's issue similar to their own experience. The BEST action is to: A. Immediately terminate with the client, B. Seek supervision or consultation, C. Ignore the feelings and continue treatment, D. Disclose personal experiences to the client

Answer: B. Seek supervision or consultation

Recognizing countertransference requires seeking supervision to process feelings and ensure they don't interfere with client care.

Question 40: Kohlberg's theory addresses development of: A. Cognitive abilities, B. Moral reasoning, C. Emotional regulation, D. Motor skills

Answer: B. Moral reasoning

Lawrence Kohlberg's theory describes stages of moral reasoning development from childhood through adulthood.

Question 41: A client exhibits excessive fear of social situations, avoids gatherings, and fears negative evaluation. This suggests: A. Agoraphobia, B. Social Anxiety Disorder, C. Panic Disorder, D. Specific Phobia

Answer: B. Social Anxiety Disorder

Social Anxiety Disorder involves marked fear of social situations where the person fears negative evaluation or scrutiny by others.

Question 42: The primary function of clinical supervision is to: A. Monitor billable hours, B. Ensure quality of client care and support professional development, C. Evaluate therapist for termination, D. Complete required documentation

Answer: B. Ensure quality of client care and support professional development

Clinical supervision primarily focuses on enhancing clinical skills, ensuring quality care, and supporting the supervisee's professional growth.

Question 43: A client states "I must be perfect at everything or I'm a complete failure." This represents: A. Rational thinking, B. All-or-nothing thinking, C. Healthy self-expectations, D. Appropriate goal setting

Answer: B. All-or-nothing thinking

This cognitive distortion, also called black-and-white thinking, involves viewing situations in extreme categories without middle ground.

Question 44: When documenting in client records, social workers should: A. Include subjective opinions and judgments, B. Record objective observations and relevant clinical information, C. Document only positive progress, D. Avoid mentioning risk factors

Answer: B. Record objective observations and relevant clinical information

Documentation should be objective, factual, relevant, and focused on clinical observations and interventions.

Question 45: A strength-based approach focuses on: A. Pathology and deficits, B. Client resources, resilience, and capabilities, C. Only past trauma, D. Medication management

Answer: B. Client resources, resilience, and capabilities

Strength-based practice emphasizes client strengths, resources, and resilience rather than focusing solely on problems or deficits.

Question 46: The Mental Status Exam assesses: A. Only cognitive functioning, B. Current psychological functioning across multiple domains, C. Only mood and affect, D. Medical conditions only

Answer: B. Current psychological functioning across multiple domains

The MSE systematically assesses appearance, behavior, speech, mood, affect, thought process, thought content, cognition, insight, and judgment.

Question 47: A client diagnosed with Obsessive-Compulsive Disorder would MOST likely exhibit: A. Flashbacks and avoidance, B. Recurrent intrusive thoughts and repetitive behaviors, C. Grandiosity and flight of ideas, D. Auditory hallucinations

Answer: B. Recurrent intrusive thoughts and repetitive behaviors

OCD is characterized by obsessions (intrusive thoughts) and compulsions (repetitive behaviors) performed to reduce anxiety.

Question 48: When a client expresses suicidal ideation, the social worker must assess: A. Only the presence of a plan, B. Ideation, plan, means, intent, and protective factors, C. Only past suicide attempts, D. Family history exclusively

Answer: B. Ideation, plan, means, intent, and protective factors

Comprehensive suicide risk assessment includes ideation, specific plan, access to means, intent to act, prior attempts, and protective factors.

Question 49: Person-centered therapy, developed by Carl Rogers, emphasizes: A. Directive interventions, B. Unconditional positive regard, empathy, and genuineness, C. Interpretation of unconscious conflicts, D. Behavioral modification

Answer: B. Unconditional positive regard, empathy, and genuineness

Rogers' person-centered therapy emphasizes core conditions of unconditional positive regard, empathy, and genuineness to facilitate growth.

Question 50: A social worker should terminate services when: A. The client misses one appointment, B. Goals are achieved, services are no longer needed, or referral is appropriate, C. The social worker feels bored with the case, D. The client requests more frequent sessions

Answer: B. Goals are achieved, services are no longer needed, or referral is appropriate
Termination is indicated when treatment goals are met, services are no longer beneficial, or the client needs services outside the worker's scope.

Question 51: Domestic violence screening should occur: A. Only when abuse is suspected, B. Routinely with all clients in a safe, private setting, C. Only with female clients, D. Never, to avoid offending clients

Answer: B. Routinely with all clients in a safe, private setting

Best practice includes universal screening for domestic violence conducted privately and routinely with all clients.

Question 52: A social worker receives a subpoena for client records. The FIRST step is to: A. Immediately release all records, B. Consult with the client and legal counsel, C. Ignore the subpoena, D. Destroy the records

Answer: B. Consult with the client and legal counsel

Upon receiving a subpoena, consult with the client, seek legal guidance, and determine appropriate response to protect client confidentiality.

Question 53: Cognitive distortions in depression commonly include: A. Realistic thinking patterns, B. Negative views of self, world, and future, C. Excessive optimism, D. Grandiose beliefs

Answer: B. Negative views of self, world, and future

Beck's cognitive triad in depression includes negative views of self, the world, and the future, contributing to depressive symptoms.

Question 54: When working with involuntary clients, the social worker should: A. Refuse to provide services, B. Acknowledge the involuntary nature and work to establish rapport, C. Use only confrontational techniques, D. Report all behaviors to the court

Answer: B. Acknowledge the involuntary nature and work to establish rapport

Effective engagement with involuntary clients includes acknowledging their situation, validating feelings, and working to build a collaborative relationship.

Question 55: The Americans with Disabilities Act (ADA) requires: A. Discrimination against people with disabilities, B. Reasonable accommodations for individuals with disabilities, C. Mandatory medication for all mental illnesses, D. Segregated services

Answer: B. Reasonable accommodations for individuals with disabilities

The ADA prohibits discrimination and requires reasonable accommodations for individuals with disabilities in employment, public services, and accommodations.

Question 56: A client presents with depressed mood, insomnia, and concentration difficulties lasting 18 months. This suggests: A. Major Depressive Disorder, B. Persistent Depressive Disorder (Dysthymia), C. Bipolar Disorder, D. Cyclothymic Disorder

Answer: B. Persistent Depressive Disorder (Dysthymia)

Persistent Depressive Disorder involves depressed mood for at least 2 years in adults (1 year in children) with additional symptoms.

Question 57: Trauma-informed care principles include: A. Re-traumatizing clients to process experiences, B. Safety, trustworthiness, peer support, collaboration, and empowerment, C. Confrontation and reality testing only, D. Ignoring trauma history

Answer: B. Safety, trustworthiness, peer support, collaboration, and empowerment

Trauma-informed care is guided by principles of safety, trustworthiness, peer support, collaboration, empowerment, and cultural sensitivity.

Question 58: A social worker discovers their client is being treated by another therapist for the same issues. The appropriate action is to: A. Continue treatment without addressing it, B. Discuss with the client and coordinate care or clarify treatment roles, C. Immediately report the other therapist, D. Terminate without explanation

Answer: B. Discuss with the client and coordinate care or clarify treatment roles

Multiple providers require discussion with the client about treatment coordination to ensure integrated, non-duplicative care.

Question 59: Play therapy is MOST appropriate for: A. Elderly clients with dementia, B. Young children who have difficulty verbalizing, C. Adult clients with depression, D. Adolescents with conduct disorder only

Answer: B. Young children who have difficulty verbalizing

Play therapy is developmentally appropriate for young children who express and process experiences through play rather than verbal discussion.

Question 60: A social worker must report suspected elder abuse: A. Only with the elder's permission, B. When there is reasonable suspicion, regardless of client consent, C. Only if the elder requests it, D. Never, to maintain confidentiality

Answer: B. When there is reasonable suspicion, regardless of client consent

Social workers are mandated reporters and must report suspected elder abuse when there is reasonable cause to believe it has occurred.

Question 61: Motivational Interviewing uses which key strategy? A. Confrontation, B. Rolling with resistance, C. Authoritative advice-giving, D. Arguing for change

Answer: B. Rolling with resistance

MI principles include rolling with resistance, expressing empathy, developing discrepancy, and supporting self-efficacy rather than confrontation.

Question 62: A client with Antisocial Personality Disorder would MOST likely display: A. Excessive fear of abandonment, B. Disregard for others' rights and lack of remorse, C. Social anxiety and avoidance, D. Perfectionism and rigidity

Answer: B. Disregard for others' rights and lack of remorse

Antisocial Personality Disorder is characterized by pervasive disregard for and violation of others' rights, deceitfulness, and lack of remorse.

Question 63: The therapeutic alliance is BEST defined as: A. The therapist's theoretical orientation, B. The collaborative relationship between therapist and client, C. The treatment setting, D. The fee structure

Answer: B. The collaborative relationship between therapist and client

The therapeutic alliance encompasses the collaborative, trusting relationship between therapist and client, a key predictor of treatment outcomes.

Question 64: When a client requests records be sent to another provider, the social worker should: A. Refuse to protect confidentiality, B. Obtain written authorization and send relevant records, C. Send all personal notes, D. Verbally confirm without documentation

Answer: B. Obtain written authorization and send relevant records

Releasing records requires written client authorization specifying what information is released, to whom, and for what purpose.

Question 65: Ego defense mechanisms serve to: A. Increase anxiety, B. Protect the ego from anxiety and threat, C. Eliminate all psychological conflicts, D. Create psychopathology

Answer: B. Protect the ego from anxiety and threat

Defense mechanisms are unconscious psychological processes that protect the ego from anxiety, conflict, and threat.

Question 66: A social worker learns a client is non-compliant with court-ordered treatment. The worker should: A. Immediately report to the court, B. Explore barriers to compliance and document, determine reporting obligations, C. Terminate services, D. Ignore the non-compliance

Answer: B. Explore barriers to compliance and document, determine reporting obligations
Address non-compliance therapeutically, explore barriers, document, and clarify legal reporting obligations based on court order terms.

Question 67: Substance Use Disorder severity is determined by: A. The type of substance used, B. Number of DSM-5 criteria met, C. Only the duration of use, D. Client's income level

Answer: B. Number of DSM-5 criteria met

DSM-5 specifies severity based on the number of criteria met: mild (2-3), moderate (4-5), or severe (6 or more symptoms).

Question 68: A client expresses homicidal ideation toward a public figure. The social worker's duty is to: A. Maintain confidentiality absolutely, B. Assess risk and consult; duty to warn may not apply to public figures, C. Immediately contact the public figure, D. Post on social media to warn others

Answer: B. Assess risk and consult; duty to warn may not apply to public figures

While assessing risk is essential, duty to warn typically applies to identifiable, specific individuals; consultation and risk management are needed.

Question 69: Family sculpting is a technique used in: A. Individual psychoanalysis, B. Family therapy to represent family dynamics physically, C. Cognitive-behavioral therapy, D. Art therapy only

Answer: B. Family therapy to represent family dynamics physically

Family sculpting is an experiential family therapy technique where family members physically arrange themselves to represent family relationships and dynamics.

Question 70: A comprehensive suicide risk assessment includes all EXCEPT: A. Access to lethal means, B. Guaranteeing the client won't attempt suicide, C. Prior suicide attempts, D. Protective factors

Answer: B. Guaranteeing the client won't attempt suicide

No-suicide contracts or guarantees are not clinically sound; comprehensive assessment focuses on risk and protective factors to inform safety planning.

Question 71: Psychoeducation in mental health treatment involves: A. Withholding information to reduce anxiety, B. Educating clients about their condition, treatment options, and coping skills, C. Only discussing medication side effects, D. Avoiding discussion of diagnosis

Answer: B. Educating clients about their condition, treatment options, and coping skills
Psychoeducation provides clients with information about their condition, treatment options, and skills to enhance understanding and self-management.

Question 72: A client discloses past childhood sexual abuse for the first time. The social worker should: A. Immediately report to authorities, B. Validate the disclosure, assess current safety, and process appropriately, C. Minimize the importance to reduce distress, D. Change the subject

Answer: B. Validate the disclosure, assess current safety, and process appropriately

Respond with validation, assess current safety and functioning, and process the disclosure at the client's pace; past abuse of adults is not mandatorily reportable.

Question 73: Behavioral activation for depression focuses on: A. Analyzing childhood experiences, B. Increasing engagement in valued activities, C. Medication management only, D. Avoiding all stressful situations

Answer: B. Increasing engagement in valued activities

Behavioral activation combats depression by increasing engagement in meaningful, valued activities to improve mood and break the cycle of withdrawal.

Question 74: When making a referral, the social worker should: A. Simply provide a phone number, B. Assess client needs, provide appropriate referral information, and follow up, C. Make the appointment without client input, D. Terminate immediately after referral

Answer: B. Assess client needs, provide appropriate referral information, and follow up
Effective referrals involve assessing needs, providing appropriate resources, supporting the transition, and following up on outcomes.

Question 75: A client with Panic Disorder experiences: A. Gradual onset of worry over days, B. Sudden, intense fear with physical symptoms peaking within minutes, C. Persistent low mood, D. Chronic anger issues

Answer: B. Sudden, intense fear with physical symptoms peaking within minutes Panic attacks involve sudden onset of intense fear or discomfort with physical and cognitive symptoms that peak within minutes.

Question 76: Boundaries in the therapeutic relationship: A. Should be flexible based on social worker preference, B. Protect both client and therapist and maintain professional relationship, C. Are unnecessary with cooperative clients, D. Only apply to fee arrangements

Answer: B. Protect both client and therapist and maintain professional relationship

Professional boundaries protect the therapeutic relationship, ensure ethical practice, and safeguard both client and therapist welfare.

Question 77: A social worker's personal values conflict with a client's decision. The worker should: A. Impose their values on the client, B. Recognize the conflict, maintain client self-determination, seek consultation if needed, C. Terminate immediately, D. Argue with the client about values

Answer: B. Recognize the conflict, maintain client self-determination, seek consultation if needed

Social workers must recognize personal value conflicts, maintain client self-determination, and seek supervision when conflicts interfere with practice.

Question 78: Grief counseling is MOST helpful when: A. Immediately forcing the bereaved to move on, B. Supporting the mourning process and adjustment to loss, C. Encouraging avoidance of grief feelings, D. Prescribing medication only

Answer: B. Supporting the mourning process and adjustment to loss

Grief counseling supports the natural mourning process, facilitates healthy expression of grief, and assists in adjusting to life after loss.

Question 79: A client reports being followed, monitored by cameras, and believes coworkers are plotting against them. This suggests: A. Generalized Anxiety Disorder, B. Persecutory delusions, C. Social Anxiety Disorder, D. Obsessive-Compulsive Disorder

Answer: B. Persecutory delusions

Persecutory delusions involve fixed false beliefs of being targeted, followed, or conspired against, seen in psychotic disorders.

Question 80: When treating adolescents, confidentiality: A. Never applies to minors, B. Should be discussed with both teen and parents, with limitations explained, C. Is absolute regardless of risk, D. Only involves parents, not the teen

Answer: B. Should be discussed with both teen and parents, with limitations explained
Adolescent treatment requires clarifying confidentiality boundaries with both teen and parents, including limitations regarding safety and legal requirements.

Question 81: Mindfulness-based interventions focus on: A. Analyzing past events, B. Present-moment awareness without judgment, C. Future planning only, D. Avoiding all thoughts

Answer: B. Present-moment awareness without judgment

Mindfulness involves purposeful, present-moment awareness with acceptance and non-judgment, used in various therapeutic approaches.

Question 82: A social worker practices outside their area of competence. This violates: A. No ethical standards, B. NASW Code of Ethics regarding competence, C. Only agency policy, D. No standards if the client consents

Answer: B. NASW Code of Ethics regarding competence

The NASW Code requires social workers to practice only within their areas of competence and obtain necessary training or make appropriate referrals.

Question 83: Expressing empathy in clinical practice means: A. Agreeing with everything the client says, B. Understanding and communicating understanding of the client's experience, C. Sharing personal similar experiences, D. Feeling sorry for the client

Answer: B. Understanding and communicating understanding of the client's experience
Empathy involves accurately understanding the client's emotional experience and effectively communicating that understanding.

Question 84: A client in recovery from alcohol use is considering attending a party where alcohol will be served. The social worker should: A. Forbid attendance, B. Explore risks, coping strategies, and help develop a safety plan, C. Encourage attendance to build confidence, D. Ignore the situation

Answer: B. Explore risks, coping strategies, and help develop a safety plan

Support the client in identifying risks, exploring coping strategies, and developing a concrete plan to maintain sobriety if they choose to attend.

Question 85: Research shows the MOST important factor in therapy outcome is: A. The therapist's credentials, B. The therapeutic relationship, C. The office environment, D. The therapist's theoretical orientation

Answer: B. The therapeutic relationship

Research consistently demonstrates that the quality of the therapeutic relationship is the most significant predictor of positive treatment outcomes.

Question 86: When documenting a client's suicidal ideation, the record should include: A. Only that ideation was present, B. Detailed assessment of risk factors, interventions, and safety plan, C. Personal opinions about the client's intentions, D. Minimal information to protect privacy

Answer: B. Detailed assessment of risk factors, interventions, and safety plan

Documentation must thoroughly detail risk assessment, clinical reasoning, interventions implemented, and safety planning for continuity of care and legal protection.

Question 87: A client with Schizophrenia would MOST likely experience: A. Only mood symptoms, B. Hallucinations, delusions, and disorganized thinking, C. Excessive worry, D. Compulsive behaviors only

Answer: B. Hallucinations, delusions, and disorganized thinking

Schizophrenia involves positive symptoms (hallucinations, delusions) and negative symptoms (flat affect, avolition) along with cognitive impairments.

Question 88: Reflective listening involves: A. Giving advice immediately, B. Paraphrasing and reflecting the client's message and feelings, C. Interrupting to ask questions, D. Focusing only on facts

Answer: B. Paraphrasing and reflecting the client's message and feelings

Reflective listening involves accurately paraphrasing content and reflecting underlying emotions to demonstrate understanding and facilitate exploration.

Question 89: A social worker accepts an expensive gift from a client. This: A. Is always appropriate, B. May constitute a boundary violation and should be carefully considered, C. Is required to maintain the relationship, D. Has no ethical implications

Answer: B. May constitute a boundary violation and should be carefully considered

Accepting gifts, especially expensive ones, may create boundary violations, conflicts of interest, or exploitation and requires careful ethical consideration.

Question 90: Displacement as a defense mechanism involves: A. Denying reality, B. Redirecting emotions from the original source to a safer target, C. Reverting to earlier developmental behaviors, D. Blocking memories completely

Answer: B. Redirecting emotions from the original source to a safer target

Displacement involves redirecting feelings from a threatening target to a less threatening one, such as anger at boss redirected toward family.

Question 91: When a client poses a danger to themselves or others, the social worker's FIRST priority is: A. Completing paperwork, B. Ensuring safety through appropriate intervention, C. Maintaining confidentiality at all costs, D. Scheduling the next appointment

Answer: B. Ensuring safety through appropriate intervention

Safety is always the first priority; appropriate interventions may include hospitalization, crisis services, or notifying authorities when necessary.

Question 92: A client diagnosed with Bipolar II Disorder experiences: A. Only manic episodes, B. Hypomanic episodes and major depressive episodes, C. Only depressive episodes, D. Psychotic symptoms exclusively

Answer: B. Hypomanic episodes and major depressive episodes

Bipolar II Disorder involves at least one hypomanic episode and one major depressive episode (no full manic episodes).

Question 93: Cultural humility differs from cultural competence by emphasizing: A. Mastery of all cultures, B. Lifelong learning, self-reflection, and addressing power imbalances, C. Avoiding cultural discussions, D. Expertise in specific cultures

Answer: B. Lifelong learning, self-reflection, and addressing power imbalances

Cultural humility involves ongoing self-reflection, recognizing power dynamics, and commitment to lifelong learning rather than claiming cultural expertise.

Question 94: A social worker suspects a colleague is impaired due to substance use. The appropriate action is to: A. Ignore it if client care seems adequate, B. Follow agency and ethical reporting procedures, C. Confront the colleague publicly, D. Wait until harm occurs

Answer: B. Follow agency and ethical reporting procedures

Suspected impairment requires following established reporting procedures to protect clients and support the impaired colleague in getting help.

Question 95: Exposure therapy is MOST effective for treating: A. Schizophrenia, B. Anxiety disorders and PTSD, C. Bipolar Disorder, D. Personality disorders

Answer: B. Anxiety disorders and PTSD

Exposure therapy, involving gradual confrontation with feared stimuli, is highly effective for anxiety disorders, specific phobias, and PTSD.

Question 96: A client struggles to identify and express emotions. This describes: A. Empathy, B. Alexithymia, C. Narcissism, D. Projection

Answer: B. Alexithymia

Alexithymia involves difficulty identifying, describing, and expressing one's own emotions, often associated with trauma or certain disorders.

Question 97: When working with clients who have experienced trauma, the social worker should: A. Force immediate trauma processing, B. Establish safety and stabilization before trauma processing, C. Avoid discussing trauma entirely, D. Focus only on current symptoms

Answer: B. Establish safety and stabilization before trauma processing

Trauma-informed practice requires establishing safety, building coping skills, and stabilizing functioning before direct trauma processing.

Question 98: A client's insurance denies coverage for additional sessions. The social worker should: A. Terminate services immediately, B. Explore options including appeals, sliding scale, or referral, C. Continue without payment, D. Threaten the client

Answer: B. Explore options including appeals, sliding scale, or referral

Address payment challenges through appeals, alternative payment arrangements, community resources, or appropriate referral to ensure continuity of care.

Question 99: Harm reduction approaches in substance use treatment: A. Require immediate abstinence, B. Meet clients where they are and reduce negative consequences, C. Enable continued use without limits, D. Focus only on detoxification

Answer: B. Meet clients where they are and reduce negative consequences

Harm reduction accepts the client's current level of use and works to minimize associated harms and risks while supporting change at the client's pace.

Question 100: A social worker finds themselves attracted to a client. The MOST appropriate action is: A. Pursue a relationship after termination, B. Seek immediate supervision and consider referral, C. Ignore the feelings, D. Disclose feelings to the client

Answer: B. Seek immediate supervision and consider referral

Attraction to clients requires immediate supervision to address countertransference, maintain boundaries, and determine if referral is necessary.

Question 101: Intergenerational trauma refers to: A. Trauma affecting only one generation, B. Trauma effects transmitted across generations, C. Trauma occurring in childhood only, D. Only biological inheritance

Answer: B. Trauma effects transmitted across generations

Intergenerational trauma describes how trauma impacts are passed through families across generations through biological, psychological, and social mechanisms.

Question 102: A client with hoarding disorder would display: A. Excessive cleaning and organizing, B. Persistent difficulty discarding possessions regardless of value, C. Frequent handwashing, D. Fear of contamination only

Answer: B. Persistent difficulty discarding possessions regardless of value

Hoarding Disorder involves persistent difficulty discarding items, resulting in accumulation that clutters living spaces and causes distress or impairment.

Question 103: When terminating with a client who shows strong dependence, the social worker should: A. Terminate abruptly to promote independence, B. Process termination gradually, reinforce gains, and provide resources, C. Continue indefinitely to prevent distress, D. Avoid discussing termination

Answer: B. Process termination gradually, reinforce gains, and provide resources

Dependent clients benefit from gradual termination processing, reinforcement of skills and progress, and connection to ongoing support resources.

Question 104: A mandated reporter's obligation applies: A. Only during work hours, B. At all times when they encounter suspected abuse, C. Only in the office setting, D. Only if they witnessed abuse directly

Answer: B. At all times when they encounter suspected abuse

Mandated reporter status is continuous; social workers must report suspected abuse whenever and wherever they encounter it.

Question 105: Validation in DBT involves: A. Agreeing with all client behaviors, B. Acknowledging the client's experience as understandable in context, C. Minimizing client concerns, D. Ignoring emotional responses

Answer: B. Acknowledging the client's experience as understandable in context

Validation in DBT communicates that the client's responses are understandable given their experiences and context, even if not effective.

Question 106: A client experiencing a panic attack should be helped by: A. Telling them to calm down, B. Using grounding techniques and controlled breathing, C. Leaving them alone, D. Increasing environmental stimulation

Answer: B. Using grounding techniques and controlled breathing

Panic attacks are managed through grounding techniques, controlled breathing, reassurance, and helping the client recognize the temporary nature of symptoms.

Question 107: Supervision of clinical social workers should include: A. Only administrative tasks, B. Clinical skill development, ethical guidance, and case consultation, C. Punishment for mistakes, D. Only documentation review

Answer: B. Clinical skill development, ethical guidance, and case consultation

Effective supervision addresses clinical skills, ethical decision-making, case conceptualization, self-awareness, and professional development.

Question 108: A client with Avoidant Personality Disorder typically exhibits: A. Disregard for others' rights, B. Social inhibition, feelings of inadequacy, and hypersensitivity to rejection, C. Grandiosity and need for admiration, D. Unstable relationships and identity

Answer: B. Social inhibition, feelings of inadequacy, and hypersensitivity to rejection

Avoidant Personality Disorder involves pervasive social inhibition, feelings of inadequacy, and extreme sensitivity to negative evaluation.

Question 109: Evidence-based practice in social work involves: A. Using only the newest interventions, B. Integrating best research evidence with clinical expertise and client values, C. Following only agency protocols, D. Ignoring research findings

Answer: B. Integrating best research evidence with clinical expertise and client values

EBP combines the best available research evidence with clinical expertise and client preferences/values to inform practice decisions.

Question 110: A social worker learns their client is HIV-positive and has not disclosed to their partner. The worker should: A. Immediately inform the partner, B. Explore disclosure with client, assess risk, and consult regarding legal obligations, C. Maintain absolute confidentiality with no discussion, D. Terminate services

Answer: B. Explore disclosure with client, assess risk, and consult regarding legal obligations
Address HIV disclosure therapeutically, understand state-specific laws, encourage client disclosure, and consult regarding duty to warn applicability.

Question 111: Relapse prevention planning includes: A. Guaranteeing no relapse will occur, B. Identifying triggers, warning signs, and coping strategies, C. Focusing only on past relapses, D. Avoiding discussion of high-risk situations

Answer: B. Identifying triggers, warning signs, and coping strategies

Relapse prevention involves identifying personal triggers, recognizing early warning signs, and developing specific coping strategies for high-risk situations.

Question 112: A client shows extreme mood swings, impulsivity, unstable relationships, and fear of abandonment. This suggests: A. Bipolar Disorder, B. Borderline Personality Disorder, C. Major Depressive Disorder, D. Schizophrenia

Answer: B. Borderline Personality Disorder

BPD is characterized by instability in relationships, self-image, affect, and marked impulsivity, along with frantic efforts to avoid abandonment.

Question 113: When practicing from a feminist perspective, social workers: A. Only work with female clients, B. Address power dynamics and promote equality and empowerment, C. Ignore gender issues, D. Blame all problems on patriarchy

Answer: B. Address power dynamics and promote equality and empowerment

Feminist practice examines power structures, addresses gender and social inequalities, and promotes client empowerment and social justice.

Question 114: A social worker discovers they made an error in treatment. The ethical response is to: A. Hide the error from the client, B. Acknowledge the error, inform the client, and take corrective action, C. Blame the client, D. Change documentation to cover the mistake

Answer: B. Acknowledge the error, inform the client, and take corrective action

Ethical practice requires acknowledging errors, informing affected parties, taking steps to rectify the situation, and preventing future occurrences.

Question 115: Cognitive restructuring in CBT involves: A. Accepting all thoughts as true, B. Identifying and challenging maladaptive thought patterns, C. Suppressing unwanted thoughts, D. Avoiding thinking about problems

Answer: B. Identifying and challenging maladaptive thought patterns

Cognitive restructuring helps clients identify distorted thinking patterns and develop more balanced, realistic thoughts.

Question 116: A client expresses hopelessness but denies suicidal ideation. The social worker should: A. Accept the denial without further assessment, B. Assess further for passive ideation and risk factors, C. Immediately hospitalize, D. Terminate due to low risk

Answer: B. Assess further for passive ideation and risk factors

Hopelessness is a significant risk factor; further assessment of passive ideation, risk factors, and protective factors is necessary.

Question 117: When clients are court-mandated for treatment, informed consent should: A. Not be obtained, B. Clarify voluntary vs. mandated aspects and limits of confidentiality, C. Be waived entirely, D. Only address court reporting

Answer: B. Clarify voluntary vs. mandated aspects and limits of confidentiality

Even with mandated clients, informed consent must clarify what is mandated, voluntary choices within treatment, and specific reporting requirements.

Question 118: Unconditional positive regard means: A. Agreeing with all client behaviors, B. Accepting the client without judgment while addressing problematic behaviors, C. Never setting boundaries, D. Avoiding difficult topics

Answer: B. Accepting the client without judgment while addressing problematic behaviors Unconditional positive regard involves accepting and valuing the client as a person while appropriately addressing harmful or problematic behaviors.

Question 119: A social worker's clinical notes are requested by the client. The worker should: A. Refuse all access to records, B. Provide access as required by law, with consideration for potential harm, C. Only provide highly edited versions, D. Charge excessive fees to discourage access

Answer: B. Provide access as required by law, with consideration for potential harm

Clients generally have rights to their records; provide access as legally required while considering potential harm and following applicable regulations.

Question 120: Solution-focused questions include: A. "Why do you have these problems?", B. "What will be different when this problem is solved?", C. "Whose fault is this situation?", D. "Why haven't you fixed this yet?"

Answer: B. "What will be different when this problem is solved?"

Solution-focused therapy uses future-oriented questions about desired changes, exceptions to problems, and client strengths rather than problem analysis.

Question 121: A client in an abusive relationship is not ready to leave. The social worker should: A. Force them to leave immediately, B. Respect autonomy while providing safety planning and resources, C. Terminate services, D. Contact the abuser directly

Answer: B. Respect autonomy while providing safety planning and resources

Respect client autonomy and readiness while providing education, safety planning, resources, and ongoing support for when they are ready to change.

Question 122: Acting out as a defense mechanism involves: A. Direct verbal expression, B. Expressing unconscious conflicts through behavior rather than words, C. Complete honesty, D. Healthy emotional expression

Answer: B. Expressing unconscious conflicts through behavior rather than words

Acting out involves expressing unconscious emotional conflicts or feelings through actions rather than words or conscious awareness.

Question 123: A client with Social Anxiety Disorder would benefit MOST from: A. Isolation and avoidance, B. Cognitive restructuring and gradual exposure, C. Immediate exposure to large crowds, D. Medication only

Answer: B. Cognitive restructuring and gradual exposure

Social Anxiety Disorder is effectively treated with CBT including cognitive restructuring of feared negative evaluations and gradual exposure to social situations.

Question 124: When a client's goals differ from the social worker's treatment recommendations, the worker should: A. Insist on their own goals, B. Collaboratively explore differences and work toward mutually agreed goals, C. Terminate immediately, D. Ignore the client's preferences

Answer: B. Collaboratively explore differences and work toward mutually agreed goals

Client self-determination requires collaborative exploration of different perspectives and negotiation of mutually acceptable treatment goals.

Question 125: A biopsychosocial formulation integrates: A. Only medication effects, B. Biological, psychological, and social factors in case conceptualization, C. Only family dynamics, D. Exclusively psychological theories

Answer: B. Biological, psychological, and social factors in case conceptualization
Biopsychosocial formulation comprehensively integrates biological, psychological, and social factors to understand the client's presentation.

Question 126: Countertransference is BEST managed by: A. Ignoring personal reactions, B. Self-awareness, supervision, and personal therapy when needed, C. Acting on all feelings, D. Avoiding self-reflection

Answer: B. Self-awareness, supervision, and personal therapy when needed

Managing countertransference requires ongoing self-awareness, regular supervision, consultation, and personal therapy to address unresolved issues.

Question 127: A client diagnosed with Illness Anxiety Disorder (Hypochondriasis) would exhibit: A. Deliberate production of symptoms, B. Preoccupation with having a serious illness despite medical reassurance, C. Actual medical illness, D. Lack of concern about health

Answer: B. Preoccupation with having a serious illness despite medical reassurance

Illness Anxiety Disorder involves excessive worry about having a serious illness despite appropriate medical evaluation and reassurance.

Question 128: When making clinical decisions, social workers should prioritize: A. Personal preferences, B. Client welfare and safety, C. Agency convenience, D. Financial considerations only

Answer: B. Client welfare and safety

The primary obligation is client welfare and safety; other factors may be considered but cannot supersede this fundamental ethical duty.

Question 129: A client with Narcissistic Personality Disorder typically displays: A. Low self-esteem and social withdrawal, B. Grandiosity, need for admiration, and lack of empathy, C. Excessive dependence on others, D. Pervasive distrust and suspicion

Answer: B. Grandiosity, need for admiration, and lack of empathy

Narcissistic Personality Disorder involves grandiose sense of self-importance, need for excessive admiration, and lack of empathy for others.

Question 130: Risk assessment for violence should include: A. Only past violence history, B. Past violence, current threats, access to weapons, and protective factors, C. Only demographic factors, D. Astrological signs

Answer: B. Past violence, current threats, access to weapons, and protective factors
Comprehensive violence risk assessment examines historical violence, current threats/intent, access to means, mental state, and protective factors.

Question 131: A social worker practices within their scope of competence by: A. Treating any presenting problem, B. Practicing within areas of education, training, and experience, C. Only using one theoretical approach, D. Avoiding professional development

Answer: B. Practicing within areas of education, training, and experience

Ethical practice requires working within one's competence boundaries defined by education, training, supervised experience, and credentials.

Question 132: Empowerment-based practice focuses on: A. Creating dependency, B. Building on client strengths and facilitating control over their lives, C. Social worker as expert, D. Focusing only on deficits

Answer: B. Building on client strengths and facilitating control over their lives

Empowerment practice recognizes client strengths, promotes self-determination, and helps clients gain control over factors affecting their lives.

Question 133: A client reports hearing a voice commenting on their actions throughout the day. This describes: A. An illusion, B. A running commentary hallucination, C. A delusion, D. Normal experience

Answer: B. A running commentary hallucination

Running commentary is a type of auditory hallucination where voices provide ongoing commentary on the person's actions, common in schizophrenia.

Question 134: When a client threatens to file a complaint against the social worker, the appropriate response is to: A. Become defensive and argumentative, B. Listen to concerns, document, and consult with supervisor/legal counsel, C. Immediately admit fault, D. Threaten the client

Answer: B. Listen to concerns, document, and consult with supervisor/legal counsel

Respond professionally by listening to concerns, documenting the interaction, and seeking appropriate consultation and legal guidance.

Question 135: Systematic desensitization for phobias involves: A. Immediate intense exposure, B. Gradual exposure paired with relaxation techniques, C. Avoidance of the feared stimulus, D. Medication only

Answer: B. Gradual exposure paired with relaxation techniques

Systematic desensitization gradually exposes clients to feared stimuli while in a relaxed state, using a hierarchy from least to most anxiety-provoking.

Question 136: A social worker should terminate services when continuing would: A. Be slightly inconvenient, B. Not benefit the client or when services are outside scope of competence, C. Require any effort, D. Last more than three months

Answer: B. Not benefit the client or when services are outside scope of competence

Termination is indicated when services are no longer beneficial, outside the worker's competence, or when another provider is more appropriate.

Question 137: Regression as a defense mechanism involves: A. Moving forward in development, B. Reverting to earlier developmental behaviors under stress, C. Aggressive behavior, D. Complete memory loss

Answer: B. Reverting to earlier developmental behaviors under stress

Regression involves returning to earlier, more primitive patterns of behavior and thinking, typically in response to stress or threat.

Question 138: A client diagnosed with Separation Anxiety Disorder would experience: A. Fear of social situations, B. Excessive anxiety about separation from attachment figures, C. Fear of specific objects, D. Generalized worry about everything

Answer: B. Excessive anxiety about separation from attachment figures

Separation Anxiety Disorder involves excessive fear or anxiety about separation from attachment figures, beyond what is developmentally appropriate.

Question 139: Advocacy in social work includes: A. Only individual client advocacy, B. Representing client interests and promoting social justice at multiple levels, C. Avoiding systemic issues, D. Only political activities

Answer: B. Representing client interests and promoting social justice at multiple levels

Social work advocacy addresses individual client needs, systemic barriers, policy change, and social justice across micro, mezzo, and macro levels.

Question 140: A client reports decreased need for sleep, increased goal-directed activity, and risky behaviors for 4 days. This suggests: A. Major Depressive Episode, B. Possible hypomanic episode, evaluate further, C. Normal stress response, D. Anxiety Disorder

Answer: B. Possible hypomanic episode, evaluate further

These symptoms lasting at least 4 days suggest a hypomanic episode (Bipolar II); full manic episodes require 7 days or hospitalization.

Question 141: Professional liability insurance protects social workers from: A. All ethical violations, B. Financial costs of malpractice claims and legal defense, C. Criminal charges, D. Licensing board sanctions

Answer: B. Financial costs of malpractice claims and legal defense

Professional liability insurance covers costs associated with malpractice claims and legal defense, though it doesn't prevent ethical or legal violations.

Question 142: When using interpreters, social workers should: A. Speak directly to the interpreter, B. Speak to the client while the interpreter translates, C. Only use family members as interpreters, D. Avoid using interpreters

Answer: B. Speak to the client while the interpreter translates

Best practice involves speaking directly to the client, maintaining eye contact with them, and using professional interpreters rather than family members.

Question 143: A client with Dependent Personality Disorder exhibits: A. Pervasive distrust, B. Excessive need to be taken care of and fear of separation, C. Grandiosity, D. Social detachment

Answer: B. Excessive need to be taken care of and fear of separation

Dependent Personality Disorder involves pervasive need to be cared for, leading to submissive, clinging behavior and fear of separation.

Question 144: The "miracle question" in Solution-Focused Therapy asks: A. About past traumas, B. "If a miracle happened and your problem was solved, what would be different?", C. "Why do you have this problem?", D. "Who is responsible for your problems?"

Answer: B. "If a miracle happened and your problem was solved, what would be different?"
The miracle question helps clients envision their preferred future and identify concrete signs that their problem has been resolved.

Question 145: Self-care for social workers is: A. Selfish and unprofessional, B. Essential for preventing burnout and maintaining competence, C. Only needed for new practitioners, D. A luxury, not a necessity

Answer: B. Essential for preventing burnout and maintaining competence

Self-care is an ethical imperative to prevent burnout, maintain competence, and ensure quality client care through managing personal well-being.

Question 146: A client diagnosed with Agoraphobia fears: A. Only open spaces, B. Situations where escape might be difficult or help unavailable, C. Only closed spaces, D. Social interactions exclusively

Answer: B. Situations where escape might be difficult or help unavailable

Agoraphobia involves fear of situations where escape might be difficult or embarrassing, or help might not be available during panic symptoms.

Question 147: Clinical documentation serves to: A. Create busy work for therapists, B. Ensure continuity of care, legal protection, and treatment accountability, C. Only fulfill insurance requirements, D. Replace supervision

Answer: B. Ensure continuity of care, legal protection, and treatment accountability
Documentation ensures treatment continuity, provides legal protection, demonstrates accountability, facilitates communication, and supports quality care.

Question 148: A client in a manic episode may require: A. Outpatient therapy only, B. Hospitalization if a danger to self/others or gravely disabled, C. No intervention, D. Only medication management

Answer: B. Hospitalization if a danger to self/others or gravely disabled

Severe manic episodes may require psychiatric hospitalization for safety and stabilization, especially if judgment is severely impaired.

Question 149: Parallel process in supervision refers to: A. Supervisor and supervisee working separately, B. Dynamics between client and clinician reflected in supervision, C. Two supervision sessions occurring simultaneously, D. Using identical techniques with all clients

Answer: B. Dynamics between client and clinician reflected in supervision

Parallel process occurs when relationship dynamics between client and clinician are unconsciously recreated in the supervisory relationship.

Question 150: A social worker maintains multiple current relationships with a former client. This: A. Is always appropriate after termination, B. May constitute a boundary violation depending on circumstances, C. Is required for good practice, D. Has no ethical implications

Answer: B. May constitute a boundary violation depending on circumstances

Post-termination relationships require careful consideration of exploitation potential, power dynamics, and client vulnerability; many are ethically problematic.

Question 151: Psychotropic medications are PRIMARILY prescribed by: A. Social workers, B. Psychiatrists and other medical professionals, C. Psychologists in all states, D. Case managers

Answer: B. Psychiatrists and other medical professionals

While some psychologists can prescribe in certain states, psychiatrists and other medical professionals (physicians, nurse practitioners) primarily prescribe psychotropic medications.

Question 152: A comprehensive treatment plan includes: A. Only the diagnosis, B. Problems, goals, objectives, interventions, and progress measures, C. Only the social worker's opinions, D. Insurance information only

Answer: B. Problems, goals, objectives, interventions, and progress measures

Effective treatment plans identify problems, establish measurable goals and objectives, specify interventions, and include methods for measuring progress.

Question 153: When a client is at imminent risk of harm, the social worker may need to: A. Wait for the next scheduled session, B. Breach confidentiality to protect the client or others, C. Maintain absolute confidentiality regardless, D. Ignore the risk

Answer: B. Breach confidentiality to protect the client or others

Imminent risk of serious harm constitutes an exception to confidentiality; social workers must take appropriate action to prevent harm.

Question 154: A client with specific phobia of dogs would benefit from: A. Avoiding all dogs permanently, B. Gradual exposure therapy (in vivo or imaginal), C. Psychoanalysis only, D. Medication without therapy

Answer: B. Gradual exposure therapy (in vivo or imaginal)

Specific phobias are effectively treated with exposure therapy, either in vivo (real-life) or imaginal, using gradual systematic desensitization.

Question 155: Vicarious trauma affects social workers who: A. Never hear about client trauma, B. Are repeatedly exposed to clients' traumatic material, C. Only work with children, D. Have personal trauma history exclusively

Answer: B. Are repeatedly exposed to clients' traumatic material

Vicarious trauma results from cumulative exposure to clients' traumatic experiences, potentially affecting the helper's worldview, spirituality, and functioning.

Question 156: A social worker disagrees with a supervisor's clinical recommendation. The worker should: A. Ignore the supervisor and do what they want, B. Discuss concerns professionally and document if unresolved, C. Immediately report to licensing board, D. Follow blindly without question

Answer: B. Discuss concerns professionally and document if unresolved

Professional disagreement requires respectful discussion, consideration of supervisor's perspective, and documentation if concerns about client welfare remain.

Question 157: When assessing for domestic violence, the social worker should: A. Ask only in the presence of the partner, B. Screen privately and assess safety, resources, and readiness to change, C. Never ask about abuse, D. Only ask if visible injuries are present

Answer: B. Screen privately and assess safety, resources, and readiness to change

Domestic violence screening must occur privately, assess current safety, explore available resources, and determine the client's readiness for change.

Question 158: A social worker receives a friend request from a client on social media. The appropriate response is: A. Accept to build rapport, B. Decline and discuss professional boundaries with the client, C. Accept but don't interact, D. Ignore without addressing

Answer: B. Decline and discuss professional boundaries with the client

Professional boundaries require declining social media connections with clients and discussing the importance of maintaining the therapeutic relationship.

Question 159: A client with Obsessive-Compulsive Personality Disorder typically exhibits: A. Obsessive thoughts and compulsive rituals, B. Perfectionism, rigidity, and excessive devotion to work, C. Fear of abandonment, D. Grandiose self-image

Answer: B. Perfectionism, rigidity, and excessive devotion to work

OCPD involves preoccupation with orderliness, perfectionism, and control at the expense of flexibility and efficiency, distinct from OCD.

Question 160: When conducting a mental status exam, the social worker assesses: A. Only the client's mood, B. Appearance, behavior, speech, mood, affect, thought process, thought content, cognition, insight, and judgment, C. Only cognitive functioning, D. Medical conditions exclusively

Answer: B. Appearance, behavior, speech, mood, affect, thought process, thought content, cognition, insight, and judgment

The MSE systematically evaluates all aspects of current mental functioning to inform diagnosis and treatment planning.

Question 161: A client experiencing mania is MOST likely to exhibit: A. Psychomotor retardation, B. Decreased need for sleep and increased energy, C. Social withdrawal, D. Excessive sleeping

Answer: B. Decreased need for sleep and increased energy

Manic episodes are characterized by decreased need for sleep, increased energy, rapid speech, racing thoughts, and increased goal-directed activity.

Question 162: Informed consent is considered valid when the client: A. Signs any form presented, B. Understands, is competent, and voluntarily agrees, C. Is coerced into agreeing, D. Has no other options

Answer: B. Understands, is competent, and voluntarily agrees

Valid informed consent requires the client has capacity to understand, comprehends the information, and voluntarily agrees without coercion.

Question 163: A social worker learns confidential client information will be subpoenaed. The FIRST step is to: A. Release all information immediately, B. Assert privilege and consult with attorney, C. Destroy the records, D. Ignore the subpoena

Answer: B. Assert privilege and consult with attorney

When records are subpoenaed, assert privilege on the client's behalf, consult legal counsel, and only release information as legally required.

Question 164: Eye Movement Desensitization and Reprocessing (EMDR) is primarily used to treat: A. Schizophrenia, B. Post-Traumatic Stress Disorder, C. Intellectual disabilities, D. Substance use disorders exclusively

Answer: B. Post-Traumatic Stress Disorder

EMDR was developed specifically for PTSD treatment and uses bilateral stimulation to help process traumatic memories and reduce distress.

Question 165: A client demonstrates lack of insight into their mental illness. This means they: A. Are dishonest, B. Don't recognize or understand they have a mental health condition, C. Are always dangerous, D. Cannot benefit from treatment

Answer: B. Don't recognize or understand they have a mental health condition

Lack of insight (anosognosia) involves inability to recognize one's mental illness, often seen in psychotic disorders and requiring adapted treatment approaches.

Question 166: Professional boundaries exist to: A. Punish social workers, B. Protect clients and maintain the therapeutic relationship, C. Make therapy less effective, D. Create distance from all clients

Answer: B. Protect clients and maintain the therapeutic relationship

Boundaries protect the therapeutic relationship, prevent exploitation, maintain professional roles, and ensure the focus remains on client needs.

Question 167: A client reports command hallucinations to harm others. The social worker's immediate duty is to: A. Maintain confidentiality absolutely, B. Assess risk, ensure safety, and warn potential victims if necessary, C. Schedule a follow-up appointment, D. Refer to another provider

Answer: B. Assess risk, ensure safety, and warn potential victims if necessary

Command hallucinations to harm others require immediate risk assessment, safety planning, possible hospitalization, and warning identifiable victims per Tarasoff.

Question 168: Rational Emotive Behavior Therapy (REBT) focuses on: A. Unconscious conflicts, B. Identifying and disputing irrational beliefs, C. Behavioral conditioning only, D. Family dynamics exclusively

Answer: B. Identifying and disputing irrational beliefs

REBT, developed by Albert Ellis, identifies and challenges irrational beliefs that lead to emotional disturbance and maladaptive behaviors.

Question 169: A social worker practices cultural competence by: A. Treating all clients identically, B. Continuously learning about diverse cultures and examining personal biases, C. Making assumptions based on ethnicity, D. Avoiding clients from different backgrounds

Answer: B. Continuously learning about diverse cultures and examining personal biases

Cultural competence is an ongoing process of self-examination, learning about diverse cultures, and adapting practice to honor client cultural values.

Question 170: When a treatment approach is not effective after reasonable trial, the ethical response is to: A. Continue indefinitely, B. Reassess, consult, modify approach, or refer to another provider, C. Blame the client for lack of progress, D. Terminate without explanation

Answer: B. Reassess, consult, modify approach, or refer to another provider

Ineffective treatment requires reassessment, consultation with colleagues, modification of interventions, or referral to ensure clients receive appropriate care.

End of Practice Exam 1

Total Questions: 170

Scoring Guide:

- 128+ correct (75%+): Strong preparation, likely to pass
- 119-127 correct (70-74%): Fair preparation, review weak areas
- Below 119 (Below 70%): Additional study needed, focus on content gaps

Next Steps:

1. Review all incorrect answers and explanations
2. Identify content areas needing additional study
3. Review relevant chapters in the study guide
4. Complete Practice Exam 2 for continued assessment

References

Achenbach, T. M., & Rescorla, L. A. (2001). Manual for the ASEBA School-Age Forms & Profiles. Burlington, VT: University of Vermont, Research Center for Children, Youth, & Families.

Ainsworth, M. D. S., Blehar, M. C., Waters, E., & Wall, S. (1978). Patterns of attachment: A psychological study of the strange situation. Hillsdale, NJ: Erlbaum.

American Association for Marriage and Family Therapy. (2015). AAMFT Code of Ethics. Alexandria, VA: American Association for Marriage and Family Therapy.

American Psychiatric Association. (2013). Diagnostic and statistical manual of mental disorders (5th ed.). Arlington, VA: American Psychiatric Publishing.

American Psychiatric Association. (2022). Diagnostic and statistical manual of mental disorders (5th ed., text rev.). Arlington, VA: American Psychiatric Publishing.

Arredondo, P., Toporek, R., Brown, S. P., Jones, J., Locke, D. C., Sanchez, J., & Stadler, H. (1996). Operationalization of the multicultural counseling competencies. Journal of Multicultural Counseling and Development, 24(1), 42-78.

Association of Social Work Boards. (2023). ASWB clinical examination candidate handbook. Author.

Association of Social Work Boards. (2023). Clinical practice analysis: Understanding the foundation of the ASWB clinical examination. Author.

Beck, J. S. (2020). Cognitive behavior therapy: Basics and beyond (3rd ed.). New York: Guilford Press.

Bentley, K. J., & Walsh, J. F. (2020). The social worker and psychotropic medication: Toward effective collaboration with mental health clients, families, and providers (5th ed.). Cengage Learning.

Bernard, J. M., & Goodyear, R. K. (2018). Fundamentals of clinical supervision (6th ed.). Boston: Pearson.

Bordin, E. S. (1983). A working alliance based model of supervision. The Counseling Psychologist, 11(1), 35-42.

Bowen, M. (1978). Family therapy in clinical practice. New York: Jason Aronson.

Bowlby, J. (1969). Attachment and loss: Vol. 1. Attachment. New York: Basic Books.

Bride, B. E., Radey, M., & Figley, C. R. (2007). Measuring compassion fatigue. Clinical Social Work Journal, 35(3), 155-163.

Bronfenbrenner, U. (1979). The ecology of human development: Experiments by nature and design. Cambridge, MA: Harvard University Press.

Bryan, C. J., Mintz, J., Clemans, T. A., Leeson, B., Burch, T. S., Williams, S. R., ... & Rudd, M. D. (2017). Effect of crisis response planning vs. contracts for safety on suicide risk in U.S. Army Soldiers: A randomized clinical trial. Journal of Affective Disorders, 212, 64-72.

Carter, B., & McGoldrick, M. (Eds.). (2005). The expanded family life cycle: Individual, family, and social perspectives (3rd ed.). Boston: Allyn & Bacon.

Christensen, A., Doss, B. D., & Jacobson, N. S. (2020). Reconcilable differences: Rebuild your relationship by rediscovering the partner you love (2nd ed.). New York: Guilford Press.

Conners, C. K. (2008). Conners 3rd Edition (Conners 3). Toronto: Multi-Health Systems.

Crenshaw, K. (1989). Demarginalizing the intersection of race and sex: A Black feminist critique of antidiscrimination doctrine, feminist theory and antiracist politics. University of Chicago Legal Forum, 1989(1), Article 8.

Cross, T. L., Bazron, B. J., Dennis, K. W., & Isaacs, M. R. (1989). Towards a culturally competent system of care: A monograph on effective services for minority children who are severely emotionally disturbed. Washington, DC: Georgetown University Child Development Center.

Erikson, E. H. (1950). Childhood and society. New York: Norton.

Felitti, V. J., Anda, R. F., Nordenberg, D., Williamson, D. F., Spitz, A. M., Edwards, V., ... & Marks, J. S. (1998). Relationship of childhood abuse and household dysfunction to many of the leading causes of death in adults: The Adverse Childhood Experiences (ACE) Study. American Journal of Preventive Medicine, 14(4), 245-258.

Figley, C. R. (Ed.). (1995). Compassion fatigue: Coping with secondary traumatic stress disorder in those who treat the traumatized. New York: Brunner/Mazel.

Foa, E. B., Hembree, E. A., & Rothbaum, B. O. (2007). Prolonged exposure therapy for PTSD: Emotional processing of traumatic experiences. New York: Oxford University Press.

Folstein, M. F., Folstein, S. E., & McHugh, P. R. (1975). Mini-mental state: A practical method for grading the cognitive state of patients for the clinician. Journal of Psychiatric Research, 12(3), 189-198.

Gabbard, G. O. (2016). Long-term psychodynamic psychotherapy: A basic text (3rd ed.). Washington, DC: American Psychiatric Publishing.

Germain, C. B., & Gitterman, A. (1980). The life model of social work practice. New York: Columbia University Press.

Gottman, J. M. (1999). The marriage clinic: A scientifically based marital therapy. New York: Norton.

Gottman, J. M., & Gottman, J. S. (2017). The natural principles of love. Journal of Family Theory & Review, 9(1), 7-26.

Gottman, J. M., & Silver, N. (2015). The seven principles for making marriage work (2nd ed.). New York: Harmony Books.

Griner, D., & Smith, T. B. (2006). Culturally adapted mental health intervention: A meta-analytic review. Psychotherapy: Theory, Research, Practice, Training, 43(4), 531-548.

Haley, J. (1987). Problem-solving therapy (2nd ed.). San Francisco: Jossey-Bass.

Hayes, J. A., Gelso, C. J., & Hummel, A. M. (2011). Managing countertransference. Psychotherapy, 48(1), 88-97.

Hayes, S. C., Strosahl, K. D., & Wilson, K. G. (2011). Acceptance and commitment therapy: The process and practice of mindful change (2nd ed.). New York: Guilford Press.

Hendrix, H., & Hunt, H. L. (2019). Getting the love you want: A guide for couples (3rd ed.). New York: St. Martin's Griffin.

Hofmann, S. G., Asnaani, A., Vonk, I. J., Sawyer, A. T., & Fang, A. (2012). The efficacy of cognitive behavioral therapy: A review of meta-analyses. Cognitive Therapy and Research, 36(5), 427-440.

Hook, J. N., Davis, D. E., Owen, J., Worthington, E. L., Jr., & Utsey, S. O. (2013). Cultural humility: Measuring openness to culturally diverse clients. Journal of Counseling Psychology, 60(3), 353-366.

Jacobson, N. S., & Christensen, A. (1996). Integrative couple therapy: Promoting acceptance and change. New York: Norton.

Johnson, S. M. (2004). The practice of emotionally focused couple therapy: Creating connection (2nd ed.). New York: Brunner-Routledge.

Johnson, S. M. (2019). Attachment theory in practice: Emotionally focused therapy (EFT) with individuals, couples, and families. New York: Guilford Press.

Kerr, M. E., & Bowen, M. (1988). Family evaluation: An approach based on Bowen theory. New York: Norton.

Klerman, G. L., Weissman, M. M., Rounsaville, B. J., & Chevron, E. S. (1984). Interpersonal psychotherapy of depression. New York: Basic Books.

Kohlberg, L. (1981). Essays on moral development, Vol. I: The philosophy of moral development. San Francisco: Harper & Row.

Kroenke, K., Spitzer, R. L., & Williams, J. B. (2001). The PHQ-9: Validity of a brief depression severity measure. Journal of General Internal Medicine, 16(9), 606-613.

Lambert, M. J. (2010). Prevention of treatment failure: The use of measuring, monitoring, and feedback in clinical practice. Washington, DC: American Psychological Association.

Lee, J. J., & Miller, S. E. (2013). A self-care framework for social workers: Building a strong foundation for practice. Families in Society, 94(2), 96-103.

Levinson, D. J. (1978). The seasons of a man's life. New York: Knopf.

Linehan, M. M. (2014). DBT skills training manual (2nd ed.). New York: Guilford Press.

Madanes, C. (1981). Strategic family therapy. San Francisco: Jossey-Bass.

Main, M., & Solomon, J. (1986). Discovery of an insecure-disorganized/disoriented attachment pattern. In T. B. Brazelton & M. W. Yogman (Eds.), Affective development in infancy (pp. 95-124). Norwood, NJ: Ablex.

Marcia, J. E. (1980). Identity in adolescence. In J. Adelson (Ed.), Handbook of adolescent psychology (pp. 159-187). New York: Wiley.

Maslach, C., & Leiter, M. P. (2016). Understanding the burnout experience: Recent research and its implications for psychiatry. World Psychiatry, 15(2), 103-111.

Maslach, C., Schaufeli, W. B., & Leiter, M. P. (2001). Job burnout. Annual Review of Psychology, 52, 397-422.

McGoldrick, M., Gerson, R., & Petry, S. (2008). Genograms: Assessment and intervention (3rd ed.). New York: Norton.

Meyer, I. H. (2003). Prejudice, social stress, and mental health in lesbian, gay, and bisexual populations: Conceptual issues and research evidence. Psychological Bulletin, 129(5), 674-697.

Miller, W. R., & Rollnick, S. (2012). Motivational interviewing: Helping people change (3rd ed.). New York: Guilford Press.

Minuchin, S. (1974). Families and family therapy. Cambridge, MA: Harvard University Press.

Minuchin, S., & Fishman, H. C. (1981). Family therapy techniques. Cambridge, MA: Harvard University Press.

Nasreddine, Z. S., Phillips, N. A., Bédirian, V., Charbonneau, S., Whitehead, V., Collin, I., ... & Chertkow, H. (2005). The Montreal Cognitive Assessment, MoCA: A brief screening tool for mild cognitive impairment. Journal of the American Geriatrics Society, 53(4), 695-699.

National Alliance on Mental Illness. (2020). NAMI Family-to-Family: A free, 8-session educational program for family, significant others and friends of people with mental health conditions. Arlington, VA: NAMI.

National Association of Social Workers. (2015). Standards and indicators for cultural competence in social work practice. Washington, DC: NASW Press.

National Association of Social Workers. (2021). Code of ethics of the National Association of Social Workers. Washington, DC: NASW Press.

Newell, J. M., & MacNeil, G. A. (2010). Professional burnout, vicarious trauma, secondary traumatic stress, and compassion fatigue: A review of theoretical terms, risk factors, and preventive methods for clinicians and researchers. Best Practices in Mental Health, 6(2), 57-68.

Norcross, J. C., & Guy, J. D. (2007). Leaving it at the office: A guide to psychotherapist self-care. New York: Guilford Press.

Pearlman, L. A., & Saakvitne, K. W. (1995). Trauma and the therapist: Countertransference and vicarious traumatization in psychotherapy with incest survivors. New York: Norton.

Piaget, J. (1952). The origins of intelligence in children. New York: International Universities Press.

Posner, K., Brown, G. K., Stanley, B., Brent, D. A., Yershova, K. V., Oquendo, M. A., ... & Mann, J. J. (2011). The Columbia-Suicide Severity Rating Scale: Initial validity and internal consistency findings from three multisite studies with adolescents and adults. American Journal of Psychiatry, 168(12), 1266-1277.

Putnam, R. D. (2000). Bowling alone: The collapse and revival of American community. New York: Simon & Schuster.

Resick, P. A., Monson, C. M., & Chard, K. M. (2016). Cognitive processing therapy for PTSD: A comprehensive manual. New York: Guilford Press.

Roberts, A. R. (2005). Crisis intervention handbook: Assessment, treatment, and research (3rd ed.). New York: Oxford University Press.

Roberts, L. W., & Dyer, A. R. (2004). Concise guide to ethics in mental health care. Washington, DC: American Psychiatric Publishing.

Ronnestad, M. H., & Skovholt, T. M. (2003). The journey of the counselor and therapist: Research findings and perspectives on professional development. Journal of Career Development, 30(1), 5-44.

Satir, V. (1988). The new peoplemaking. Mountain View, CA: Science and Behavior Books.

Shapiro, F. (2017). Eye movement desensitization and reprocessing (EMDR) therapy: Basic principles, protocols, and procedures (3rd ed.). New York: Guilford Press.

Shonkoff, J. P., & Garner, A. S. (2012). The lifelong effects of early childhood adversity and toxic stress. Pediatrics, 129(1), e232-e246.

Sidell, N. L. (2019). Social work documentation: A guide to strengthening your case recording (2nd ed.). NASW Press.

Skovholt, T. M., & Trotter-Mathison, M. (2016). The resilient practitioner: Burnout and compassion fatigue prevention and self-care strategies for the helping professions (3rd ed.). New York: Routledge.

Spitzer, R. L., Kroenke, K., Williams, J. B., & Löwe, B. (2006). A brief measure for assessing generalized anxiety disorder: The GAD-7. Archives of Internal Medicine, 166(10), 1092-1097.

Stamm, B. H. (2010). The concise ProQOL manual (2nd ed.). Pocatello, ID: ProQOL.org.

Stanley, B., & Brown, G. K. (2012). Safety planning intervention: A brief intervention to mitigate suicide risk. Cognitive and Behavioral Practice, 19(2), 256-264.

Substance Abuse and Mental Health Services Administration. (2014). SAMHSA's concept of trauma and guidance for a trauma-informed approach. HHS Publication No. (SMA) 14-4884. Rockville, MD: SAMHSA.

Sue, D. W., & Sue, D. (2015). Counseling the culturally diverse: Theory and practice (7th ed.). Hoboken, NJ: Wiley.

Sue, D. W., Capodilupo, C. M., Torino, G. C., Bucceri, J. M., Holder, A. M. B., Nadal, K. L., & Esquilin, M. (2007). Racial microaggressions in everyday life: Implications for clinical practice. American Psychologist, 62(4), 271-286.

Tervalon, M., & Murray-García, J. (1998). Cultural humility versus cultural competence: A critical distinction in defining physician training outcomes in multicultural education. Journal of Health Care for the Poor and Underserved, 9(2), 117-125.

Tuckman, B. W. (1965). Developmental sequence in small groups. Psychological Bulletin, 63(6), 384-399.

Tuckman, B. W., & Jensen, M. A. C. (1977). Stages of small-group development revisited. Group & Organization Studies, 2(4), 419-427.

Turner, F. J. (Ed.). (2017). Social work treatment: Interlocking theoretical approaches (6th ed.). Oxford University Press.

U.S. Department of Health and Human Services. (2013). HIPAA privacy rule and sharing information related to mental health. Author.

van der Kolk, B. A. (2014). The body keeps the score: Brain, mind, and body in the healing of trauma. New York: Viking.

van Dernoot Lipsky, L., & Burk, C. (2009). Trauma stewardship: An everyday guide to caring for self while caring for others. San Francisco: Berrett-Koehler.

von Bertalanffy, L. (1968). General system theory: Foundations, development, applications. New York: George Braziller.

Watkins, C. E., Jr. (2011). Does psychotherapy supervision contribute to patient outcomes? Considering thirty years of research. The Clinical Supervisor, 30(2), 235-256.

Weathers, F. W., Litz, B. T., Keane, T. M., Palmieri, P. A., Marx, B. P., & Schnurr, P. P. (2013). The PTSD Checklist for DSM-5 (PCL-5). National Center for PTSD. www.ptsd.va.gov

Weissman, M. M., Markowitz, J. C., & Klerman, G. L. (2018). The guide to interpersonal psychotherapy (updated and expanded edition). New York: Oxford University Press.

Worden, J. W. (2018). Grief counseling and grief therapy: A handbook for the mental health practitioner (5th ed.). New York: Springer.

Yalom, I. D., & Leszcz, M. (2005). The theory and practice of group psychotherapy (5th ed.). New York: Basic Books.

Yehuda, R., & Lehrner, A. (2018). Intergenerational transmission of trauma effects: Putative role of epigenetic mechanisms. World Psychiatry, 17(3), 243-257.

Made in United States
North Haven, CT
26 October 2026

21184086R00313